A CULTURAL HISTORY OF MEDICINE

VOLUME 2

A Cultural History of Medicine
General Editor: Roger Cooter

Volume 1
A Cultural History of Medicine in Antiquity
Edited by Laurence Totelin

Volume 2
A Cultural History of Medicine in the Middle Ages
Edited by Iona McCleery

Volume 3
A Cultural History of Medicine in the Renaissance
Edited by Elaine Leong and Claudia Stein

Volume 4
A Cultural History of Medicine in the Enlightenment
Edited by Lisa Wynne Smith

Volume 5
A Cultural History of Medicine in the Age of Empire
Edited by Jonathan Reinarz

Volume 6
A Cultural History of Medicine in the Modern Age
Edited by Todd Meyers

A CULTURAL HISTORY
OF MEDICINE

IN THE
MIDDLE
AGES

Edited by Iona McCleery

BLOOMSBURY ACADEMIC
LONDON · NEW YORK · OXFORD · NEW DELHI · SYDNEY

BLOOMSBURY ACADEMIC
Bloomsbury Publishing Plc
50 Bedford Square, London, WC1B 3DP, UK
1385 Broadway, New York, NY 10018, USA
29 Earlsfort Terrace, Dublin 2, Ireland

BLOOMSBURY, BLOOMSBURY ACADEMIC and the Diana logo are trademarks
of Bloomsbury Publishing Plc

First published in Great Britain 2021
This paperback edition first published 2024

Copyright © Bloomsbury Publishing, 2021

Iona McCleery has asserted her right under the Copyright, Designs and Patents Act,
1988, to be identified as Editor of this work.

Cover image: Florence, Biblioteca Nazionale Centrale, MS Magliabechiano II. VI.16, fol. 48v
© Leemage / Getty Images

All rights reserved. No part of this publication may be reproduced or transmitted
in any form or by any means, electronic or mechanical, including photocopying,
recording, or any information storage or retrieval system, without prior
permission in writing from the publishers.

Bloomsbury Publishing Plc does not have any control over, or responsibility for, any third-party
websites referred to or in this book. All internet addresses given in this book were correct at
the time of going to press. The author and publisher regret any inconvenience caused if
addresses have changed or sites have ceased to exist, but can accept no responsibility
for any such changes.

A catalogue record for this book is available from the British Library.

Library of Congress Cataloging-in-Publication Data
Names: Cooter, Roger, editor.
Title: A cultural history of medicine / general editor, Roger Cooter.
Description: London ; New York : Bloomsbury Academic, 2021. |
Series: The cultural histories series | Includes bibliographical references and index. |
Identifiers: LCCN 2020051490 | ISBN 9781472569936 (hardback)
Subjects: LCSH: Medicine–History.
Classification: LCC R131 .C78 2021 | DDC 610.9—dc23
LC record available at https://lccn.loc.gov/2020051490

ISBN: HB: 978-1-4725-6992-9
        Set: 978-1-4725-6987-5
        PB: 978-1-3504-5149-0
        Set: 978-1-3504-5164-3

Series: The Cultural Histories Series

Typeset by RefineCatch Limited, Bungay, Suffolk
Printed and bound in Great Britain

To find out more about our authors and books visit www.bloomsbury.com
and sign up for our newsletters.

CONTENTS

LIST OF ILLUSTRATIONS   vii

GENERAL EDITOR'S PREFACE   xii
Roger Cooter

Introduction: The Cultural History of Health   1
Iona McCleery

1   Environment: Managing Urban Sanitation for *Sanitas*   21
Dolly Jørgensen

2   Food: From Healthy Regimen to Consumption and Supply   39
Iona McCleery

3   Disease: Confronting, Consoling and Constructing the
Afflicted Body   63
Justin Stearns

4   Animals: Their Use and Meaning in Medieval Medicine   87
Kathleen Walker-Meikle

5   Objects: The Archaeology of Medieval Healing   107
Gemma L. Watson and Roberta Gilchrist

6   Experiences: Feeling Unhealthy in the Middle Ages   131
Naama Cohen-Hanegbi

7	Mind/Brain: Medieval Concepts *Wendy J. Turner*	155
8	Authority: Trusting the Text in the Early Middle Ages *F. Eliza Glaze*	177

BIBLIOGRAPHY	203
NOTES ON CONTRIBUTORS	245
INDEX	247

ILLUSTRATIONS

INTRODUCTION

0.1 Ibn Butlan, *Tacuinum sanitatis* (Tables of Health) (late-fourteenth century). Vienna, Österreichische Nationalbibliothek, Codex Vindobonensis Series Nova 2644, fol. 4. Credit: Österreichische Nationalbibliothek, Vienna.   2

0.2 Food preparation *Tacuinum sanitatis* (Tables of Health) (late-fourteenth century). Vienna, Österreichische Nationalbibliothek, Codex Vindobonensis Series Nova 2644, fol. 81. Credit: Österreichische Nationalbibliothek, Vienna.   3

0.3 The four temperaments, The *Kalender of Shepherdes* (early-sixteenth century), reprinted in H. Oskar Sommer's edition of 1892. London, Wellcome Library. Credit: Wellcome Collection/ Public Domain.   14

0.4 Miracle cure, *Le Livre des faiz monseigneur saint Loys* (fifteenth century). Paris, Bibliothèque Nationale, MS Français 2829, fol. 101. Credit: Getty Images.   16

0.5 Sleep, *Tacuinum sanitatis* (Tables of Health) (late-fourteenth century). Vienna, Österreichische Nationalbibliothek, Codex Vindobonensis Series Nova 2644, fol. 100. Credit: Österreichische Nationalbibliothek, Vienna.   17

CHAPTER 1

1.1 The senses, Augustine, *De spiritu et anima* (early-thirteenth century). Trinity College Cambridge MS O.7.16, fol. 47. Credit: Master and Fellows of Trinity College Cambridge.   25

viii ILLUSTRATIONS

1.2 Sheep butchery, *Tacuinum sanitatis* (Tables of Health)
(late-fourteenth century), Vienna, Österreichische
Nationalbibliothek, Codex Vindobonensis Series Nova 2644,
fol. 72v. Credit: Österreichische Nationalbibliothek, Vienna.   28
1.3 Latrine and latrine pit, Boccaccio, *Decameron* (mid-fifteenth
century). Paris, Bibliothèque de l'Arsenal, MS 5070 réserve, fol.
50v. Credit: Bibliothèque Nationale de France.   32
1.4 Paver, Nuremburg Hausbuch (mid-fifteenth century). Nuremburg,
Stadtbibliothek Nürnberg, MS Amb. 317.2°, fol. 77. Credit:
Stadtbibliothek Nürnberg.   34

CHAPTER 2

2.1 Royal feast, *Queen Mary Psalter* (early-fourteenth century).
London, British Library, MS Royal 2 B VII, fol. 71v (detail).
Credit: British Library/Public Domain.   48
2.2 Fresh fish, *Tacuinum sanitatis* (Tables of Health) (late-fourteenth
century), Vienna, Österreichische Nationalbibliothek, Codex
Vindobonensis Series Nova 2644, fol. 82. Credit: Getty Images.   49
2.3 Salted fish, *Tacuinum sanitatis* (Tables of Health) (late-fourteenth
century), Vienna, Österreichische Nationalbibliothek, Codex
Vindobonensis Series Nova 2644, fol. 82v. Credit: Getty Images.   51
2.4 Church stall bench end (fifteenth century), originally from the
chapel of St Nicholas, Kings Lynn, England. Credit: Victoria and
Albert Museum, London.   53
2.5 A representation of Matthew 17: 27, English Gospel Book of
unknown origin (c.1000). The J. Paul Getty Museum, Los Angeles,
MS 9, fol. 2. Credit: Getty Open Content programme.   55
2.6 Cure of Juliana Puintel, stained glass window (early-thirteenth
century). Canterbury Cathedral, Trinity Chapel, North
Ambulatory, no. nIV. Credit: Getty Images.   57

CHAPTER 3

3.1 Taking the pulse, Avicenna, *al-Qānūn* (The Canon). Binding board
of manuscript of 1632. Wellcome Library, London, Or Arabic MS
155. Credit: Wellcome Collection/Public Domain.   67
3.2 Bishop instructing clergymen with leprosy, James le Palmer,
Omne bonum (late-fourteenth century). London, British Library,
MS Royal 6.E.VI, vol 2, fol. 301 (detail). Credit: British Library/
Public Domain.   77

ILLUSTRATIONS ix

3.3 St Vincent Ferrer preaching, part of an altar piece originally in
S. Domenico, Modena, by Bartolomeo degli Erri and his brother
Agnolo (late fifteenth-century), now Ashmolean Museum,
Oxford. Credit: Getty Images. 79

CHAPTER 4

4.1 Planet man, Book of Hours (late-fifteenth century). Oxford,
Bodleian Library, MS Douce 311, fol. 1v. Credit: Bodleian Library. 92
4.2 Urban pigs, Marco Polo, *Le livre des merveilles* (early-fifteenth
century). Paris, Bibliothèque Nationale, MS français 2810, fol. 7.
Credit: Getty Images. 95
4.3 Snake bite, Pseudo-Apuleius Platonicus, *De medicaminibus
herbarum* (late-twelfth century). London, British Library, MS
Harley 5294, fol. 42 (detail). Credit: British Library/Public Domain. 96
4.4 Zodiac horse, Manuel Díes, *Libre de cavalls* (late-fifteenth
century). Beinecke Rare Book and Manuscript Library, Yale
University, Beinecke MS 454 fol. 1. Credit: Beinecke Rare Book
and Manuscript Library, Yale University. 103

CHAPTER 5

5.1 Distillation vessel (ceramic alembic, fourteenth century,
height 290mm) from St Mary Spital, London. Credit:
Museum of London Archaeology. 113
5.2 Reconstruction of the Barber-surgeon's chest and contents as
found on the Tudor warship the *Mary Rose*, with other
equipment from the cabin. Credit: Mary Rose Trust. 115
5.3 Drawing of a reversible, ash-wood double bowl excavated from
St Mary Spital, London (diameter 170mm, height 56mm).
Credit: Museum of London Archaeology. 118
5.4 Mercury droplets as found on the skeleton of a young female
buried in Exeter Cathedral Green. Credit: Royal Albert
Memorial Museum and Art Gallery, Exeter. 119
5.5 Copper-alloy plate associated with the humerus of a woman
from the cemetery of St Mary Magdalene leper hospital,
Reading. Credit: Reading Museum Service. 121
5.6 Jet bowl from Trig Lane, London (diameter 130mm, height
27mm). Credit: Museum of London Archaeology. 122
5.7 Scratched marks on redware from St Claire monastery of
Petegem, Belgium. Credit: Flanders Heritage Agency. 125

5.8 Hernia truss as found in the grave of a mature-adult male in the north transept of the church of St Mary Merton, Surrey. Credit: Museum of London Archaeology. 127

CHAPTER 6

6.1 Death of Fernando of Castile in 1252, *Chroniques de France* (late-fourteenth century). London, British Library, MS Royal 20 C VII, fol. 11 (detail). Credit: British Library/Public Domain. 136

6.2 Administering the Last Rites, Matins of the Office of the Dead, *The Dunois Hours* (mid-fifteenth century). London, British Library, MS Yates Thompson 3, fol. 211 (detail). Credit: British Library/Public Domain. 137

6.3 Sick man's bedside, Jean Froissart, *Chroniques* (late-fifteenth century). London, British Library, MS Harley 4379, fol. 125v (detail). Credit: British Library/Public Domain. 141

6.4 Dental specialist, James Le Palmer, *Omne bonum* (late-fourteenth century). London, British Library, MS Royal 6 E VI, Vol. 2, fol. 503v (detail). Credit: British Library/Public Domain. 146

CHAPTER 7

7.1 Ibn Sīna (Avicenna)'s brain theory in his *De generatione embryonica* (dated 1347). Cambridge University Library, MS Gr.g.I.I, fol. 490v. Credit: The Syndics of Cambridge University Library. 161

7.2 Disease man, *Petits traités d'hygiène et de médecine* (fifteenth century). Paris, Bibliothèque Nationale, MS Latin 11229, fol. 37v. Credit: Bibliothèque Nationale de France. 162

7.3 Cerebral ventricles, Gregor Reisch, *Margarita philosophica* (Freiburg: Johann Schott, 1503), book 10, tractate 2, signature Hii. Credit: Wellcome Collection/Public Domain. 163

CHAPTER 8

8.1 Cautery illustration (*c.*1100). London, British Library MS Sloane 2839, fol. 1v. Credit: British Library/Public Domain. 187

8.2 Photograph of the medieval medical books of Monte Cassino. Credit: F. Eliza Glaze. 189

ILLUSTRATIONS   xi

8.3   Crowsfoot and dog bite, Pseudo-Apuleius Platonicus,
      De medicaminibus herbarum (late-twelfth century). London,
      British Library, MS Harley 5294, fol. 25. Credit: British Library/
      Public Domain.   191
8.4   Constantine the African judging urines, *Various medical treatises*
      (fourteenth century), Oxford, Bodleian Library, MS Rawlinson C.
      328,
      fol. 3. Credit: Bodleian Library.   197
8.5   Trota, *Miscellanea Medica XVIII* (early-fourteenth century).
      London, Wellcome Library, MS 544, p. 65. Credit:
      Wellcome Library/Public Domain.   200

GENERAL EDITOR'S PREFACE

ROGER COOTER

The cultural history of medicine is all embracing. Virtually nothing can be excluded from it – the body in all its literary and other representations over time, ideas of civilization and humankind and the sociology, anthropology and epistemology of health and welfare, not to mention the existential experiences of pain, disease, suffering and death and the way professionals have endeavoured to deal with them. To contain much of this vastness, the volumes in this Series focus on eight categories, all of contemporary relevance: Environment, Food, Disease, Animals, Objects, Experience, Mind/Brain, and Authority. From the ancient through to the postmodern world these themes are pursued with critical breadth, depth and novelty by dedicated experts. Transnational perspectives are widely entertained. Above all these volumes attend to and illuminate what exactly is a *cultural* history of medicine, a category of investigation and an epistemological concept that has its emergence in the 1980s.

Introduction: The Cultural History of Health

IONA McCLEERY

In late-fourteenth century northern Italy, four illuminated manuscripts were produced of the *Tacuinum sanitatis* or 'Tables of Health'. Originally a non-illustrated work in Arabic by Ibn Butlan, a mid-eleventh-century Christian of Baghdad, the elite Latin manuscripts range in topic from shopping for food and pharmaceutical items through to idealistic representations of hunting, agriculture, dining, cooking, sex and coping with the weather. The many scenes are accompanied by short texts that explain the health benefits and harmful aspects of foodstuffs, activities or seasons (see Figures 0.1, 0.2, 0.5, 1.2, 2.2, 2.3; Arano 1996; Hoeniger 2006).[1] The scope of these manuscripts reflects the scope of this volume on the cultural history of medicine: ideas about preventing disease; concerns about environmental health; experiences of illness; emotional well-being; sensory perception and conditions such as melancholy; interactions with animals, food and eating; the material culture of daily life; and medical authority. Ibn Butlan is represented at the start of each manuscript dressed as an academic authority figure. The whole text and its images are dependent on the authoritative concept of the non-naturals: six things that can cause illness or restore health: air, food and drink, exercise, sleep, excretion and the emotions (described further below).

In the *Tacuinum, sanitas* or 'health' operates as an umbrella concept that incorporates many aspects of daily life that we might not so easily see as part of healthcare today. Taking a very broad cultural approach to the history of

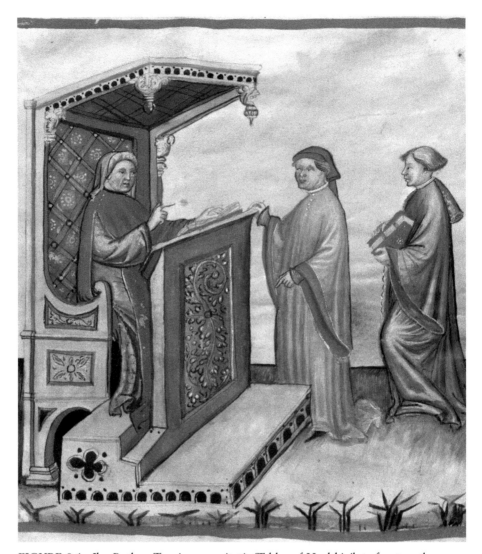

FIGURE 0.1: Ibn Butlan, *Tacuinum sanitatis* (Tables of Health) (late-fourteenth century). Vienna, Österreichische Nationalbibliothek, Codex Vindobonensis Series Nova 2644, fol. 4. Credit: Österreichische Nationalbibliothek, Vienna.

medieval medicine might seem to be a fairly radical way of opening up the field as it could include everything that might affect well-being. The matter of what should be included in a cultural history of medieval medicine and why is the subject of this introductory chapter. The wide variety of topics reflects not only current research interests, but also older cultural concepts of medicine.

INTRODUCTION 3

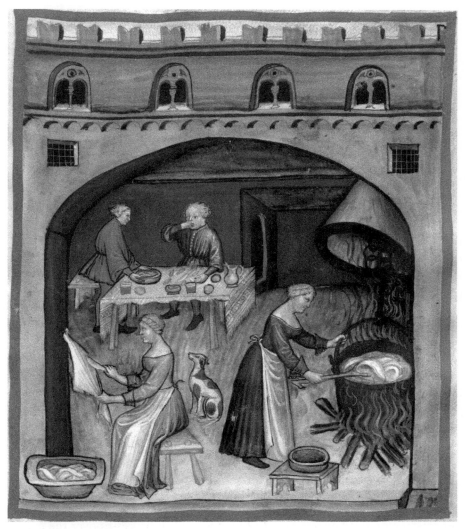

FIGURE 0.2: Food preparation, *Tacuinum sanitatis* (Tables of Health) (late-fourteenth century). Vienna, Österreichische Nationalbibliothek, Codex Vindobonensis Series Nova 2644, fol. 81. Credit: Österreichische Nationalbibliothek, Vienna.

Inspiration is drawn both from the *Tacuinum sanitatis* and from the definition of medicine provided by Bishop Isidore of Seville (d. 636):

> To medicine belong not only those things practiced by the skill of those properly called physicians [*medici*], but also matters of food and drink, clothing and shelter. Ultimately, it consists of every defense and fortification

by means of which our body is preserved [healthy] in the face of external blows and accidents.

—Isidore of Seville 2006: 109

WRITING A CULTURAL HISTORY OF MEDICINE AS A COLLABORATIVE PROJECT

The first major discussions about the content and approach of this volume began at a round table at the International Medieval Congress (IMC) held in Leeds in July 2015. Panelists and participants were invited to consider what a 'cultural' history of medicine should look like. They were invited to reflect on what medicine meant; which cultural theories, approaches and frameworks most influenced their research; and how the different disciplines, departments, institutions and countries in which they worked affected the conduct of their research and teaching on medieval medicine. Did medievalists use cultural theory differently to modernists and, if so, how did this matter? The discussion and audience responses raised several interesting issues, the most general of which was that the cultural history of medicine for the medieval period was an enterprise very much in progress. This was driven home by many of the chapter categories chosen by the general editor (for this volume as for all the other volumes in this cultural history of medicine series). 'Disease' was familiar enough, and so were 'Authority', 'Environment' and 'Experience' but 'Animals', 'Objects', 'Food' and 'Mind/Brain' presented new and exciting empirical, conceptual and methodological challenges.

Confronting the fundamental question of what a cultural history of medicine ought to be like for the Middle Ages soon led us to query all three of the concepts involved: 'Middle Ages', 'medicine' and 'the cultural'. The first of these, 'the Middle Ages' raises well-known chronological, geographical and conceptual problems, but is unavoidable within the context of a book series, even though the break-down of time into centuries and periods is often unhelpful for understanding lived experiences or broader cultural processes over the *longue durée*. There has been significant scholarship on the early Middle Ages and the Islamicate world over the last decade (e.g. Van Arsdall 2007; Horden 2011; Shefer-Mossensohn and Abou Hershkovitz 2013; Fancy 2013; Pilsworth 2014; Leja 2016; Chipman, Pormann, Shefer-Mossensohn 2017; Chipman 2018; Savage-Smith, Swain and van Gelder, eds. 2020; Burridge 2020) which meant that it was very important to include those perspectives, but most of the contributors to this volume self-identify as late medievalists who work on Europe between the thirteenth and the early-sixteenth centuries. We were nevertheless encouraged to be comparative and are very aware of the 'global turn' in Medieval Studies and of the role of Critical Race Studies in medieval research (Whitaker 2019; Heng 2018; Holmes and Standen, eds. 2018). These

INTRODUCTION

subjects have been related to health through medieval theories of human identity and difference, experiences of trade, global pandemics of plague, and the sufferings (and health practices) of enslaved people (Eliav-Feldon, Isaac and Ziegler, eds. 2009; Green 2010, 2012; Ferragud 2013; Green ed. 2014; Blumenthal 2014; McCleery 2015; Winer, 2017; Lambourn 2018; Barker 2019). Inequalities in healthcare and mortality during the COVID-19 global pandemic of 2020 were a reminder to medievalists that experiences of illness and care are always uneven, affected by politics and economics.

With regard to 'medicine', we had to decide whether we wanted this to refer simply to its practice, or to treat it as a category embracing everything from birth to death that affected health and illness. We decided on the latter, which we felt did not exclude the former, to which, indeed, a fair amount of scholarship has been devoted over the last five years. Medieval wounds and wounding and treatment of trauma in general are well covered (Kirkham and Warr, eds. 2014; Tracy and DeVries, eds. 2015; Rogge, ed. 2017; Turner and Lee, eds. 2018; Arner 2019) and there is renewed interest in military medicine and hygiene more broadly (Geltner 2019a; Phillips forthcoming). There is also a growing range of publications on hospitals, leprosaria and other pre-modern welfare institutions (Bonfield, Reinarz and Huguet-Termes, eds. 2013; Abreu and Sheard, eds. 2013; Brenner 2015; Ragab 2015; Brasher 2017; Jáuregui 2018). The history of childbirth is a vibrant field (Powell 2012; Cormack ed. 2012; Harris-Stoertz 2014; Giladi 2015; Jones and Olsan 2015; French 2016; Foscati 2019; Baumgarten 2019). Much of this scholarship is multi-national, written in or translated into English, although a great amount of research is only in German, French, Italian, Catalan and Spanish.

'Medicine', we decided, was ultimately too narrow a term, likely to lead to perspectives from modern biomedicine instead of medieval culture. 'Health' rather than 'medicine' was preferable, as indeed had been proposed by Monica Green in one of her several influential reflective articles. She defined the subject as 'threats to health and health-seeking behaviors (of which biomedicine is just one part)' (Green 2011: 7). Conceptually and pragmatically, however, biomedicine is nevertheless influential, as it is to all people who live in the twenty-first century and are familiar with modern medicine. The chapters in this volume on 'Food' and 'Objects' out of necessity show awareness of research that rests on an understanding of clinical, nutritional, biochemical and epidemiological data. Furthermore, bioarchaeology—the study of biological traces from the past—has become one of the most significant contributors to research into medieval health in the last few years, with special importance for studying the health of the anonymous poor. It cannot exist without modern scientific data and understanding.

As Eliza Glaze pointed out at the round table: '"Medicine" can be used as code for a much broader range of activities and perceptions, as long as these are further defined and explored'. We have tried throughout this volume to see 'medicine' as a multi-disciplinary catch-all term that is a useful tool in teaching and communication beyond our academic disciplines. Medieval approaches to health and illness go far beyond a narrow focus on 'patients' or medical learning, which might be seen as anachronistic or too biomedical in their framing.[2] Throughout, medieval people are seen as resilient, proactive health agents and/ or 'health-seekers' involved in personal or communal health strategies. We remain aware, however, of our textual reliance on the views and behaviours of literate elites who left evidence of their attitudes and beliefs. It is far more difficult to access the views of the poor and illiterate, although much has been done through the aforementioned analysis of bioarchaeological evidence and also through miracle narratives and legal records (Hanawalt 1986; Finucane 1997; Turner and Butler, eds. 2014; McCleery 2014a; Butler 2015).

Regarding 'culture', the round table expressed a great diversity of opinion. Most of the participants had in their heads something akin to the view presented by Mary Fissell in an influential 2004 essay on the cultural history of medicine: that cultural history is about 'how people in the past made sense of their lives, of the natural world, of social relations, of their bodies' (Fissell 2004: 364). This all-embracing definition fits the broadening of medieval medicine to include *everything* and *everyone* who might affect health. It also includes all possible sources of information for experience and practice (see Ritchey and Strocchia (2020) for a similar approach). We agreed with Fissell's (2004: 364) critique of cultural history's 'predilection for the marginal or the transgressive'. We were more inclined to the view that cultural history belongs less to the transgressive and exotic than to ordinary everyday medieval people, be they merchants, labourers, scholars, noblewomen or kings. That is to say, the preference was for what anthropologists call an *emic* approach, with a focus on explanations for health and disease that people in the Middle Ages themselves employed, thus avoiding retrospective diagnosis (Cunningham 2002; Arrizabalaga 2002). Yet, as stated above, it would be foolish to neglect valuable *etic* approaches, that is, external and modern ones, such as bioarchaeology, genetics or nutritional science—and, indeed, gender studies, climate science and linguistics—since they have explanatory power as long as they are used carefully (Mitchell 2011; Green 2014: 51–3; Foxhall 2014). Our aim of being comparative is itself an *etic* approach as it involves comparisons of individuals and communities who are unaware of each other. We would also be foolish not to recognize the tension with our own *emic* selves doing the interpreting, because we are modern people from different countries and disciplines who see through modern eyes and need to communicate with other modern people.[3]

Mary Fissell does not use the terms *emic* and *etic* in her influential essay, but she engages in similar debate about the tension between past and present, by arguing that cultural history has to be a modern intellectual exercise, while still

INTRODUCTION

being anchored in specific historical socio-economic contexts. For her 'making meaning' is to a large part what we are doing by interpreting the past. Many of the *emically* produced artefacts, bodies, images and texts that we study do not easily yield up their 'original' meanings, if indeed they ever had any with straightforward uncontested significance. 'Meaning' is therefore a highly subjective, unstable concept dependent on prior experience, education, expectations and ideological purpose: 'meanings that are made can be unmade and remade' (Fissell 2004: 365). Indeed, new generations of scholars do their best to unmake previous interpretations in order to establish themselves as innovative academics, and the methodologies that they use differ according to discipline, field and country.

There was a great deal of personal reflection at the round table on what influences us most as scholars and which ideas and methods we found most inspiring. The departments or 'tribes' that we work in, move between or with which we interact (Becher and Trowler 2001); the terms and extent of our employment – whether we have a permanent contract or tenure; are the only medievalist in the university obliged to teach everything from Ancient Assyria to the French Revolution and beyond, or are part of a collegiate centre for medieval studies; whether we work in higher education or museums and archives or as independent scholars; our life-cycle stage, ethnicity, nationality and gender; our political outlook, familial situation and personal anxieties: all these things affect how we do our research but are often not acknowledged enough.

The issue that generated most debate at the round table was whether all cultural historians must explicitly engage with theoretical approaches, and whether medievalists are less inclined than modernists to engage in theory. Although there was a consensus that it is important to reflect on what we are doing and why, we decided that this volume would not be too dominated by theory. Most of the contributors reflect on the historiographical background to their topic, and several chapters explicitly address methodology. For example, narratology, or the close analysis of especially first-person accounts of illness, described by Flurin Condrau (2007: 527) as 'the major methodological refinement of patients' history over the last twenty years' has influenced a number of medievalists seeking to understand personal experiences of illness, although it is not without its hazards (McCleery 2009; Frohne 2015; Cohen-Hanegbi 2017). This approach does not, however, necessarily allow for cultural meanings to emerge easily or without debate, since often what we have are the surviving traces of something we cannot easily understand.

One of the advantages of *etic* approaches based on big datasets or scientific analysis is that they can allow us to recover lost tacit knowledge about practices and rituals involving the human body that may never have been written down, at least not in explicit terms, requiring careful interpretation of oblique references in literature, marks on material objects, or lesions on bones (Jardine

2004: 269–70; Gilchrist 2012: 7–10). For example, a combination of methodologies drawn from literary, linguistic and material cultural research is helping to reconsider manuscripts as material not just intellectual productions, made out of parchment (animal skin), papyrus or cloth-based paper with biographies of their own and replete with lost traces of beliefs and practices worth uncovering through the close study of doodles, dirt, and indications of mobility, readership, translation and transmission (Rudy 2010; Leong 2014; Green 2018; Kozodoy 2019). The study of knowledge transmission during the Middle Ages via close scrutiny of manuscripts as cultural artefacts with lives of their own suggests that the stuff of a cultural history of medicine is much more than the content of texts. It also includes these 'slippages, misrememberings, and displacements' of the past (Fissell 2004: 379).

Medieval *historians* have tended not to engage with theory as much as literary scholars and archaeologists. Social contructivism, performativity or the 'linguistic turn' appear more rarely in medieval historical studies; personally, I did not become aware of any of these approaches until I worked in a Department of Philosophy as a post-doctoral lecturer and researcher from 2003–2007. I now find my research greatly enhanced through interdisciplinary PhD co-supervision with colleagues in other disciplines such as English and History of Art. With some exceptions, guides to researching medieval history tend to be source-led rather than reflections on why we do what we do, what relevance it has today beyond academia, and how we might communicate better with a more diverse range of scholars. As was pointed out at the round table, the fact is that many aspects of the Middle Ages still need to be dug up from the ground or identified in the archive; then have to be conserved, analysed, translated, edited and published. It may also be that there simply are not enough sources available on some topics to allow for more speculative cultural interpretations. Medieval medical historians nevertheless need to do more to integrate their subject better within studies of medieval politics and economics, as well as engage more with matters of modern concern on which we are well-qualified to comment (Green 2009). At least in our teaching, we habitually deal with the issues of relevance, historical relativism and anachronism, yet we rarely publish on these aspects in academic journals.

NEW DIRECTIONS AND DEBATES IN MEDIEVAL HEALTH AND MEDICINE

The study of medieval medicine has developed in leaps and bounds since the 1980s, although it is not clear that it has yet become an identifiable field in its own right, differentiated from the history of medieval science, daily life, natural philosophy – or 'pre-modern' medicine and healthcare more broadly. Nor perhaps should it. In a thought-provoking overview of scholarship published in

2009, Monica Green identified medieval medicine as a 'vibrant sub-discipline' (Green, 2009: 1218) and outlined some important philological, social and cultural strands of research. She did not at that time discuss bioarchaeology, which, since then, has become a major influence on medical history. Formerly, medieval scholarship depended primarily on philological and linguistic skills, leading to the fragmentation of expertise across multiple disciplines with few centres of excellence where groups of collaborators could work together *en masse*. This situation is broadly similar today. However, in the UK there are two large cross-chronological multi-disciplinary projects funded by the Wellcome Trust in which medievalists have flourished. *Hearing the Voice* at Durham University (http://hearingthevoice.org) has, since 2012, focused on voice-hearing in mental health, neuroscience, linguistics, philosophy and literature (Saunders 2015). *Generation to Reproduction* at the University of Cambridge (www.reproduction.group.cam.ac.uk/) has, since 2009, focused on the history of fertility and birth (Hopwood, Flemming and Kassel, eds. 2018).

The Wellcome Trust has long been the main funder of medical history and medical humanities in the UK, consequently shaping their interdisciplinary nature and the careers of researchers through its own agenda, albeit in a highly supportive way. The history of medieval medicine is an increasingly attractive topic to teach and research in the UK – appealing to undergraduate students (many of whom studied elements of it at school in a programme called *Medicine Through Time*) – and it appears at several themed or general medieval conferences in the UK and around the world; there has been a permanent strand for health and medicine at the International Medieval Congress in Leeds since 2018. In the USA, Monica Green is one of the most active scholars. She runs the MEDMED-L listserv, which has built and maintained a crucial virtual community for nearly 1,000 researchers around the world interested in medieval health and medicine. Green secured National Endowment for the Humanities funding for two summer schools (2009 and 2012) run in London, which were the envy of non-US nationals unable to participate. Nevertheless, despite all these highlights, medievalists often remain quite isolated and have to continually justify the value of what they do in order to survive; a problem they share, of course, with a great deal of humanities scholarship.

Since Green's overview of 2009, two publications in 2011 made it clear that there was a growing thematic diversity in medieval medicine. The *festschrift* to the influential medieval scholar Michael McVaugh – a leading light of our sub-discipline since the 1980s – includes articles on cosmetics, leprosy, dietary advice, concepts of pain and madness, medical awareness in religious writings for and by women, and medical advertising, alongside analyses of the production and circulation of manuscripts (Glaze and Nance, eds. 2011). A special issue of the *Social History of Medicine* in that same year, devoted to the Middle Ages (only the second time that this had happened in this influential journal's thirty-year history), included articles on new thinking about 'non-medical' sources for the history of medicine – legal records, ecclesiastical records, chronicles and literary texts – as well as four studies of medical recipes and translations in the early Middle Ages (Pilsworth and Banham, eds. 2011).

Since 2011, there have been several significant developments: fresh research on the Black Death (1347–1352) and other plague epidemics, including new insights from bioarchaeological sciences and genetics and from the experience of modern epidemics such as Ebola and COVID-19; renewed debates on retrospective diagnosis (to some extent a consequence of new research on disease); and, related to all of these, what could be called an 'environmental' turn, which includes animal disease and public health measures, and the health impacts of climate change, urbanization, pollution and food (in)security. The other major areas that have been developing over the last decade are medieval Disability Studies, and what could be called the 'rhetorical' or 'literary' turn in the study of medicine, health and the body.

It is not possible to go into all these topics in detail here, especially as much of this scholarship appears throughout the present volume. Before the publication of Irina Metzler's first book in 2006, medieval Disability Studies hardly existed. It is now moving towards theoretical and conceptual sophistication with a widening geographical and cultural scope, numerous intersections with the history of childcare, disease, mental health, hospitals and aging and applications for the history of technology, literary studies, gender studies and institutional history (Metzler 2006, 2013, 2016; Eyler, ed. 2010; Turner and Pearman, eds. 2010; Turner, ed. 2010; Richardson 2012; Lee, 2012; Turner 2013a; Shoham-Steiner 2014; Hsy 2015; Krötzl, Mustakallio and Kuuliala, eds. 2015; Kuuliala 2016; Nolte et al, eds. 2017, Skinner 2017; Connelly and Künzel, eds. 2018). This volume does not do full justice to the 'rhetorical' and 'literary' turns – although they are influential throughout. New ways of understanding representations, symbols and metaphors of illness, medical practice and the body in a wide variety of texts, whether medical, religious, historical – that is, chronicles – or literary, has helped to break down some of the perceived differences between these genres and the disciplines that study them (Citrome 2006; Solomon 2010; Vaught, ed. 2010; Coste, Jacquart, Pigeaud, eds. 2012; Yoshikawa, ed. 2015; Turner, ed. 2016; Langum 2016; McCann 2018; Orlemanski 2019).

Regarding disease and the environment, the main research has focused on plague epidemics, although there has been important work on parasitology and panzootics such as the animal murrains of the fourteenth century which also affected human health (Newfield 2009; Slavin 2012, forthcoming; Mitchell, ed. 2015). For plague, the primary development is the consensus amongst bioarchaeologists, epidemiologists and geneticists – and many but by no means all historians (Cohn 2013) – that the Black Death was caused by *Yersinia pestis*

INTRODUCTION

(the bacterium that causes modern bubonic plague, first recognized in 1894). Excavations of medieval plague cemeteries have yielded ancient DNA of *Yersinia pestis* and led to the complete reconstruction of its genome (Bos et al 2011). The main direction of research now is to analyze other plague epidemics in the same way, to investigate a wide range of mammalian hosts and numerous insect vectors, including human parasites, and to reconsider the spread of the disease, for example, across Africa, East Asia and the Middle Ages (Green, ed. 2014; Varlık 2015; Chouin, ed. 2018). There are still numerous pending questions: How did it move so fast across Eurasia (much faster than any other disease)? Why did it *apparently* have different effects and consequences in different regions? Innovative archival research is now shedding light on both epidemiological and historiographical patterns; for example, in new approaches to Bohemia, the Netherlands and the Iberian Peninsula (Mengel 2011; Roosen and Curtis 2019; Agresta 2020). A striking British archaeological approach is based on assessing fluctuating patterns of pottery sherds in eastern English excavations. It suggests an average population decline of 44.7 per cent, in keeping with the high mortality rates generally supported by most recent historical research, although in some areas it was much higher, while it was much lower in a few (Lewis 2016). In future, medievalists will need to explain more of these patterns: knowing what bacterium was present, however exciting the scientific research, does not necessarily help to explain the impact of disease on medieval people.

Plague research has also broken down some of the traditional exogenous (external: drought, flood, disease) *versus* endogenous (internal: war and political structures) causes for the late medieval crisis. New environmental work on animal disease, volcanic eruptions, earthquakes, food shortages, drought and flooding, in particular through pioneering research by Bruce Campbell (2016), shows that human behaviour, health and institutions were heavily affected by interconnected planetary-wide phenomena while, at the same time, human activity was already having a major impact on the planet. As yet, few scholars have argued for beginning the Age of the Anthropocene – that is, the geological age in which we live now in which humans have exerted most influence over the planet – earlier than 1492 (Bonneuil and Fressoz 2017: 14–17). However, it was startling to learn – based on analysis of an ice core sampled from an Alpine glacier – that the only time in the last 2,000 years when atmospheric lead pollution reverted back to 'natural' levels was during the Black Death, probably due to the temporary cessation of mining and smelting (More et al. 2017). What is now needed is more work on the health impacts of climate change, industrial pollution, malnutrition and changing occupational, religious and communal contexts, particularly as regards vulnerability and risk, an area in which bioarchaeologists, geographers, economists and social historians are already working together (Slavin and DeWitte 2013; Gerrard and Petley 2013; DeWitte and Kowaleski 2017; Alfani and Murphy 2017). As yet, however, most historical attention remains focused on explaining political and cultural changes during the late Middle Ages with the plague sometimes playing too large a role – the *Deus ex machina* that ushers in modernity. New ideas are needed on what medieval people did about the plague and how it affected them. In this respect, the concept of 'healthscaping' popularized by Guy Geltner (2013) as a way of describing deliberate methods of improving the urban landscape has proved very attractive for historians trying to understand human agency in tackling health problems.

KEY MEDIEVAL FRAMEWORKS: THE SIX NON-NATURALS AND THE FOUR HUMOURS

One of the key points made by Geltner and others interested in medieval public health is that its implementation at the time involved a wider understanding beyond academic circles of medical ideas about health and disease (Horden 2007; Geltner 2013, 2019b; Geltner and Coomans 2013; Rawcliffe 2013a; Rawcliffe and Weeda, eds. 2019; Coomans 2019). In particular, there was widespread awareness of the concept of the four humours – blood, phlegm, red/yellow bile, black bile – the qualities of hot, cold, wet and dry and the six non-naturals – air quality (with bad air known as *miasma*), food and drink, exercise and rest, sleep, excretion and the 'accidents of the soul'. These concepts appear everywhere from urban regulations to personal letters (Ingram 2019). In the last section of this introduction, it seems appropriate, therefore, to explain briefly some of these aspects of medieval theory.

The idea of the four humours developed over a long period of time, first appearing together in the Hippocratic work *The Nature of Man* in *c.*410 BCE:

> The human body contains blood, phlegm, yellow bile and black bile. These are the things that make up its constitution and cause its pains and health. Health is primarily that state in which these constituent substances are in the correct proportion to each other both in strength and quantity, and are well-mixed.
>
> —Lloyd, ed. 1978: 262

The relationship of this theory to Ancient Chinese and Indian theories of the flow of substances or agents in the body is unclear but they are comparable. Similar ideas about the balance of heat and fluid in the body can also be found in other global cultures. In what we tend to rather misleadingly call 'humouralism' – the qualities of hot-cold-dry-wet are more important than the individual humours themselves – every human, animal, life-cycle stage, season, plant, organ had its individual balance of qualities. For example, a naturally

INTRODUCTION   13

melancholic person was relatively colder and drier in complexion or temperament (in Latin *complexio* and *temperamentum* both mean 'balanced mixture') due to a higher level of black bile (Greek: *melas kholé*), but so was a person in middle age, a slice of dry-cured meat, a pig, the spleen, the season of autumn, the earth element, and the planet Saturn, which thereby linked each microcosm to the macrocosm of the universe. Similarly, a hotter and wetter sanguine person (Latin – *sanguis*: blood) shared this temperament with childhood, sugar, an ape, the heart, spring, air and Jupiter. Although there was some ontological understanding of illness and injury caused by specific external agents, medieval people saw illness as highly individualized resulting mainly from an internal imbalance or blockage of the flow of humours, and leading to treatments like bloodletting and cautery or the use of allopathic preparations, topically or via ingestion, the qualities of which counter-balanced the perceived cause. Humans were either sick, healthy or somewhere in between on a 'latitude' or spectrum of health. Perfect health was probably an idealized state impossible to achieve. Both the 'sick' and the 'healthy' therefore resorted to medical care and could be interested in medical theories, although this can most easily be documented at elite levels (Siraisi 1990: 78–114; van der Lugt 2011; Horden and Hsu, eds. 2013; Kaye 2014: 128–40).

Although the idea of the four humours is most closely linked to Hippocrates and his second century CE follower Galen, what medieval people knew about the humours mainly came from the systematization of Greek thought, especially the bringing together of the not-always-harmonious ideas of Galen and Aristotle, by authors from several religious traditions writing largely in Arabic in the Islamicate world during the ninth to eleventh centuries. Particularly influential was the Zoroastrian ʿAlī b. al-ʿAbbās al-Majūsī's (d. *c.* 990) *Kitāb Kāmil aṣ-ṣināʿa aṭ-ṭibbīya* (The Complete Book of the Medical Art), which was first translated into Latin by Constantine 'the African' as the *Pantegni* in the late-eleventh century (Kwakkel and Newton 2019). As explained in Glaze's chapter at the end of this volume, the Latin-speaking western half of the Roman Empire had previously retained only the most practical parts of ancient medical theory. The 'new' theoretical texts that were translated, taught and disseminated between the ninth and fifteenth centuries must therefore be seen as distinctively *medieval* constructions of knowledge that were forged in towns and centres of learning and trade across the Middle East, North Africa and Europe – it is a mistake to see this as a simple revival or survival of unchanging Greek wisdom. The old-fashioned teleological narrative which saw medieval teachers, scribes, officials, and healers of all kinds as transmitters rather than constructors of knowledge before the 'Renaissance' is one of the reasons why medieval medicine was unfairly denigrated for centuries. It is worth remembering that it was *medieval* humouralism that was continually re-constructed into the early nineteenth century (and until the present in parts of South Asia) because it was

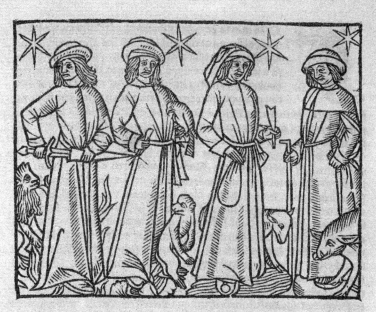

FIGURE 0.3: The four temperaments, The *Kalender of Shepherdes* (early-sixteenth century), reprinted in H. Oskar Sommer's edition of 1892. London, Wellcome Library. Credit: Wellcome Collection/Public Domain.

INTRODUCTION 15

meaningful to people (and we still talk in English about a sense of humour and catching 'cold'). Humouralism persisted because it was flexible. It could be adapted to the needs of different knowledge and faith communities through the development of persuasive discourses that allowed for the convergence of medical and religious ideals of behaviour – albeit with periods of tension or competition – while permitting pre-existing concepts about bodies, souls and places to continue. There has, for example, been extensive research on the symbiotic relationship of religious and medical concepts of healing, which allowed for continued beliefs in the evil eye, charms, demons and miracles (Nutton 1993; Ziegler 1998; Salmón and Cabré 1998; Olsan 2003; Attewell 2007; Stearns 2011: 91–105; Rider 2011; McCleery 2014a; Bhayro and Rider, eds. 2017; Page and Rider, eds. 2019; Yoeli-Tlalim 2019; Gilchrist 2020).

Another major author of the Islamicate world was Ḥunayn ibn Isḥāq (d. 873), a Christian physician of Baghdad, known in Latin as Johannitius, who wrote an introduction or *Isagoge* to the *Tegni* (Art of Medicine) of Galen. Ḥunayn not only managed to turn this fearfully complicated text into an accessible manual of medical theory, later used in European universities, but he also introduced in systematized fashion the concepts of the 'naturals,' 'contra-naturals' and 'non-naturals,' none of which had been so clearly outlined before (García Ballester 2002). The 'naturals' included the elements, the internal organs of the body, the humours and the qualities; the 'contra-naturals' were diseases and their causes and consequences; the six 'non-naturals' were described as follows:

There are six types of causes that are associated with health and sickness. The first is the air that surrounds the body, [then] food and drink, exercise and rest, sleep and waking, fasting and fullness, and incidental conditions of the mind. All these preserve health from accidents, if used with appropriate moderation as to quantity, quality, time, function, and order. But if anything is done contrary to this, diseases occur and persist.

—Wallis, ed. 2010: 150

Modern research on each of these six things has been variable for the Middle Ages. There is a lot of focus on the emotions and food, both of which are major scholarly fields in their own right and, more recently, air – which to a great extent incorporated the older Hippocratic approach in *Airs, Waters and Places* to include climate, terrain and living spaces more broadly – and plays a major role in environmental histories of the Middle Ages. Sleep, excretion ('fasting and fullness') and exercise have been better studied for the early-modern period so far (Cavallo and Storey 2013; Handley 2016), although there has been work on some aspects of medieval sleep (McLehose 2013, 2020; Gordon 2015). The fact that the non-naturals incorporated sexual activity and bathing has also

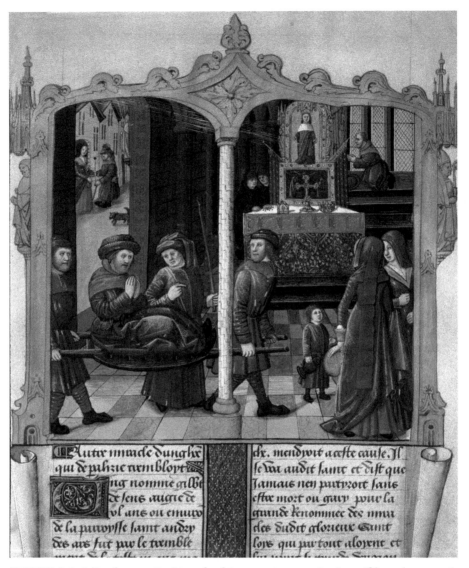

FIGURE 0.4: Miracle cure, *Le Livre des faiz monseigneur saint Loys* (fifteenth century). Paris, Bibliothèque Nationale, MS Français 2829, fol. 101. Credit: Getty Images.

brought these issues under the umbrella of health (Proctor 2008; Coomans and Geltner 2013: 63–74; Solomon 2013; Atat 2020). Nevertheless, as Sandra Cavallo (2017: 1–2) notes, considering how significant a role all six of these things played in health through until at least the eighteenth century, it is surprising how little sustained study they have received, especially as regards

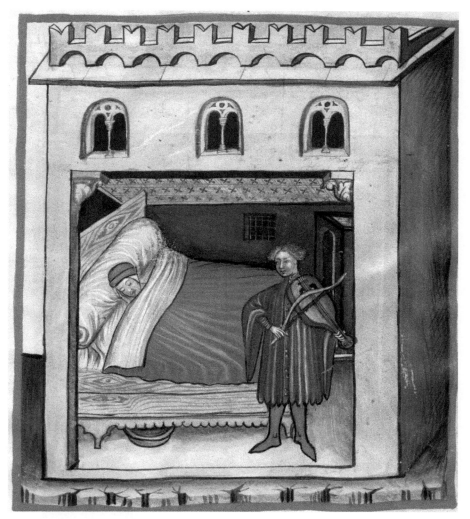

FIGURE 0.5: Sleep, *Tacuinum sanitatis* (Tables of Health) (late-fourteenth century). Vienna, Österreichische Nationalbibliothek, Codex Vindobonensis Series Nova 2644, fol. 100. Credit: Österreichische Nationalbibliothek, Vienna.

preventative medicine. Although they could have a therapeutic function in curative regimes and palliative care, the non-naturals were primarily preventative in their application. This focus meant that adjustment of diet and lifestyle required the close involvement in health of the individual, the cook, the parent, other carers and domestic helpers and the community as a whole, including religious and political authorities. Some of these groups are represented in the cover image for this volume from a Florentine manuscript of the first half of the fourteenth century. Keeping healthy through these means can therefore be seen as a medieval form of the concept of 'biopolitics' as elaborated by Michel Foucault (McCleery 2014b: 210–17; Geltner 2019b: 13–17). Health from this perspective is a matter of (self) discipline, both physical and moral, exercised from below and from above and much aided in the Middle Ages by the ways in which medicine and religion shared many ideals of moderate lifestyle and care (Langum 2016; Cohen-Hanegbi 2017; Ritchey and Strocchia, eds. 2020). Our cover image is notably not from a medical manuscript but from an Italian translation of a well-known French guide to the vices and virtues: here visiting and caring for the sick is being presented as a religious duty.[4]

CONCLUSION

Peregrine Horden (2007) has suggested that non-natural medicine could be 'medicine without doctors' but growing familiarity with medical advice also made medical practitioners of all kinds authorities in their communities. Arguably it was through widespread dissemination of medical theories such as the non-naturals that medieval societies became medicalized and, in turn, medicine was socialized according to local customs and needs, as can be seen in the richly illustrated images of the *Tacuinum sanitatis* with which this introduction began. As we have already pointed out, the cultural history of medieval health and medicine is a project still in progress with a great deal more work to be done before mappings of meaning across highly diverse global cultures and societies can be fully drawn; they will always be a matter of debate due to the equally diverse backgrounds of dedicated scholars. However, it is hoped that at least for ideas about the environment, food, disease, animals, the archaeology of health, personal experience, the workings of the brain, and medical authority this volume leads the way in opening up new avenues for research and showing what so far has been interpreted from the past.

ACKNOWLEDGEMENTS

I would like to thank all the participants of the round table at the International Medieval Congress (IMC) in Leeds in 2015 for their ideas, especially Irina Metzler and Jo Edge for their insights. Thanks go to Axel Müller, Director of the IMC, for scheduling the round table and for commenting on a draft of this introduction.

NOTES

1. The digital version of the Vienna codex of the *Tacuinum sanitatis* is available from https://search.onb.ac.at/primo_library/libweb/action/dlDisplay.do?vid=ONB&docId=ONB_alma21296213330003338&fn=permalink (accessed 29 June 2020).

INTRODUCTION

2. For example, for a discussion of the problematic concept of the term 'patient', see McCleery (2009).
3. See Metzler (2006: 10) for one of the first applications of the *emic/etic* binary to medieval health research. For the origins and still polemic usage of these terms in Linguistics, Cultural Anthropology, and History of Science, see Harris (1976) and Jardine (2004).
4. Florence, Biblioteca Nazionale Centrale, MS Magliabechiano II. VI.16, fol. 48v. See Cosnet (2015) for more on this text.

CHAPTER ONE

Environment: Managing Urban Sanitation for *Sanitas*

DOLLY JØRGENSEN

INTRODUCTION

The word *sanitation*, which has the modern connotation of cleanliness, derives from the Latin *sanitas*, meaning health. The word *sanitation* in various forms shows up in all sorts of modern conveniences from hand sanitizer to sanitary napkins/towels to sanitation departments that collect urban household trash. This kind of sanitation, which most specifically arises in the context of urban cleanliness, is a nineteenth-century innovation (Melosi 2000). Although sanitation as a word did not exist in the Middle Ages, *sanitas* certainly did. Just as their modern counterparts do, medieval urban residents also associated cleanliness with health while conversely associating filth with corruption and unhealthy living conditions.

This chapter discusses conceptions of environmental risks to health in medieval towns and cities. The investigation is divided into three parts: identifying sanitation problems, adding infrastructure to better sanitary conditions and enforcing standards. The first section shows that unhealthy urban environments were defined through sensory perceptions – noxious smells, potentially dangerous sights and foul tastes. While the humoural theory of disease shaped some of the understanding of disease transmission, evidence indicates that the senses played a more direct role in determining cleanliness versus filth. Food preparation (particularly butchery), craftwork that handled organic matter such as dyeing and leatherworking, latrine design and waste disposal all became regulated as potentially harmful activities because of their ability to offend the senses. The second section gives an overview of the sanitary infrastructures that became standard in medieval urban areas. The third section surveys the control mechanisms for enforcing sanitary standards for roads, waterways and waste disposal sites. The focus is on local-level governance including statutes, court records and other administrative documents after 1300 in England and Italy, where the majority of scholarly work on sanitation has been published, with supporting information from elsewhere including France, the Nordic countries, the Low Countries and Central Europe.

Working with medieval sources to explore urban sanitation has some inherent limitations. Urban governments became powerful civic authorities in the late medieval period, generating legal documents that provide contemporary evidence about responses to environmental problems. However, care must be taken when interpreting them as social and cultural historical sources for several reasons. First, although the availability of written sources increases dramatically after 1350, the records are still spotty and give us only small glimpses into medieval life in each city. That limitation necessitates combining evidence from various cities, as well as supplementing historical documents with archaeological evidence of physical infrastructures and waste disposal practices.

Second, regulations are promulgated by authorities, whose views may not necessarily be representative of the urban population. As a judicial body, medieval civic councils heard misdemeanour presentments, levied fines, and received capital pledges for minor offences. In the legislative arena, councils issued ordinances founded on bills presented by any individual or group who wished to voice a grievance or amend common practice. The voices heard in these documents are thus only those who either chose to complain about current conditions or those who had complaints levied against them. Because these sources come from litigation, there is always a question as to whether the sanitation deficiencies they describe are the norm or the exception. I take the view that they are exceptions – that laws and fines for sanitation misdeeds document what is considered generally unacceptable to the community at large. This interpretation is backed up in the seminal work of Marjorie McIntosh (1998) who found that crime reporting in England from 1370 to 1600 came from community members rather than top-down regulation.

The sanitary condition of medieval towns and cities has attracted a fair amount of scholarly attention in the last decade – work that revives and revises often-overlooked scholarship on the history of medieval sanitation in the early twentieth century (Thorndike 1928; Sabine 1933, 1934, 1937). This historical scholarship has been framed within the fields of either urban environmental history (Magnusson 2013) or public health history (Geltner 2012). The historical situation in England has been most written extensively written on (Rawcliffe 2013a, 2013b), including analysis of sanitation infrastructure, governmental structures, and pollution control (Carr 2008; Jørgensen 2008, 2010a, 2010b; Ciecieznski 2013). Guy Geltner (2013, 2014, 2019b) has offered several in-depth examinations of Italian city state governmental functions targeting sanitation offences in the name of public health. Although most of this work is based on textual records, some scholarship has integrated archaeological evidence to support the documentary records (Jørgensen 2008; van Oosten 2016). Literary scholars have also used medieval fiction to discuss the cultural place of filth (Morrison 2008; Bayless 2012). In general, current historical scholarship is countering claims made in the late twentieth century that the medieval urban environment was overwhelmingly filthy (e.g. Keene 1982; Zupko and Laures 1996).

The recent proliferation of studies of the medieval urban environment is part and parcel of a larger movement that has established urban environmental history as a defined research field, following in the footsteps of the American scholars Martin Melosi, Joel Tarr, and William Cronon who published key urban history works in the late 1990s (Frioux 2012). Recent interest in the medieval environment as an object of study has been strong in the English-speaking academic community, which has resulted in more studies of medieval England than elsewhere. As urban environmental history grows, we can expect more and more studies in other parts of Europe that would add to our source base, such as a recent Masters dissertation by Carr-Riegel (2016) on medieval Krakow's urban environmental issues, and a PhD thesis by Coomans (2018) on sanitation in the late medieval Low Countries.

Beyond the history discipline, archaeologists have been interested in medieval sanitation infrastructure for many years (Addyman 1989; Gläser 2004), including waste disposal practices (Keene 1982; Hooper 2006). Newer developments in environmental archaeology and archaeological-based disease investigation have spurred significant studies to identify internal and external parasites and diseases passed on through poor sanitary measures in medieval populations (e.g. King and Henderson 2014; Mitchell 2015a, 2015b). These studies show that while medieval governments and urban residents might have implemented sanitary controls, as will be discussed in this chapter, it does not mean that illnesses associated with poor cleanliness disappeared. Living in close proximity to animals and their wastes, eating food that lacked refrigeration and potentially improper preservation and drinking water taken from sources that could have faecal contamination without physical signs of degradation all contributed to ongoing struggles for public health. But critically, the continued existence of sanitation-related disease does not mean that sanitation ideas were absent in the medieval city.

THE SENSORY PERCEPTION OF
MATTER OUT OF PLACE

The anthropologist Mary Douglas (1969) famously defined uncleanliness or pollution as 'matter out of place'. A question that always arises, then, is why and how something is defined as 'out of place'. For modern health science, bacteria, viruses, environmental contaminants, and rogue human cells (in the case of cancer) are out of place – they are the agents of illness. Without knowledge of the microscopic, medieval people also developed ideas of what was out of place, but this relied on a different epistemology of illness. Within the realm of city sanitation, odoriferous and visible materials were identified as harmful because they could be sensed (Jørgensen 2013a).

In European Antiquity and the Middle Ages, sensory perception was understood by learned scholars as a form of transmission of information about an object as well as its tangible and even intangible properties (Woolgar 2006). The senses served as conduits of physical contact: eyes received/transmitted light and representations of the original object, noses channelled vapours into the brain, ears carried air that had been struck and tongues and hands gained impressions of the object through touching. Bartholomaeus Anglicus's thirteenth-century encyclopaedia *De proprietatibus rerum* stated that the physical senses (which were ranked in importance from top to bottom in the body as sight, hearing, smell, taste and touch) relayed the tangible and intangible properties of objects to 'the common sense' portion of the brain (Woolgar 2006). This was particularly the case for smell and taste, since the matters sensed by the body were composed of the four elements (fire, water, earth and air) and these elements affected the four related humours; the body would react to them based on the person's individual humours.

More than just a scholarly exercise, sensory perception of urban spaces affects how residents responded to objects and conditions they encounter. As Emily Cockayne (2007) has shown for seventeenth-century England, people became uncomfortable with other people's practices and things when they impinged upon their senses negatively. The natural reaction was then to attempt to control or remove the offence. Unsanitary conditions were sensed primarily through the nose. Organic wastes – specifically wastes that come from decaying body parts, decomposing vegetation, faeces, and urine – are highly odoriferous and do indeed carry many potential pathogens. Modern research indicates that there is a fairly consistent dislike of bodily fluid odours across human cultures, which may be linked to an evolutionary response to avoid disease (Curtis and Birna 2001). So, while interpretation of smell is certainly culturally situated (e.g. Drobnick 2006), associating organic waste odours with disease may be a typical human response.

For medical practitioners in the Middle Ages, medieval miasmic theory attributed disease to the corruption of air, which could be visible like a fog or

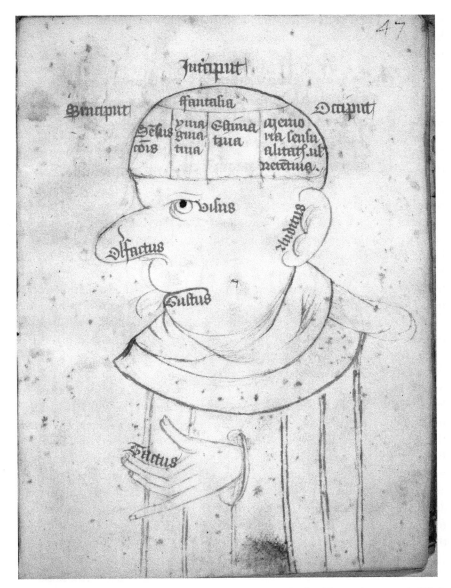

FIGURE 1.1: The senses, Augustine, *De spiritu et anima* (early-thirteenth century). Trinity College Cambridge MS O.7.16, fol. 47. Credit: Master and Fellows of Trinity College Cambridge.

invisible. Aristotelian philosophy held that odour was an immaterial quality that radiated from an object; whereas Bartholomaeus and his eleventh-century predecessor Constantine the African aligned themselves with Platonic thought that smell was a smoke or vapour (Woolgar 2006). Miasmas, based on the Greek word meaning pollution, were corrupting influences that needed to be avoided if possible. These bad smells could potentially be countered by good smells from herbs, incense or flowers, which promoted the building of enclosed gardens and perfume trades (Woolgar 2006). Miasmatic theory has been widely embraced as the root of modern sanitation measures in the West (Melosi 2000). Edwin Chadwick, the secretary of England's Poor Law Commission, who is credited with initiating the modern sanitation movement in the 1840s, claimed that 'all smell is disease', placing him squarely in a miasmatic world (Reinarz 2014).

Corruption of the air was a typical late-medieval urban complaint (Robinson 2020). The obsession with stenches as the source of harmful air would continue through the early modern period (Dobson 1997). Medieval sources often characterize the harmful nature of organic, decaying matter as stinking (*fetida*), rotting (*putrida*), or poisoning (*corrumpitur*), invoking the sense of smell as the mode of understanding pollution. Thus, the medieval medical poem *Regimen Sanitatis Salernitanum* (Salernitan Regimen of Health) encouraged readers to keep the air free of the smell of excrement: '*Aer sit mundus, habitabilis ac luminosus, nec sit infectus, nec olens foetore cloacae*' which can be literally translated as 'Let the air be pure, clear, and bright, / and let it be neither infectious nor odorous with the stink of the sewer' (Ordonaux 1870: 56).

Complaints were often based on organic wastes that had been disposed of directly on the ground, rather than being buried or otherwise controlled, and emitted strong smells. For example, in a case brought before the Norwich leet court in 1288, a man named Roger Benjamin paid a two shilling fine for setting up a muck-heap in which he buried butchery waste causing the air to be 'abominably corrupted' (Latin: *aer pessime corrumpitur*). Similar wording was used in another case that same year when William the skinner was fined for throwing dead cats into a pit whereby '*aer corrumpitur*' (Hudson 1892: 23). In November 1372, King Edward III of England commanded the local government of Gloucester to keep an area near the castle door free from animal dung heaps because: 'the air is so corrupted and infected that the constable and his household and other passers by are assailed by an abominable stench, the advantage of fresh air is prevented, the condition of the men is harmed' (Deputy Keeper of the Records 1914: 243).

Although the coming of the Black Death to Europe in 1348–49 affected European life tremendously, sanitary concerns appear consistently both before and after the event. Records from up to a century before the plague reveal that the smell of waste was considered to corrupt the air. Research on London (Jørgensen 2014) and Italy (Geltner 2019b) both show that regulations were in place, court cases were heard, and practical actions were taken to ensure sanitary conditions before the plague appeared. The same type of language is used throughout the period even after the outbreak of the disease with no significant changes in the framing of pollution. While it is true that medicinal tracts from the Middle Ages, particularly those written about plague prevention in southern Europe, highlight

ENVIRONMENT

the role of miasmas, tracts fail to directly link waste or other sanitation concerns to the disease. One exception might be the foul smell of dead bodies, which was the subject of pestilence regulation: Pistoia's 'Ordinances for Sanitation in a Time of Mortality' from 1348 required particularly deep graves for plague victim corpses to 'avoid the foul stench which the bodies of the dead give off' (Osheim 1994). The Pistoia ordinances also banned butchers from having a shop near any kind of tavern, shop, stable, or pen that 'give off a putrid smell', presumably to ensure the quality of the meat, although there is not any direct mention of wastes from these locations. In London, the return of the plague in 1391 appears to have prompted protests against butchery practices which were deemed to be infecting the air (Sabine 1933). While this could be read to mean that the plague brought about a change in thinking about sanitation and smell, we must remember that in 1343, before any outbreak of plague, the London authorities had named a spot for the butchers to dispose of waste for 'the decency and cleanliness of the city' (Sabine 1933: 343). Although some outcries for sanitation can have been prompted by particular outbreaks of disease, the fear of spreading the plague does not appear to have significantly changed the practical approaches to urban sanitation in the first hundred years of its appearance in Europe.

By the sixteenth century, things were somewhat different and indications are that plague outbreaks might have directly motivated sanitation actions. Thomas More, the author of *Utopia*, was Commissioner of the Sewers from 1515 and in 1518 was asked to enforce the first English royal plague orders (Totaro 2005: 72). Although those orders focused on crowd control and reducing contact with the dead, the link between More's two tasks was no coincidence. Writing in 1596, John Harington noted that urbanization led to 'infection', particularly because of latrines and human faeces, and was thus interested in designing and installing flush toilets (Jørgensen 2010c: 7).

Creating stagnant water bodies, particularly when combined with waste disposal in those wetted areas, was portrayed in texts as dangerous to health. Stench (*fetor*), for example, was said to emanate from a blocked drain in Bologna in 1376 (Geltner 2014: 315). An extended investigation of the danger of odours from a contaminated river occurred in Coventry, England, in 1480. The Prior of Coventry sent a letter to the city council complaining that the city dwellers were regularly throwing household waste and stable dung into the river so that a stench, or an 'evell eyre' as he labelled it, made 'he, his Brethern & all other ffolkes there be hurte' (Harris 1907–1913: 445). The Prior argued that waste disposal of this sort was against the law. The Mayor and council made an official reply to the Prior's complaint, noting that the council was doing everything in its power to identify and punish waste disposal violations like the one the Prior brought forward. The council noted that each time the Leet court, which handled nuisance complaints, met in the city, it included inquiries about waste disposal into the river. In addition, the Aldermen of each ward made a daily search of the

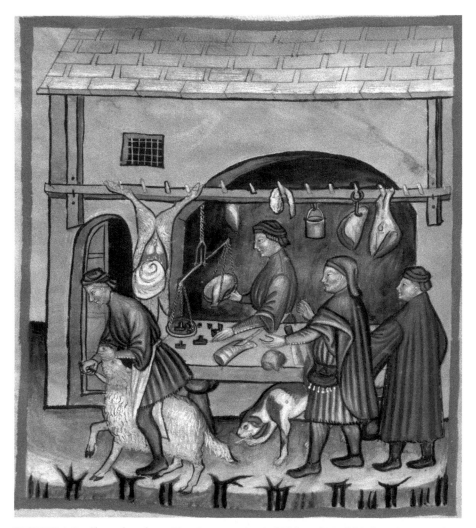

FIGURE 1.2: Sheep butchery, *Tacuinum sanitatis* (Tables of Health) (late-fourteenth century), Vienna, Österreichische Nationalbibliothek, Codex Vindobonensis Series Nova 2644, fol. 72v. Credit: Österreichische Nationalbibliothek, Vienna.

property adjoining the river. But although the council was working with great diligence to find people throwing filth into the river, few specific offenders could be identified, so cleaning up the smelly problem proved difficult.

Butchery wastes could be particularly troublesome for creating odours if they were disposed of incorrectly (Sabine 1933; Carr 2008). The case of the butchers of London is instructive in this regard. In 1368, the Mayor and Aldermen of London held an inquest into the disposal of butchery waste in the Thames

ENVIRONMENT

'whereby the water was rendered corrupt and generated fetid smells'. As also discussed further below by Kathleen Walker-Meikle in her chapter on animals, the jury found that the butchers of St Nicholas Shambles were disposing of waste in the Thames, so they recommended the relocation of all animal slaughter outside the city walls. In 1371, the issue was still ongoing and the butchers were still disposing of carcasses in the river. The King ordered London's mayor to remove the 'Butchers' Bridge' where the butchers regularly threw offal into the Thames because of 'the corruption, the grevious stench and the loathsome sight' of the waste disposal practices. In a follow-up statement ordering the cessation of the butchery disposal practices the King made it clear that the waste was causing smells which, in turn, were causing illness:

> Whereas of late, by reason of the slaughtering of great beasts in the city aforesaid, from the putrefied blood of which running in the streets, and the entrails thereof thrown into the water of Thames, the air in the same city has been greatly corrupted and infected, and whereby the worst of abominations and stenches have been generated, and sicknesses and many other maladies have befallen persons dwelling in the same city.
>
> —Riley 1868: 356

In this case, animal blood and entrails, particularly when disposed of in water, were blamed for corruption of the air through smell. It is interesting to note that corruption of the water itself – water that otherwise might be consumed as drinking water or in other products such as beer – was not a concern. The air as a primary disease vector appears to have been most worrisome to the London city leaders, although sight of the bloody carcasses and dirty entrails does also appear in the complaint. The same focus on air is evident when King Charles VI of France ordered the demolition of the meat market near his palace in Paris because of 'the corruption and infection of the air and the harm to the human body' (de Lespinasse 1886: 275).

Other craftspeople working with organic materials including tanners, candlemakers, and leatherworkers were also singled out as culprits creating foul smells (Leguay 1999: 54). Tanners, for example, used bird guano, dog dung, oak bark and urine in their processes, creating stinking wastewaters (Jørgensen 2010b). In Nottingham, England, the local court noted that the city's professional dyers were harming 'the common people with the stench from the residues of their waters dropping and falling on the King's highway' and that the dye wastewaters caused 'corruption of the whole people passing' (Corporation of Nottingham 1882: 273, 275).

Latrine pits emitted strong faecal odours as the waste decomposed, and complaints about the potential danger of these odours also appear in the medieval record. Latrine nuisances in Lucca and Bologna, Italy were described as 'putrid' and 'fetid' (Geltner 2013, 2014), an indication that odour was the chief worry. In 1487, when the city of Malmö was granted privileges as a Danish town, the law stated that latrines had to be dug into the ground such that wastes did not flow out and spread a 'bad smell' over the streets and neighbouring plots (Anders 1986: 265). London court records give an indication of the type of complaints that arose. In 1341, the London Assize of Nuisance investigated odours entering the house of a widow named Isabel from her neighbour Henry's cesspit (Chew and Kellaway 1973: Misc. Roll DD, no. 365). The smell was wafting through a window and several smaller openings into her tenement. Henry was ordered to remove the nuisance. In 1355, there were complaints about the degraded state of the ditch surrounding the Fleet Prison in London affecting the prisoners (Riley 1868: 279–280). Waste from latrines directly built over the ditch as well as tanning waste was causing an 'infection of the air'. The result of this 'abominable stench' was that 'many of those there imprisoned are often affected with various diseases and grievous maladies, not without serious peril unto them'. Concern about the sanitary condition of the Fleet River had even appeared the year before, in 1354, when butchery waste dumped in the Fleet was also blamed for odours harming the health of the prisoners (Sharpe 1905: fol. xxviii). All this evidence indicates that the smell from both solid and liquid organic waste materials was understood in the Middle Ages to be generally unhealthy.

Sight should, however, not be dismissed as a motivator for identifying unhealthy situations in the medieval city. As noted in the case of the London butchers and the Thames, the sight of the butchery offal was also singled out as a concern. A similar conjunction of smell and sight appeared in a complaint by the Friars Minor in York, England, in 1372 (Deputy Keeper of the Records 1911: 438). The air takes centre stage in their grievance in which the friars noted that 'the air in their church is poisoned by the stench there generated as well around the altars where the Lord's body is daily ministered as in their other houses, and flies and other vermin are thereby bred and enter their church and houses'. But they also mention that the parishioners refused to attend mass because of both 'the stench and the horrible sights'. The remedy commanded by the King of England was to dispose of the waste where it could be 'covered up' – a fix that addressed both the smell and sight problem. Town statutes often forbade butchers from having visual signs of contamination. For example, in Seni, Croatia, butchers could not have unfinished skins hanging outside their shops (Azman et al. 2006) and in Coventry. England, butchers had to keep their doors clean of 'bloode and other fylthis' (Harris 1907–1913: 42–3).

It is possible that optical theories of intromission, in which the eye can absorb an object's qualities, played a part in wanting to avoid seeing waste (Geltner 2013: 10; Geltner 2014: 315). In the theory of intromission, the object gives off a light, which is transmitted to the eye through a process of replication of the original as a likeness or representation (Woolgar 2006: 21).

In this theory, the visible object has tangible contact with the eye and can change the essence of the soul through that contact. This led to the belief that the sight of a thing could physically affect the viewer. Yet even without invoking optical disease transmission, visual evidence of waste was a sure way to identify where a potentially lethal smell was coming from.

Taste could also have played a role in identifying the unclean, especially as the sense of taste is closely related to smell. A Parisian ordinance from 1374 declared food inedible if it was around waste of any kind, and the quality of water in drinking fountains in Paris was said to be questionable because of contact with waste (Leguay 1999: 44). In other instances, blood and butchery waste show up as direct agents of water pollution. In fourteenth-century Lucca, Italy, for example, allowing animal blood to flow into a public space was punishable by a fine; and slaughtering animals above a well or washing them near a well was forbidden (Geltner 2013). This restriction likely had to do with the potential for the blood to make the water undrinkable. The same concern holds true for a regulation in Narbonne, France, from 1315 which forbade the dyers of the city from disposing of their foul-smelling blue or red madder into the water except in the early evening so that the water would be drinkable in the morning (Leguay 1999: 58). The same kind of nighttime-only disposal regulation for blue madder was passed in Winchester, England (Bailey 1856: 97–8) and for tanners' waste in Verona (Zupko and Laures 1996: 82). Food hygiene could also be directly affected by waste disposal – for instance, the York government banned the washing of tanned skins in the area of the riverfront where the butchers prepared sausages (Sellers 1912–15, 1: 15).

INFRASTRUCTURE FOR SANITATION

The concerns about sensing waste material led medieval town governments to regulate the building of sanitation infrastructure. These developments appear in many different locales at roughly the same time in the city records. This congruence of approaches to sanitation issues is likely the result of similar population pressures in the rapidly urbanizing cities of the fourteenth century and the availability of a common set of tools and management techniques. As urban populations grew in the Middle Ages, local governments became more vested in maintaining peace among neighbours which, in turn, required legally defining what constituted nuisance behaviours and what building standards should be followed. The growth of sanitation infrastructure as instruments of enforcement is part and parcel of the growth of the power of urban governments (Jørgensen 2010a).

However, we should be wary of attributing too much novelty to medieval building rules and nuisance law that are first recorded in great numbers in the fourteenth century – it may be that some of the regulations were common practice before the late medieval period, but are only recorded in writing because city-level records were becoming more systematized and complete. For example, local sanitation-related ordinances are recorded in the 1200s in several Italian cities, including Bassano in 1259, Verona in 1276, Ferrara in 1287 and Spoleto in 1296 (Zupko and Laures 1996). On the other side of Europe, the Scottish Statutes of the Guild, originally adopted in Berwick in 1249, levied a fine against anyone putting filth or household ashes into the street, marketplace, or river bank (Innes 1868: 72). Yet the number of surviving documents certainly proliferates over time; by the fifteenth century, sanitation issues are regularly recorded in urban records.

Infrastructure standards for latrine construction were set up in many cities. General city laws regulated where latrines, privies and cesspits could be located, often in reference to the homeowner's property line. The German Magdeburg civic law code, first compiled in 1188, specified that cesspits had to be three feet away from the property fence and had to be enclosed (Carr-Riegel 2016: 49). A 1269 city law from Ribe, Denmark, required latrines to be built at least fourteen feet from cemeteries, at least ten feet from the nearest street and at least six feet from the nearest neighbour (Økland and Høiaas 2000: 9). The 1487 city privileges of Bergen, Norway, stated that latrines had to be at least two feet from the street and neighbouring property and could not have an overflow (Økland and Høiaas 2000: 10). Regulations passed in 1463 and 1464

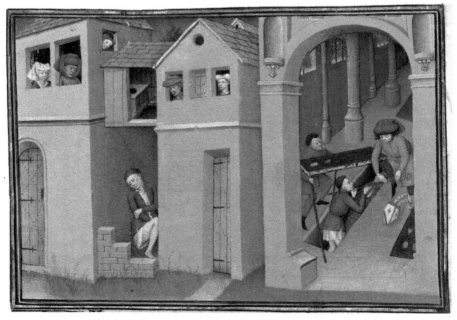

FIGURE 1.3: Latrine and latrine pit, Boccaccio, *Decameron* (mid-fifteenth century). Paris, Bibliothèque de l'Arsenal, MS 5070 réserve, fol. 50v. Credit: Bibliothèque Nationale de France.

ENVIRONMENT

in Leiden, Netherlands, mandated the provision of cesspits for all tenants and prohibited drainage of cesspits into overflows or canals (van Oosten 2016: 712). In Bologna, five men who had open latrines in 1295 were ordered to close them off from those passing by (Geltner 2018).

Some cities provided city-owned and operated latrines, which were often strategically placed in market areas which had many visitors. For example, the York government owned and maintained public latrines in an arch of the bridge over the river Ouse below the *maison dieu* in 1367. In 1400, the Ouse Bridge financial records attest to the city paying 13s 8d for its annual maintenance, in addition to repair works that had to be undertaken from time to time (Stell 2003: 122, 208, 257). Several entries in the bridgemaster's accounts indicate that the city paid 6s 4d annually for oil to light the latrines at night, a move that would have made using a damp, dingy public latrine more comfortable. London had a similar large public latrine house on London Bridge by 1306 which served both the merchant and resident community of the bridge as well as visitors to the area (Sabine 1934: 307). In fact, medieval London had at least thirteen public latrines; often these were latrine complexes that could accommodate many simultaneous users (Sabine 1934: 309).

Waste collection services were publicly organized. Collecting taxes to provide a public service may seem like a relatively new development, yet medieval governments collected taxes to build and maintain sanitary system infrastructure (Jørgensen 2008). In Coventry, for example, waste collection services are recorded in 1420 when the council gave William Oteley the right to collect one penny from every resident and shopholder on a quarterly basis for his weekly street cleansing and waste removal services (Harris 1907–1913: 21). The constable of each ward had to ensure that a weekly cart service was provided. The cart service appears to have made regular rounds every Saturday, as inhabitants were told to put out their muck and sweepings only on a Friday night because the cart would come the next morning. Many cities appear to have had similar systems. York had a dung cart 'in every ward and a place assigned without the barre or postern wher al such dung as shalbe caried out of every ward shalbe layd so that husbands of the contre may come ther to and have it away' (Raine 1940: 165). The city of Norwich had two public carts for the removal of 'ffilthie and vile matter' (Hudson and Tingey 1908–10: 2: 110) and also paid John the Common Sergeant for cleansing the common marketplace several times and Austyn Bange for carrying muck out of the city-run lepers' house (Hudson and Tingey 1908–10: 2: 53, 61). The waste collection services were intended to pick up waste from the streets and the gutters before they could begin to smell strongly. Weekly service helped promote prompt removal.

Paved streets and drainage gutters also served as sanitary infrastructures (Jørgensen 2008). Streets paved with stones with some kind of drainage gutter

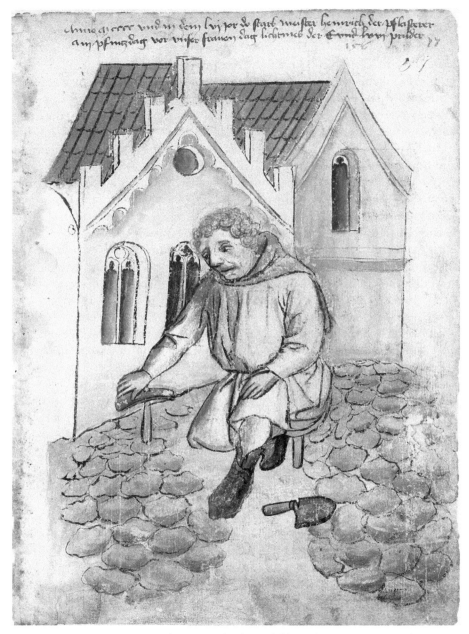

FIGURE 1.4: A paver, Nuremburg Hausbuch (mid-fifteenth century). Nuremburg, Stadtbibliothek Nürnberg, MS Amb. 317.2°, fol. 77. Credit: Stadtbibliothek Nürnberg.

in the middle were common in many medieval towns and cities. For example, Siena, Italy, mandated paving both streets and alleyways in 1262 to avoid mud accumulating in the streets (Armstrong 1900). Professional pavers who were often employed to maintain the paving of major thoroughfares and markets appear in medieval budgetary records, such as in Krakow, Poland, where payments are attested from 1390 onwards (Carr-Riegel 2016: 24). Pavement and gutters would have facilitated runoff from the street, avoiding the accumulation of mud and stagnant water, which would have been seen as unhealthy. Street sweepers appear to have been employed by some city governments: Coventry paid for cleaning of the marketplace (Harris 1907–1913: 217), Norwich appointed two people in each ward to clean the streets in 1496 (Hudson and Tingey 1908–10: 1: 288), and London had designated street cleaners called 'rakiers' (Sharpe 1909: fol. cxliv). Street cleaners probably came from the lowest classes: in Central European records, hired street cleaners were often vagrants, paupers, and prisoners (Havlíček et al. 2017: 273).

ENFORCEMENT OF SANITATION

Building infrastructure to minimize odoriferous wastes, and thereby remove matter that was dangerous to health, was only the first step toward *sanitas* in the medieval city. The use of those infrastructures also had to be enforced. Records indicating how sanitation was enforced come in two varieties: laws or statutes that promulgate standards and set up fines for disobedience, and court records indicating inspections carried out, cases heard and fines levied. While repeated promulgation of statutes has been read by some scholars to indicate systematic failure of the legal system to keep the medieval city clean (Zupko and Laures, 1996), more recent work has seen the reissuance of sanitary laws as an indication that sanitary violations were seen as socially unacceptable (Jørgensen 2008; Rawcliffe 2013; Geltner 2014). It may be that most provisions were written down in response to a specific petition or nuisance, rather than being formulated as a pre-emptive general law, as Kucher (2005: 512) argues for regulations in Siena. As Martha Howell remarked, social legislation assisted in defining medieval city spaces as 'clean, pure, open, propertied, risk-limited, peaceful' (2000: 17).

City sanitation statutes tend to be negative ('thou shalt not') proclamations: waste should not be disposed of in the street or gutter, on a neighbouring property, or in the river, and latrines should not leak. These proclamations tend to attach some kind of fine to the forbidden activity, such as Magnus Eriksson's Swedish city law of 1353 which levied a six-mark fine for building a latrine closer than three feet from the property line (Holmsbäck and Wessen 1966) or an order from Coventry in 1444 that no manure was to be swept into the gutter or the perpetrator would receive a 4d. fine (Harris 1907–1913: 208).

There are also positive, actionable laws that address how often to clean the streets, where to take waste for disposal, and how to report sanitary violators. In Krakow, for example, a statute on road cleaning from 1373 required that residents had to sweep the street clean up to the road's central gutter within a certain distance from their door (Carr-Riegel 2016: 43). Such a command was designed to make sure that the street cleaning labour would be divided between the residents, a common feature of medieval sanitation control (Jørgensen 2008).

Specific job titles were designated for sanitation duties in the medieval city (Jørgensen 2010a). In the late thirteenth century, London had four men in each ward jurisdiction designated to keep up the pavements, remove obstructions such as dung in the street and levy non-compliance fines (Sharpe 1899: fol. 88b). These men were collectively known as 'scavangers' or 'rakers' (Sharpe 1905: fol. clxv). In Bologna, the *fango* notary was the official in charge of all 'dirt'-related things from 1256 (Geltner 2014). The *fango* notary performed inspections, noting both compliance and non-compliance with sanitation rules affecting waterways, streets, ditches, bridges and pavements. The oath of parish representatives in 1288 included reporting:

> filth and wells that are not cleaned and lack chains and buckets, or if the latter are broken; and those keeping un-walled ditches; and those who throw feces or dung in public roads; or those cooking fat or grease, during the day or the night, in that parish or neighborhood; and those burying bones or having them buried in the city or rural settlements of Bologna; and those placing or leaving cloths to soften in a non-draining ditch; [. . .] and those having clogged ditches; and those throwing dung or carcasses into public ditches or who keep buckets or any other vessel containing putrid or otherwise dangerous matter.
>
> —Geltner 2014: 314

In Coventry, the sergeant served as the primary officer enforcing waste laws through the 1400s (Harris 1907–1913: 91). The sergeant had the responsibility to search for people throwing waste into the river or heaping it up at one of the city's market crosses and to inspect a large city ditch for illegal latrines. The sergeant organized the removal of waste piles with city funds, found labourers to clean the ditch, and went through the city streets every Sunday afternoon and Monday to verify that the residents had performed their weekly street sweeping on Saturday.

There are court records indicating some level of sanitary enforcement. Lucca's *Curia viarum* and London's Assize of Nuisance both fined people for unsanitary acts such as improper waste disposal, damage to waterways and failing to construct approved latrines (Geltner 2013). The Assize of Nuisance,

ENVIRONMENT

which dealt primarily with building law, recorded 24 cases dealing with latrine construction or placement in the period 1301 to 1346 (Jørgensen 2015: 227). These complaints typically focused on smelly or leaking latrines that neighbours considered a nuisance. The court officials heard evidence about the latrines and often visited the site before issuing the judgment, which often ordered repairs or the removal of the latrine. The *Curia viarum* records, as well as those of similar offices in other Italian cities, give detailed insights into enforcement by recording the proceedings of the court, outcomes of hearings and financial data, which all show a concerted effort to maintain a clean city (Geltner 2019b). The *concinc der ribauden* in Ghent likewise managed a wide range of sanitary issues, from waste disposal to keeping pigs off the streets (Coomans 2019). The scope of sanitary enforcement is also evident in the court records for Nottingham, England, in 1395, which cited 33 offenders of sanitary violations (Corporation of Nottingham 1882: 268–83). These included three men who threw dung into the Saturday marketplace, a woman who threw dung into a ditch, a group of dyers who emptied out their dyeing water into the street, and a butcher who blocked up a lane with blood and entrails. Norwich's Leet also levied fines for throwing waste in the river (Jørgensen 2010b).

CONCLUSION: CLEANLINESS AND HEALTHINESS

As this chapter demonstrates, uncleanliness in the medieval urban space was defined by what a person could see or smell. Strong odours from decomposing organic material were shunned as dangerous under the prevailing miasmic disease theory. This meant that bulky and organic waste such as butchery offal, latrine excrement, animal manure and tannery liquids were common targets of sanitary controls. In general, the laws and their enforcers attempted to get these kinds of wastes off the streets and into contained disposal or reuse locations. Legal structures that prevailed in Europe considered public spaces as public goods (Howell 2000), so sanitation restrictions in streets, markets and waterways were a natural development. Clean streets became a civic virtue because it made citizens healthier and the city more beautiful (Kucher 2005). Violation of sanitary norms was not considered acceptable behaviour. On top of regulations, city governments established and maintained public works, including paved roads, weekly trash carts and common latrines, to minimize urban dirt. While this means that medieval streets were not filled to the brim with waste, the health of the urban dwellers was probably still affected by what are today considered diseases linked to poor sanitation. Contact with excrement was commonplace – daily city life included hauling manure, cleaning animal intestines and industrial processes such as dyeing and tanning that used both faeces and urine as ingredients. All of these were potential pathogen sources. Latrines, while generally not leaking onto the street, could be leaking bacteria into groundwater sources, something which the medieval residents had no way of knowing. In addition, houses tended to be damp and have little airflow, increasing the likelihood of respiratory infections. This means that medieval notions of sanitation – removing those things with strong decomposition odours from under one's nose – did not always equate to healthiness. What was sensed in the medieval environment as matter out place was controlled, but it was not necessarily the only unhealthy thing in the city.

CHAPTER TWO

Food: From Healthy Regimen to Consumption and Supply

IONA McCLEERY

INTRODUCTION

The close relationship between food and medicine is recognized by historians of food and has been studied by medical historians who focus on regimens of health (Weiss Adamson 1995; Nicoud 2007; Albala 2002; Proctor 2005). Yet nutrition is not as well established as one might expect in either medical or food histories (Pennell 2013; Lewicka 2014: 606; Gentilcore 2016: 3–4; Pennell and Rich 2016: 6).[1] Food is not yet a mainstream topic in medieval or early-modern studies; its cultural significance often playing second fiddle to its economic role (Woolgar 2010: 1–2; Woolgar 2016: 5). Its relative neglect is surprising considering the significance of diet in public health today. This chapter will explore the role of food in health, focusing on fish as a way to introduce medieval theories of regimen and the practices of consumption and supply. The chapter will consider debates about the gap between theory and practice in daily life. Medieval people were probably aware of medical advice but, as today, often did not act on it for a variety of reasons. One major reason to be discussed below was religious practices, but fashion, taste, cost, social status and regional variations were also significant. It is important to remember that what people eat in all time periods is only partly related to health.

DEBATES AND THEORIES

There are many debates in the history of medieval food that lie beyond the health focus of this chapter. The study of food is, to a large extent, polarized between food production (agriculture and the economics of supply and demand) and food consumption (recipes, cooking methods, cooks, and the cultural contexts of dining and cuisine), with much more of a focus on production, while studies of consumption mainly looked at elite feasting (Woolgar 2010). As far as the huge existing historiography of food is concerned, health emerges mainly in the study of dearth and famine, on the one hand (Jordan 1996; Franklin-Lyons 2009; Benito i Monclús, ed. 2013; McCleery 2016; Slavin 2019) and, on the other hand, in study of regimen texts, debates about the use of sugar and spices—about which more below—dishes specifically for the sick and convalescent, and hospital diets (Scully 1992; 1995; Weiss Adamson 1995, 2004; Laurioux 2006a; Albala 2012; Flandrin 2013; Rodrigues and Sá 2015; Pitchon 2016). In other contexts, the pleasures of the table and dietary health are sometimes seen as diametrically opposed topics for the Middle Ages, at least until the publication in c.1470 of *De honesta voluptate et valetudine* (On Right Pleasure and Good Health). This first printed cookbook by Bartolomeo Sacchi (d. 1481), known as Platina (1998), is a hybrid text, a combination of humanist scholarship, lifestyle advice and the recipes of Martino of Como, cook to the Duke of Milan. It is often seen as the beginning of modern gastronomic cuisine, but can be compared to earlier writings that, as we shall see, also paid attention to flavour, appetite and 'that pleasure which derives from continence in food' (Platina 1998: 101; Laurioux 2006b: 45–52, 327–6; Nicoud 2007: 367–78).

More recently some historians have brought together the two poles of production and consumption by focusing on how urban authorities regulated the supply, sale and consumption of food and drink, and the disposal of food and food waste as ways of maintaining communal health (Geltner 2012; Rawcliffe 2013a: 229–90; García Marsilla 2013; Kelleher 2013; Litzenburger 2016). To some extent, these new approaches are beholden to the work of archaeologists, who for many years studied both the production and consumption of food through excavations of fields, storage, water supply and sewage drains, latrines, middens, fishponds, gardens, hearths and serving areas. Bioarchaeological analyses of pot residues, seeds and pollen and human and animal skeletons have transformed understanding of food consumption, cooking processes, malnutrition, obesity and the relationships between diet and disease via osteological analysis and laboratory-based techniques (e.g. stable isotope analysis) (Woolgar, Serjeantson and Waldron, eds. 2006; DeWitte and Slavin 2013; Patrick 2014; Alexander et al 2015; Toso 2018).

Also relevant is research on pharmacy. It has been calculated that 85 per cent of pharmaceutical ingredients were plant-based in the Middle Ages (Ausécache 2006: 249). Many of these were also foodstuffs: vinegar, wine, olive oil and

FOOD 41

most garden herbs and spices; the latter a category that includes sugar as well as substances derived from long-distance trade such as cloves and nutmeg from Indonesia (Freedman 2008; Lev and Amar 2008).[2] Things that we would view entirely as food, like spinach, appear mainly in dishes for the sick or are found as topical treatments (e.g. a wash for a breast tumour made of coriander, lettuce and other leaves) (Scully 2008: 69–70; Wallis 2010: 350). It is often not possible to know how substances mentioned in financial records were used (e.g. spices in the early sixteenth-century accounts of the Hospital do Pópulo in Caldas da Rainha in Portugal could have been for both kitchen and pharmacy) (Rodrigues and Sá 2015). Comfits (sugar-coated seeds) may have been seen by the wealthy as both food and medicine; fashionable sweets consumed at the end of meals to aid digestion and sweeten the breath (Scully 2005: 129–30).

For the purposes of this chapter, the definitions of food and medicine will be those proposed by the Persian physician al-Majūsī (d. *c.*990):

> Remedies in the absolute sense are the materials which the body at first changes but which then change the body and transform it into their temperament; deadly poisons are those materials which change the body and gain power over it without the body being able to resist them; remedial food materials (*medicinales cibi*) are those which at first change the body until the body gains power over them and transforms them into its own nature ... finally, the (pure) foods are those which the body changes and transforms into itself
>
> —Weiss Adamson 1995: 17

Falling under this definition of 'medicinal foods' are substances such as garlic and vinegar. Al-Majūsī also developed the idea that food stuffs were believed to have a particular mix of qualities – hot, cold, dry, wet – up to four degrees of intensity in each. Medicinal foods tended to be at the extremes: black pepper and garlic were both hot and dry in the fourth degree; lettuce varied from cold and wet in the third degree to the second (Scully 2008: 62–4; Arano, ed. 1996, color plate XVIII, black & white images 181–2). It helps us to understand why there was such ambiguity about fruit. In regimen texts, fruit was mainly viewed as a medicinal aid to digestion rather than as a form of nourishment; this does not mean that it was not seen as tasty but that its 'digestibility' was limited (Arnau de Vilanova 1999: 158–9).

The problem was that fruit was seen as too cold and watery to be nourishing. Digestion was a form of cooking, with the stomach sometimes identified as an oven or furnace. All foodstuffs were 'cooked' three times; the first time in the stomach to produce what was called 'chyle', which was then cooked in the liver to produce blood; the third 'cooking' created the humours and brought blood and 'spirit' to the whole body. Things not easily digested became superfluities, evacuated as vomit or faeces. A stomach that was not warm enough in the first place would be unable to 'cook' cold and wet foods or, as was often thought to be the case with viscous or fatty substances, foods could get stuck and cause corruption within the body. It was therefore important that foods were eaten in the right order depending on the season – colder foods were better later in the meal or in summer, although theories on this vary according to the foodstuff and the author – and those with stomachs that were cold due to complexion or illness should pay particular attention to what they ate (Arnau de Vilanova 1999: 162, 172; Brabant 2002; Demaitre 2013: 249–50; Gentilcore 2016: 18–20; Nicoud 2007: 671–80; Nicoud 2017). Many medieval medical treatises devote space to eating disorders and conditions of the stomach and gut, caused in numerous cases by excessive eating or failure to regulate diet properly (Demaitre 2013: 239–81). These conditions are all deserving of much more study than they have hitherto received. Indeed, it would be possible to write a cultural history of the stomach that looks closely at its medieval physiology, anatomy, injuries and pathologies, but also considers its metaphorical role, for example, in the medieval 'body politic'. In the political model of cleric John of Salisbury (d. 1180), the stomach and intestines represented the financial advisors of a state; both were prone to corruption if not regulated (John of Salisbury 1990: 67, 135–6).

To return to fruit: eating it became a moral minefield as medical theories disseminated beyond learned circles; not only was there a risk of ill-health or even death to the consumer, but he or she could be accused of gluttony and lacking self-discipline. There is plenty of evidence for the economic and cultural role of fruit in medieval society; apples, pomegranates, figs, pears and citrus all held a profound symbolic place in literature and religious art and were widely eaten (Dyer 2006; Montanari 2010). However, it was fully understood that too much fruit, especially if uncooked, could make one ill as it changed the body, and in excess could not ultimately be changed by it (Nicoud 2015: 162). It is difficult for modern people to appreciate – those of us lucky enough to live in a world of refrigerators and canned food – what it is like to have a glut of fruit all at once; almost certainly eating too much of it would have caused diarrhoea, but due to difficulties of preservation and the desire for sweetness, there could have been a temptation to over-consume. In two cases discussed by the present author in an earlier study (McCleery 2014c), King John of England (d. 1216) was said by chroniclers to have died from over-eating peaches. This attribution of death to gluttony was a direct comment on his lack of self-governance which, in turn, reflected on his poor government of the kingdom. In contrast, King Duarte of Portugal (d. 1438) spoke of how 'the health of the people is the health of the prince' and, in his own writings on regimen, counselled a twice-yearly purge (probably an enema) because of fish-eating during Lent and fruit-eating in the autumn. While he still ate these things, he understood how to mitigate the risks.

As Marilyn Nicoud (2015) points out, eating was always seen as potentially risky depending on one's complexion, age and state of health and the season, context, combination and timing of foods consumed. Every individual had to manage this risk, while also expected to eat according to his or her own faith, gender, location, wealth and social status. Eating was therefore a manifest sign of a great many medieval cultural issues not all of which can be gone into here since many of them have little directly to do with health, although certainly all could contribute to personal well-being.

Due to the great extent of scholarship on medieval food and the huge range of possible foodstuffs, it is difficult to draw together the rather fragmented multidisciplinary evidence. The decision, therefore, has been taken to focus on one foodstuff for the rest of this chapter: fish. It could have just as easily been fruit, bread or meat. Fish, however, are arguably less well-studied from the perspective of health, since they were invariably seen as unhealthy in the Middle Ages, and they provide an excellent case study of the complex links between dietary advice, taste, supply and demand, eating practice and religious precepts. Previous studies focus on particular aquatic environments or are written for popular audiences (Hoffman 1996; Kurlansky 1999; Fagan 2006). There has not been a great deal of research on the cultural context of fish-eating (Albala 1998; Montanari 2012: 72–8; Woolgar 2016: 112–19). In what follows, some of the excellent recent research that has been done on fish will be brought to bear on health issues.

FISH IN REGIMEN TEXTS

One of the most prominent sources for ideas about (un)healthy foods are *Regimina sanitatis* (Regimens of Health), a genre of medical writings already mentioned in passing that developed from the mid-thirteenth century in Latin and then in a variety of vernacular languages (Arnau de Vilanova 1996; Gil Sotres 1998; Weiss Adamson 2004; Nicoud 2007; Bonfield 2017). Its main impetus was the translation and assimilation in Christian Europe of the complex dietary research that had long gone on within the Islamicate world, where highly medicalized regimens – such as those by Jewish physicians Ishāq al-Isrā'īlī (d. 955) and Moses Maimonides (d. 1204) – were written much earlier based on the ancient Greek and Roman concepts of the four elements and the four humours, but formalized within Islamic and Jewish contexts, for example by the influential al-Majūsī (Waines 1999; Lewicka 2014). The format of the regimens followed the six non-naturals (see the Introduction to this volume). Therefore, these texts placed a great deal of emphasis on food and drink, but also considered relationships between the non-naturals; for example, sleeping, bathing or exercising too soon after meals was considered unwise. The complexion of the individual always had to be taken into account. Regimens were mainly seen as preventative medical texts written for the healthy to preserve them from harm. They were related to the highly individualized genre of *consilia*; personal guides for specific people who had fallen ill, often written in the form of letters (Agrimi and Crisciani 1994; Nicoud 2007: 293–338). For example, physician Gentile da Foligno (d. 1348) advised a man from Arezzo suffering from melancholy (a cold and dry condition) to avoid cheese, beans, vinegar, raw vegetables and most fruits (all either cold or dry). He could eat warm and moist things: birds of most kinds, soft eggs and various kinds of broth. He was also allowed 'occasionally rock fish, roasted or boiled, and sprinkled with a spice powder [a mixture of cinnamon, cloves, cardamom, white pepper, ginger and saffron]' (Wallis, ed. 2010: 412–13). Rock fish may have been a number of species and was recommended as a digestible fish by Galen in the late-second century (Grant, ed. 2000: 178).

The medieval authors of *consilia* and *regimina* were cautious about fish if not downright negative; where it was included, as in the above case, the type and cooking method were usually specified. In a regimen for conserving health attributed to the thirteenth-century physician Petrus Hispanus, the author stated baldly in a section on things that harm the brain: 'a meal of fish causes much phlegm' (Petrus Hispanus 1973: 457). According to this text, salty meat and fish both harmed the lungs in excess but, unlike meat products, some of which— marrow, kid, veal and hare—could be beneficial to certain organs (as discussed by Kathleen Walker-Meikle in Chapter 4), fish were never encouraged (Petrus Hispanus 1973: 461, 463, 465, 469). Fish were viewed with widespread ambivalence in texts of this kind due to their cold and watery (phlegmatic) complexion: 'most fish are bad nutrients, especially for those of humid temperament and for the aged' (Maimonides 1964: 19); older people were seen as naturally phlegmatic so should avoid further moisture. The wateriness of fish was a real problem. A shorter dietetic text, also attributed to Petrus Hispanus, which recommends foods and lifestyles according to the month of the year, advises that 'all roast fish from rivers and lakes should be eaten with oil, vinegar and cumin, since these three things consume the moisture of the fish. Fresh seafish should be eaten with wine and spices' (Petrus Hispanus 1973: 415).

This distinction between different types of fish – lake, river, sea – goes back at least to Galen and reflects concerns about the relative healthiness of moving or still/stagnant waters. Some ancient methods of preparing fish, such as the complex fish sauces garum or liquamen, seem to have almost disappeared in Western Europe by the tenth century, perhaps for economic reasons (Grant ed. 2000: 174–6; Asfora Nadler 2016: 499–511). In the early-sixth century, the Greek physician Anthimus wrote in a letter to the King of the Franks, viewed as the first medieval dietary treatise, that 'we ban the use of fish sauce from every culinary role' (Anthimus 2007: 54–5), but there is no evidence that the king listened. Anthimus seems to otherwise have approved of mainly freshwater

FOOD

fish as long as they were fresh and usually if eaten by the healthy, but the writings of Petrus Hispanus and Aldobrandino of Siena (a late-thirteenth-century royal physician) shows how the influence of Judaeo-Arabic dietary writings later problematized fish-eating in Christian Europe.

Although Mediterranean and/or Nile fish were important foodstuffs in Islamic Spain (Al-Andalus), the Middle East and North Africa, they were not highly regarded (Miller 2007: 156; Lewicka 2011: 209–25). All types of fish were seen as suitable foods for Muslims within Sunni tradition, but this was not the case within Shīʿī Muslim and Jewish traditions, both of which prohibited fish without scales (Cook 1986: 237–45; Laurioux 2002: 119; Freidenreich 2011: 53). The Hispano-Jewish physician Moses Maimonides, who died in Cairo in 1204, had as mentioned earlier, a poor opinion of fish:

The large of body among them, the salted, those that congregate in bad water, and those that abound in fat and viscidity are particularly bad. But the fish that are small of body, white and frangible of flesh, sweet of taste, from the sea or running waters, like those called mullet or pilchard, are not bad nutriments; nonetheless, one should restrict them.

—Maimonides 1964: 19

Generally sea fish seem to have been preferred by medical authors perhaps because the motion and saltiness of the waters kept them naturally preserved, less wet and less viscous (Le Cornec 2006), but fish mostly caught in rivers, such as salmon and trout, remained elite fish. Some medical authors continued to prefer freshwater fish (Arnau de Vilanova 1996: 696). Aldobrandino of Siena suggested a very complex typology of fish based on where they live, what they eat, whether they have scales, their size, whether they can live in both salt and freshwater and how they are preserved and cooked (Aldobrandino 1911: 174–7). Hardly any authors recommended the herring or stockfish that the majority of the northern European population consumed, as we shall see, including elite diners. The most suitable fish, even for Christian writers, were small with scales, which rendered unhealthy the very high-status porpoise, often described as *bestial*, for example, by Arnau de Vilanova (d. 1311) in the regimen that he wrote for the King of Aragon, because its flesh was considered 'meat-like', or sturgeon, another high-status fish, which has plates rather than scales (Arnau de Vilanova 1996: 695–9).

So, it seems that small fish were the healthiest. The oldest surviving cookery recipes from medieval England, discovered in a late twelfth-century medical manuscript that once belonged to Durham Cathedral Priory, include a sauce 'for tiny little fish' (*ad minutos pisciculos*) containing coriander, garlic and pepper (Gasper and Wallis 2016: 1384). There is no indication of the origin or type of fish, but the recipe is strikingly reminiscent of Anthimus's fried or roasted *minuti pisciunculi* in the early-sixth century. He states that they are young trout *(trucanti)*, described as good for *fastidium* – loss of appetite – which is precisely the health problem that Gasper and Wallis argue was the reason why culinary recipes were included in their twelfth-century medical compilation (Anthimus 2007: 66–7; Gasper and Wallis 2016: 1374–6).

Fish that were believed to choose to live in 'muddy and corrupt waters' such as eels and lampreys, were particularly criticized in regimens (Proctor 2007: 17). Anthimus had already explained in the sixth century:

> Do not offer lampreys to either healthy or sick people, because this fish has bad flesh that is melancholic, engendering oppressively bad humors together with black blood and harmful diseases.
>
> —Anthimus 2007: 66–7

In the fourteenth century, physician Maino de Maineri (d. *c.*1368) wrote in his Regimen of Health that:

> With all due respect to those who are habitués of the lamprey, this fish is very dangerous, even though it is tasty in the mouth. It is analogous in water to the snake on earth, and so it is to be feared that it may be venomous . . . And because of its viscosity, it is good that it be immersed alive in the best wine and remain there until dead, then prepared with a galantine [jelly] made with the best spices, just as the cooks of the great lords know how to make. I recommend, further, that it be first parboiled twice in wine and water and then thoroughly cooked.
>
> —Scully 2005: 45

De Maineri also provided a sauce for lampreys and moray eels, alongside equally complex ones for porpoise, sturgeon, salmon, trout, crab, oysters and other fish: 'for giant roasted lampreys and moray eels take white ginger, cloves, galangal, and grains of paradise, three drams of each, and toasted bread soaked in vinegar. Mix with fish oil and verjuice and boil' (Thorndike 1934: 188; Scully 1985: 196). It is easy to see from these culinary recipes that Maino de Maineri assumed his patients were going to eat these foods regardless of his advice.

CONSUMPTION AND SUPPLY OF FISH

Maino de Maineri's advice on how to cook lamprey raises a number of issues to do with everyday elite life. He refers to how something could taste good, even if was deemed unhealthy; to the fact that a person could become accustomed to a certain foodstuff through habit or fashion; and to his familiarity with the cooks of great lords. This was a physician who worked for King Robert of Scotland in the 1320s, and later for the Visconti rulers of Milan. The research of Caroline Proctor (2007) has shown that King Robert enjoyed moray eels and kept his household well-stocked with both eels and lampreys. We know that there were physicians such as Maino in many royal, episcopal and noble households responsible for advising their elite patients on how to live healthily, as well as restoring them to health if necessary. The late-fourteenth-century *Forme of Cury*, the fullest collection of medieval English cookery recipes, was compiled for King Richard II of England (1377–1399) by the 'chef mayster cokes . . . by assent of maysters of physyk and of Phylosophye'; this reference suggests that cooks and physicians worked together to devise a healthy diet for their lord. Christopher Woolgar (2007) discusses evidence for physicians advising on diet at the English and Burgundian courts. We do not know for sure, however, if any patients listened to a word of their dietary advice. Gentilcore (2016: 21–2) suggests that medical complaints about renaissance courtiers who endangered their health by failing to listen might have been a rhetorical device, intended to boost sales in the age of print. There are earlier examples of such complaints, but should we view them so cynically (Laurioux 2002: 145; Proctor 2005: 102; Bonfield 2017: 119; Freedman 2008: 57–60)?

This, therefore, is one of the biggest debates about regimen texts. If fish were deemed to be so unhealthy why were they eaten in such enormous and luxurious quantities throughout the late Middle Ages, described in such detail in the cookery books, and depicted in illustrations of medieval feasts? There are dishes of salmon, pike, haddock, eel, mackerel, tench, plaice, oysters, mussels and porpoise in *The Forme of Cury*. For example, one recipe for mussels or oysters involved boiling them and then mixing in bread, vinegar, chopped onion, salt, saffron and 'powdour fort' (a prepared mixture of sharper spices, usually black pepper, ginger, cloves and nutmeg) (Hieatt and Butler, eds. 1985: 126). In contrast, the regimen books are ambiguous about shellfish; if they mention such food at all they usually saw it as low-status, but we know that shellfish was eaten by some elites during Lent (Woolgar 2000: 43) and even at other times of the year (García Marsilla 2018: 582). Platina's *On Right Pleasure and Good Health* includes recipes for several eel and fish pies, baked variously with figs, raisins, cinnamon, ginger, saffron and almonds, but he adds to Martino of Como's recipes the comment that they are all harmful; two of them could be served to enemies 'for [there is] nothing good in it' (Platina 1998: 372–81). One has to ask why he included them; or was the warning enough to alert the eater to the risks of eating too many? Was the implication always that only the healthy would eat these things? The only aquatic item included in dishes by Chiquart, the fifteenth-century cook of the Duke of Savoy, specifically for the sick was crayfish, which was, in fact, considered to be warm and dry in the second degree (Chiquart 1992: 136). The fourteenth-century French royal cook known as Taillevent would only allow the sick a perch soup (*couleis*), cooked in almond milk, sugar and white wine (Taillevent 1988: 165).

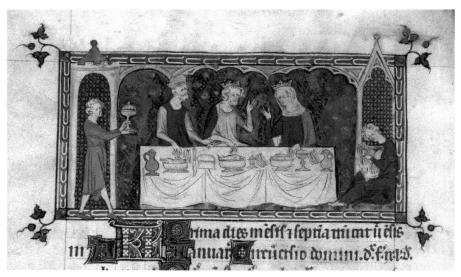

FIGURE 2.1: Royal feast, *Queen Mary Psalter* (early-fourteenth century). London, British Library, MS Royal 2 B VII, fol. 71v (detail). Credit: British Library/Public Domain.

The courtly cookery books of Taillevent and Chiquart have nothing to say about risk: Chiquart mentions thirty-seven types of fish; Taillevent has over sixty including, in addition to those already mentioned, mullet, hake, sole, tuna, flounder, turbot, lobster, whale, sardines, john dory, ray, squid and anchovies (Taillevent 1988; Chiquart 2010). One of Chiquart's inter-course entertainments or *entremets* included a large fire-breathing pike cooked in three ways along its length (fried, boiled and roasted) and each section was served with orange, green and sorrel sauces, respectively. This might not have been intended for eating. He also offered a sauce for sturgeon made with parsley, onions and vinegar (Scully, ed. 2010: 109, 138, 184). In most European kingdoms, sturgeon was reserved for the king; in 1321, King Dinis of Portugal (d. 1325) was presented with a sturgeon the size of a dolphin found far up the river Tagus by the Chief Rabbi Guedelha. It was such a wonder that a document was drawn up to describe it, signed by numerous witnesses including a German physician, Master Heinrich.[3] Both royalty and monasteries kept well-stocked freshwater fish ponds for bream, roach and pike, all of which were elite fish (Serjeantson and Woolgar 2006: 125; Woolgar 1999: 120–1; Aston, ed. 1988). As can be seen in Figure 2.2, freshwater fish caught in rivers or ponds could be kept alive in buckets until they were ready to be cooked. Management of these waters was taken very seriously. Some English manorial records tell us about illegal fishing by lower-status people. In Wakefield, Yorkshire, in March 1314, four men of Alverthorpe were fined forty pence each 'for fishing at night in

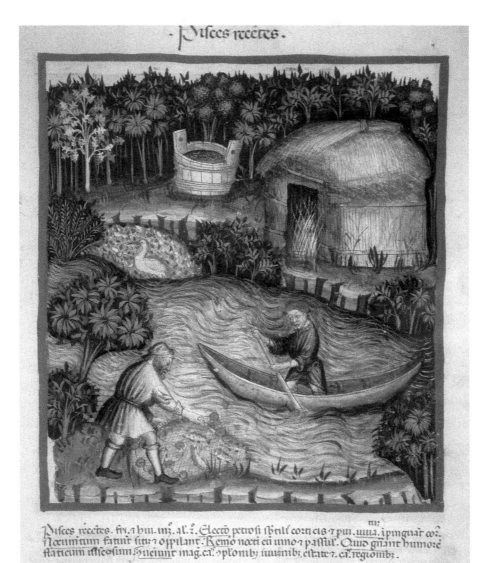

FIGURE 2.2: Fresh fish, *Tacuinum sanitatis* (Tables of Health) (late-fourteenth century), Vienna, Österreichische Nationalbibliothek, Codex Vindobonensis Series Nova 2644, fol. 82. Credit: Getty Images.

forbidden waters and taking water-wolves [pike]' (Lister, ed. 1917: 36). In January 1333, Henry Dyker was fined the very large amount of two shillings for fishing in the River Calder; perhaps a disguised farm of licenses just as the salmon started to run (Walker, ed. 1983: 151).

What European populations ate in increasing amounts from the eleventh century onwards was not, however, freshwater fish, but marine fish such as cod and herring – the former preserved as 'stockfish' by drying and salting; the latter dried or smoked. As can be seen in Figure 2.3, marine fish were rarely depicted in the sea but ready for sale in barrels. Woolgar's research shows that aristocratic English households also consumed herring, sometimes in enormous amounts. In 1296–1297, Joan de Valence, Countess of Pembroke, purchased 52,530 herrings. In 1431–1432, John de Vere, Earl of Oxford purchased 26,640 (Woolgar 1999: 113, 119). By the late Middle Ages the elites of cities hundreds of miles from the sea, such as Vienna, were eating these fish (Kunst 2017: 11) even though, as pointed out earlier, they are barely mentioned by regimen books and infrequently in elite cookery books. Chiquart (2010: 109, 195, 283, 285) mentions herring four times. Taillevent (1988: 196) has one fresh cod recipe and one for salt cod.

Marine fish may have made a substantial contribution to lower-status medieval diets, although quite how much is difficult to ascertain; in food payments to English harvest workers, there are just a few herrings compared to large amounts of bread, meat and ale, probably because those were seen as much more filling and therefore more desirable (Birrell 2015). The main evidence for the wider impact of fish-eating comes from archaeology, as described below, and from the urban regulation of fishing and fishmongering, which has received less scholarly attention than the regulation of bread or meat. In many urban areas, fish seem to be seen as a staple food, alongside bread/grain, meat, oil and wine, to be tightly regulated for taxation purposes, and to maintain the health of the body politic. In Porto, northern Portugal, in January 1391, there was an investigation of the sale of sardines 'maliciously' marketed for more than the regulated price and in March that year (during Lent) the export of lampreys was banned (Basto, ed. 1937: 47, 52–3). The Portuguese banned the sale of netted fish as more prestigious line-caught fish or salted fish as fresh; regulated the proper disposal of fish waste; and resolved complaints about odour and contamination (Gomes 2011: 51–7). In Oviedo, in northern Spain, there were prosecutions for the selling of rotten or otherwise unsuitable fish in the early-sixteenth century (Fernández 2009: 77). Carole Rawcliffe (2013: 251–3) and Christopher Bonfield (2017: 113) report similar regulations and prosecutions for late medieval England. The young wife of the well-to-do *Ménagier* of late-fourteenth-century Paris was advised by her husband how to choose fresh produce at market: for eels she is told 'those with small, pointed heads, fine shiny, iridescent, and glistening skin, small eyes, fat body, and white belly are fresh. The others have a

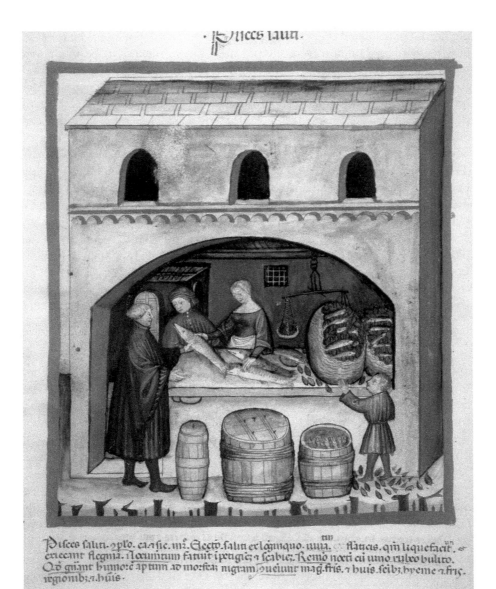

FIGURE 2.3: Salted fish, *Tacuinum sanitatis* (Tables of Health) (late-fourteenth century), Vienna, Österreichische Nationalbibliothek, Codex Vindobonensis Series Nova 2644, fol. 82v. Credit: Getty Images.

big head, tan belly and thick brown skin' so presumably should not be for sale. She is also advised on how to freshen up dried salted stockfish by beating it and soaking it overnight to remove the salt and restore the moisture (Greco and Rose, eds. 2009: 303, 305). Research on late medieval Portugal suggests that urban authorities were worried about fish supplies, perhaps due to the impact of the plague on fisher families (Pereira 2012: 14–15). These same concerns can also be suggested for eastern England, perhaps because of the higher cost of labour post-plague and international warfare (Childs and Kowaleski 2000: 22, 34–5; Kowaleski 2016). The complexities of catching and preserving a highly perishable product led to intense commercialization that required skilled labour; even minor fluctuations in the populations of fisher folk along the Atlantic seaboard may have had wider nutritional repercussions.

The main focus in the history of fish eating has, until fairly recently, been the pious fasting of elite diners rather than food for the majority of the population. In contrast, archaeologists have excavated ponds and weirs, carefully sieved the contents of medieval latrines to uncover tiny bones and applied sophisticated laboratory techniques. In the case of stable isotope analysis, high carbon and nitrogen values in human bones are usually interpreted as resulting from a marine diet; larger fish bones can themselves be analysed. The results seem to be – for medieval England at least – that there was a 'fish event horizon' around the year 1000; few marine fish remains can be found before the eleventh century, but thereafter the remains of fish, especially cod, increase exponentially to a late medieval high after which they drop off again. Cod were also brought to England from increasingly further away as time went on, with heavier exploitation of waters around Iceland and Norway (Serjeantson and Woolgar 2006; Barrett et al 2011; Barrett and Orton 2016; Galloway 2017; Dufeu 2018).

Archaeologists have proposed both supply and demand reasons for these patterns; on the supply side, warmer weather and improved shipping, fishing and salting technologies encouraged people to follow the fish further into the ocean while still managing to bring them back in edible form. On the demand side, a larger, more commercialized, population in the process of urbanization needed more food. Great attention is paid to Christian dietary practices prohibiting the consumption of meat during Lent and Advent, on other holy days, and in England at least, also on Wednesday, Fridays and Saturdays, which adds up to around half the year. Much of the visual culture of fishing and shipping survives in medieval ecclesiastical contexts (e.g. see Figure 2.4). All this demand may have exhausted inshore and freshwater supplies of fish already affected by pollution and industrial processes (Hoffman 1996; Woolgar 2000; Barrett, Locker and Roberts 2004; Serjeantson and Woolgar 2006; Barrett et al 2011; Barrett and Orton eds. 2016). Historians have debated some of these explanations, although without disputing the evidence for a major increase in cod in the late Middle Ages. They point out that freshwater fish were always

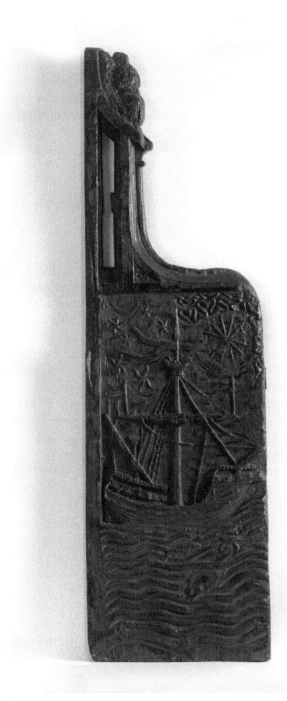

FIGURE 2.4: Church stall bench end (fifteenth century), originally from the chapel of St Nicholas, Kings Lynn, England. Credit: Victoria and Albert Museum, London.

elite, so stocks are likely to have been more tightly controlled rather than exhausted over time, and that herring may have been heavily fished earlier than the tenth century. Historians tend to be less convinced about the role of Christian dietary abstinence as a spur to fish-eating, as discussed below. They also point to the much-debated but very apparent growth in European population from the tenth century onwards, which could have been a cause rather than a consequence of greater specialization and more labour-intensive fishing and salting methods, but it is impossible to explore this aspect here (Campbell 2002; Frantzen 2014: 232–45; Kowaleski 2016; Galloway 2017).

RELIGIOSITY VERSUS DIGESTIBILITY IN FISH EATING

In the last section of this chapter, it seems appropriate to discuss in more detail the claim that Christian beliefs impacted on medieval fish eating and therefore affected ideas about an (un)healthy diet. Fish and fishing appear throughout the Bible and were symbolic of Christian identity from the earliest period of the faith. The idea that some of the Apostles started out as poor fishermen and went on to become fishers of souls was influential for centuries (see Figure 2.5). One wonders whether the 'tiny little fish' in the twelfth-century Durham culinary recipes mentioned above – part of a medical text but bound up at some stage in the late-twelfth or early-thirteenth century with theological texts – would have resonated in clerical ears as the *pisciculos* of Mark 8:7, one of the several descriptions of Jesus feeding thousands of people in the Gospels (Biblia Vulgata 1965: 999). Arnau de Vilanova, a physician known for his theological interests, was quick to point out in his early-fourteenth-century treatise *De esu carnium* (On Meat Eating) – which justified why the Carthusian Order of monks chose not to eat meat at all (seen as medically dangerous and at odds with the advice in his own regimens) – that when Jesus fed the crowd in Mark 8 it was with fish and bread, not meat (Arnau de Vilanova 1999: 129). He did not try to explain why these monks did not eat fish either.

The usual perspective is that fish were the main food of fasting in the Middle Ages. Fasting probably began in early monasticism as a method of self-discipline to reduce lust and the temptation to sin, but there is little evidence that it involved more than bread and water, despite Fagan's (2006: 13–23) attempts to link fasting and fish-eating at an early stage. Why they were eventually linked has not been fully studied. By the thirteenth-century, the Christian theologian Thomas of Aquinas (d. 1274) argued in his *Summa theologiae* (Summary of Theology, II-II, Q147, A8) that meat-eating and wine-drinking were warming and therefore likely to induce lust, but he does not say anything explicitly about the cooling properties of fish as understood in humoural medicine, although this might be implied. Instead, he suggested that fish were 'generally' less

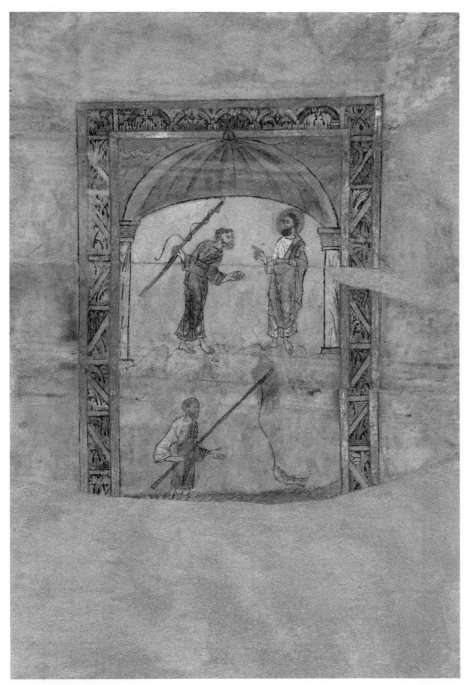

FIGURE 2.5: A representation of Matthew 17: 27, English Gospel Book of unknown origin (c.1000). The J. Paul Getty Museum, Los Angeles, MS 9, fol. 2. Credit: Getty Open Content programme.

pleasurable than meat so it was better to give up meat 'although this is not always the case.' He was aware that some fish were 'delectable' (Aquinas 1921: 70–2). Quite when fish-eating on certain days and periods of the year became widespread inside *or* outside of monastic communities is unclear and needs much more research. In England, Barrett et al (2004) suggest that a tenth-century religious reform movement was key, but Kowaleski (2016) and Frantzen (2014) dispute this, arguing that the use of fish in monasteries was closely related to patterns of secular lordship over land and resources. Fish-eating by monks was modelled on aristocratic conspicuous consumption. For France and the Iberian Peninsula, where the previously described 'fish event horizon' is not visible in the archaeological record until later and ecclesiastical rules on dietary abstinence might have varied (Clavel 2001; 143: Morales Muñiz, Roselló Izquierdo and Morales Muñiz 2009: 151–2) it may be that pious fish-eating only became more widespread once the majority of a population was less permanently hungry and more able to be selective with diet. Fish could only become a food of denial if some types were deemed cheaper than meat (Montanari 2012: 78). We should not be too quick to assume that fish-eating had the same cultural significance in all medieval times and places, but there is not yet enough non-English research to say for sure. In the sixteenth century, dietary practices became a matter of debate between Catholics and Protestants, some of whom, on both sides, still saw abstinence as a useful curb to lust, while others assumed that fish-eating was only done out of piety, not pleasure and would easily decline (Gentilcore 2016: 99–101). As noted above, scholars have already seen a decline in fifteenth-century England, which suggests that dietary change had multiple causes. Whether there was a similar decline in other regions of Europe that remained firmly Catholic is unclear.

The issue to be explored here is whether the fact that medieval people continued to eat something considered unhealthy affected *how* they ate it, regardless of whether it was done out of pleasure or piety. By the late Middle Ages, elaborate fish dinners with tasty sauces were themselves a sign of gluttony, whereas formerly vegetarian Cistercian monks who ate old boiled beef were probably not in moral decline, as used to be argued, but much more penitential in spirit than their elite neighbours who made piety itself fashionable (Thomason 2015). Medieval people seem to have *liked* fish with acidic sauces or in vinegary pies. What is not clear is whether eating in this way was originally done to temper the perceived un-healthiness of something that some of them may have felt they were obliged or thought risky to eat; that is, did medieval people take the advice of the regimen texts described earlier and apply it to their cookery recipes, and if so, when did this happen? What is clear is that a great deal of dietetic knowledge circulated quite early through religious writings. Among the hundreds of twelfth-century miracles attributed to Archbishop Thomas Becket of Canterbury (d. 1170) are several in which eating fish was the cause of illness.

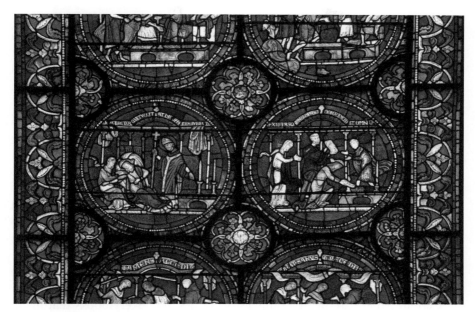

FIGURE 2.6: The cure of Juliana Puintel, Stained glass window (early-thirteenth century). Canterbury Cathedral, Trinity Chapel, North Ambulatory, no. nIV. Credit: Getty Images.

For example, a novice monk of Pontefract Priory in Yorkshire went blind from eating salmon; Roger of Middleton worsened his dropsy (an intrinsically watery condition) by eating cod; and Juliana Puintel ate fish too soon after childbirth (Robertson, ed. 1876, vol 1, 381–2, 184–7, vol 2, 92–3). These miracles predate the Latin regimens by some decades and may be an early example of a new convergence of medical and theological ideas about temperance (Cohen-Hanegbi 2017: 100–33; Nicoud 2017: 63).

Historians of medieval culinary texts have long been inclined to take cookery texts at face value as the main evidence for elite cuisine. There is a major debate over whether physicians who wrote regimens just copied what cooks were doing anyway. Food historians recognize that culinary books share underlying dietary precepts with medical texts, and that many contain a section on dishes specifically for the sick (over 20 per cent of Chiquart's recipes fall into this category); mostly fairly bland soups involving chicken and sugar (Scully 1992). It may be the case that this practice explains why a woman brings a chicken to the sick man in this volume's cover image from a Florentine manuscript of the first half of the fourteenth century.[4] However, some historians – most recently, Giles Gasper and Faith Wallis (2016) –argue that there is little evidence that the majority of the culinary texts pay much attention to health; taste and fashion were more significant. Johanna Van Winter (2007: 341–54) firmly agrees with this view. Ken Albala (2002: 247) is quite scathing about Platina's claim to be interested in health. Laurioux (2002: 144–52; 2006a; 2006b; 2016) is often cited as similarly arguing for the limited influence of medicine on cookery, but his approach is more nuanced. He is much more aware of wider cultural contexts, including the probably limited literacy of most cooks and the uneven survival of both medical and culinary manuscripts.

Terence Scully (1992, 1995, 2008) is the historian most closely associated with the opposite extreme, that all medieval cooking was 'dietetics in action'. Ria Jansen-Sieben (1994), Paul Freedman (2008), Jean-Louis Flandrin (2013), Wanessa Asfora (2011) and Melitta Weiss Adamson (1995, 2004: 205–29) largely share Scully's view that recipes were made more digestible by careful attention to sugar and spices used deliberately to warm or dry foodstuffs like fish to make them healthier and less risky according to the advice of the learned regimens. The cooking method may also have been relevant; boiling fish moistens them further, whereas roasting warms and dries – for Arnau de Vilanova (1996: 458), fish should only be roasted in winter. These scholars firmly argue that culinary recipes originated within the context of healthcare.

Certainly there are many examples of recipes in cookery books that might suggest the tempering of fish with herbs, sugar and spices, reflecting the advice given above by physicians Arnau de Vilanova, Aldobrandino of Siena, Maino de Maineri, Petrus Hispanus and Gentile da Foligno in their regimens. Fish dishes in cookery books are invariably accompanied by at least some of the following: sugar, almond milk, nuts, saffron, galingal, mace, garlic, onions, wine, vinegar and *powdour fort*, all of which would warm them up. Gasper and Wallis (2016: 1380) argue that vinegar was cold so it could hardly have warmed up cold fish, but if we suggest that compilers of recipes were aware, to some extent, of the system of degrees of qualities –unfortunately never explicitly stated, which is half the problem, but then most of these texts contain no measurements or cooking times—then it could be the case that vinegar (cold in the first degree, dry in the second) was seen as warmer and dryer than fresh fish which was cold and wet in the third degree (Arano 1996: black & white images 59–61). It is also worth remembering that in regimens, fish had other problems besides coldness and moisture. Some of the ingredients and processes in preparing fish dishes may have tackled viscosity, fattiness, or the waters of origin, as described earlier. Joel Kaye (2014: 216–8) notes in his major study of balance in the thirteenth and fourteenth centuries that moisture, dryness, coldness and heat were all relative concepts that could result in contradictory combinations. Michael Solomon (2018) also argues that medieval food intake was subject to 'hygenic relativity' and 'radical individuality;' recipes suitable for one person and their individual circumstances might not be appropriate for another.

It is possible to argue that some sauces to go with fish may have mainly livened up the dish by adding colour. Ingredients such as alkanet and sanders or saffron would have made the food red or yellow, which might just have been a matter of fashion although they could also have had a humoural resonance (Woolgar 2018). One of the most common fish sauces was 'green sauce' made with fresh green herbs, spices, vinegar and breadcrumbs (Hieatt and Butler, eds. 1985: 130; Taillevent 1988: 223; Chiquart 2010: 139, 184). This could have been a symbolic reminder of the fish's watery home, as Woolgar suggests (2018: 10), but it would also have made the dish more digestible *because* it looked and tasted nicer. Any visitor to Portugal will be aware of the vast array of recipes still used today to make reconstituted air-dried *bacalhau* (cod) palatable. Here, Gasper and Wallis (2016: 1362) are surely on the right track when they argue that sauces 'were medical *because* they were gastronomical'. Maino de Maineri admitted that his sauces had more to do with pleasure than with health, but he still included them in a regimen because they reduced the risk of eating other things (Thorndike 1934: 186). Sauces, therefore, fitted al-Majūsī's concept of medicinal foods, cited at the start of this chapter.

CONCLUSION

It is not possible here to fully reconcile these divergent viewpoints about food, although one way forward might be to make more comparisons with the present. It is strange that historians are doubtful about medieval people's ability to follow medical advice, given that modern people also struggle to do so. Nutrition looms large in modern healthcare for good reason – diet plays an enormous role in disease and disability – yet medical advice can seem contradictory (often because of how it is reported in the media) (Ladher 2016). At the same time, we purchase elaborate cookery books or watch television programmes that describe expensive and heart-attack inducing meals that few of us will ever make, often because, like medieval people, we are bound by constraints of cost and access (Cooke 2016). Enjoying these things is aspirational; it need not imply that the risks of eating such foods are not known. Future historians and archaeologists will no doubt find twenty-first-century evidence for diet very confusing to interpret, not least because the supply lines of our food and our relationship to the lands and seas that provide it have become blurred and mysterious. Relying on public health leaflets as a guide would be as misleading as only using medieval regimens. This chapter has argued that medieval people had a keen understanding of where food came from and how it was preserved and transported; understanding this infrastructure is important to understanding medieval health.

What also might be very clear from this chapter is that there is still a great deal to do on the history of food. Too many questions remain unanswered, and not all of them can be pursued in a history of health. Perhaps most importantly: how were recipes of any kind read and used, and by whom? Most manuscripts show no signs of usage, and certainly few marks that might imply they had been anywhere near the kitchen or sick bed: Chiquart (2010: 97–8) claimed that he had never used a cookbook until he was asked to write one by the duke for whom he worked ('for his consideration and pleasure'). This problem is shared by many kinds of medieval practical texts, whether pharmaceutical, metallurgical, culinary, medical or alchemical, but the nature of recipes and their purpose needs to be scrutinized much more as multi-layered productions (Lewicka 2011: 30–35; DiMeo and Pelling, ed. 2013; Govantes-Edwards et al. 2016: 179–81). Until we question why it was necessary to write down such a simple recipe as a 'green sauce' for fish in elite manuscripts in the first place, we cannot begin to understand the dietary health work of either cooks or medics, let alone how readers, whoever they were, consumed these books.

Although culinary recipes may well have flourished in a separate oral culture for centuries, as opponents of Scully argue, the fact that they were written down in the same courtly contexts in which regimens were produced is surely important to analyse more fully. At the same time, only a few physicians included extensive culinary recipes in their medical texts, even if many cookery books were copied or collected by physicians. It would be a mistake to view Maino de Maineri as a typical author, although Fernando Salmón (2011) may be right to suggest that culinary recipes should be understood in the same light as *experimenta* or other empirical insertions in medical texts. The problem is that too many scholars focus on a small number of texts and images, something that this chapter also has to do for reasons of space. This chapter (and book) also uses images from a fourteenth-century manuscript of the *Tacuinum sanitatis* as if they were representative of daily life. Catherine Hoeniger (2006: 81) is doubtful, seeing them more 'as an assertion of power and class . . . eating well and healthily was [a] privilege'. These images do at least show that supply and marketing were seen as intrinsic to health. Marilyn Nicoud (2007: 529–681) has explored the dissemination of dietetic manuscripts beyond medical contexts, but she urges further research on this topic.

The history of medicine can be all-embracing, as explained in the introduction to this volume: health and well-being can be incorporated into every part of daily life, or it can focus narrowly on theories, recipes, practitioners and procedures. The cultural history of food can also seem comparatively narrow – the study of recipes, feasts, cooks and kitchens – but it has also grown recently to embrace the previously separate histories of agricultural production, fishing and famine. In both cases archaeology has played a key role in providing new questions and evidence. The result is that study of the role of food in medicine is not yet very coherent, often caught between very divergent agenda, with sometimes polarizing debates between scholars and disciplines. It is certainly full of promise for future research. This chapter presents the multiplicity of ways in which medieval wellbeing was caught up in food supply and consumption.

ACKNOWLEDGEMENTS

I would like to thank Chris Woolgar for reading a draft of this chapter and providing helpful commentary. I would also like to thank the audience of my paper on medieval fish-eating at the Yorkshire Archaeological and Historical Society for their useful questions in November 2017.

NOTES

1. Although Melitta Weiss Adamson, Marilyn Nicoud, Terence Scully, Jean-Louis Flandrin and Bruno Laurioux are very active in this area, their work on dietetics – often difficult to access due to publishing costs or exhausted print-runs – has had a relatively limited effect on the rich historiographies of pre-modern food and medicine. As Pennell (2013) and Pennell and Rich (2016) explain, food is a very diverse field of research – much of it taking place outside of universities in museums, re-enactment groups and independent scholarship – with multiple methodologies, disciplinary, institutional and national perspectives and sources.
2. The myth that medieval people used spices to hide the taste of rotten food is still pervasive in popular culture. Let us counter it very simply: people who could afford to buy spices from South-East Asia could afford to buy the best local meat and fish. See Freedman (2008).
3. Lisbon, Arquivos Nacionais da Torre do Tombo, *Gavetas,* gaveta 2, maço 1, document 4. This physician may be the same individual documented in Aragon and Castile between 1310 and 1316 by McVaugh (1994: 17), apparently specializing in royal births.
4. Florence, Biblioteca Nazionale Centrale, MS Magliabechiano II. VI.16, fol. 48v. It is, however, a rather a mature-looking bird , perhaps even a cockerel, which would not normally be recommended to somebody as sick as this individual because it would be too old and tough. For an alternative theory of its purpose, see the section on cancer and lupus in Chapter 4 on animals by Kathleen Walker-Meikle where chickens are used in cases of 'wolfish' cancer.

CHAPTER THREE

Disease: Confronting, Consoling and Constructing the Afflicted Body

JUSTIN STEARNS

INTRODUCTION

In early-fifteenth-century Cairo, Ibn Ḥajar al-ʿAsqalānī (d. 852/1448), a prominent Muslim jurist and scholar, lost three of his daughters to successive waves of the plague. Fāṭima and ʿĀliya died in 819/1416 and Zayn Khātūn, his oldest daughter, died in 833/1429–30 while pregnant (al-ʿAsqalānī 1990: 9). In the years between these deaths, Ibn Ḥajar authored his book-length treatise on the plague, *Badhl al-māʿūn fī faḍl al-ṭāʿūn* (*An Offering of Kindness on the Virtue of the Plague*), in which, drawing on medical, legal and theological sources, he argued at length that pious Muslims who died of the plague were martyrs and that the plague itself was transmitted by jinn (Stearns 2011: 86–9). At the other end of the Mediterranean in the decades preceding the deaths in Ibn Ḥajar's family, the Catholic preacher Vincent Ferrer (d. 1419) was acquiring fame through his copious sermons in which he frequently drew on the metaphor of disease, especially leprosy, to argue for the danger of good Christians associating with heretics, Jews, and Muslims (Daileader 2016; Stearns 2011: 54–65). In both cases these scholars were less interested in the nature of the diseases they discussed than in what meanings they possessed more broadly and, as such, they provide a productive opening to a discussion of how to write the cultural history of disease in the Middle Ages.

My choice of Ibn Ḥajar and Vincent Ferrer to introduce and frame this chapter has other implications as well. Including this Muslim scholar in a narrative of medieval medicine is unusual if only because histories of the Middle Ages generally only record those Muslim voices (Avicenna, Averroes, etc.) who become known in Latin in Christian Europe, and because the Middle Ages is an awkward period to use to frame the Muslim world and its intellectual and social history.[1] Not only was Ibn Ḥajar unknown to pre-modern European scholars, he was also not a physician, but primarily a religious scholar (Jacques 2009). In this he was similar to Vincent Ferrer, a Valencian Dominican priest who, during his final two decades, became an itinerant preacher who believed the apocalypse was imminent (Daileader 2016; Smoller 2014). In approaching the history of disease in the Middle Ages through these two figures, this chapter not only looks to the broader social and intellectual significance of its subject matter, as one would expect of a cultural history, but also reframes the geographic area under discussion to include the eastern and southern littorals of the Mediterranean. This is, then, a cultural history of disease among communities following Abrahamic faiths in a Mediterranean world that emerged out of the Hellenized Roman Empire that had shaped Late Antiquity.[2]

CATEGORIES

As problematic as the concept of culture is, it is useful in this context in that it pushes us to consider the significance of disease beyond the medieval scholarly medical reception of the corpus of writings linked to the second/third-century CE Greek physician Galen. Anthropologists have debated the danger of the concept of culture encouraging an essentialized understanding of human difference, replacing, in effect, earlier terms such as race or civilization as an organizing principle that linked geography, language or phenotype to a static set of characteristics (Abu-Lughod 1991; Brumann 1999). The concept has remained productive, however, especially since it gestures beyond the purely intellectual, economic, or political to some broader set of socially transmitted patterns of thought that characterize a given population. For our purposes here, a cultural history of disease pushes us, on the one hand, to reflect on how medieval communities experienced disease at the intersection of, specifically, social, religious and medical discourses and practices. On the other hand, in light of the Mediterranean scope of both Hellenism and Abrahamic monotheism, it suggests bringing Christian and Muslim scholarship and social history into closer conversation as components of a common cultural space (along with Judaism, which for reasons of space and the expertise of the author, is unfortunately neglected in the following).[3]

DISEASE 65

Considering a Mediterranean cultural sphere, the littorals of which were in constant and dynamic conversation with hinterlands that connected this enclosed sea with the lands beyond the various mountain ranges (e.g. Atlas, Pyrenees, Alps), desert regions, and highlands, has the additional benefit of provincializing Christian Europe (Chakrabarty 2007), and allowing the Muslim world consideration in its own right and not simply as space of transmission.[4] It also challenges the tendency to frame the Middle Ages teleologically as antecedent to a subsequent modernity centred in Europe that may have drawn on its interactions with other parts of the world but which would subsequently eclipse the intellectual and cultural production of the rest of the globe.[5] It presents, instead, a religiously and linguistically diverse world that was nonetheless united through its ongoing interaction with Roman, Hellenistic, and Abrahamic legacies.

GENEALOGIES OF KNOWLEDGE

What was disease for the inhabitants of the medieval Mediterranean? It is easiest to answer this question by referring to a series of authoritative discourses, all of them representative of different intellectual elites, be they physicians, religious scholars of various specializations, or authors of literary works. Since literacy rates throughout this period were low, these sources are limited in what they can tell us about the views of the broader population, but at the very least they lay out the understandings that social and religious authorities propagated and at times they contain anecdotal reference to the beliefs of the non-literate population.

From a medical perspective, at its most basic, disease was the absence of health. As such, it was an abnormal state resulting from the imbalance of a body's internal humours. This view, articulated at length in the writings of Galen, who lived much of his life in Rome, drew, in turn, upon the earlier writings of Hippocrates (d. *c.*380 BCE). Galen's authority in the Middle Ages cannot be overestimated, although it would be reductionist to assume that subsequent scholars interpreted his work equally or refrained from contesting this authority or presenting alternate views.[6] Still, Galen's prolific writings and the later medieval selections from them proved to be the prism through which the work of his predecessors, especially Hippocrates, passed to the medieval world.[7] Whatever disagreements may have previously existed on the question of disease, physicians now agreed broadly that the human body contained three physiological systems based in the brain, heart, and liver, the correct working of which was predicated on a balance of the four humours each of which was characterized by a combination of qualities, either hot or cold, dry or wet (see volume introduction).[8] The body itself could be divided into two: the uniform aspects that are present throughout the body – Galen listed here 'arteries, veins, nerves, bones, cartilages, ligaments, membranes and flesh' – and the individual organs with their specific functions: 'brain, heart, lung, liver, stomach, spleen, eyes, and kidneys' (Johnston 2006: 137). Within this framework, Galen outlined three basic types of disease: (1) those affecting uniform aspects that resulted from an imbalance of humours; (2) those affecting the organs that resulted from 'abnormal morphology'; and (3) those resulting from a 'dissolution of continuity' in either the uniform features of the body or its organs. These diseases can, in turn, be combined, and can then afflict either the uniform features or organs (Johnston 2006: 70–2).

If much of health depended on preserving a proper balance of the humours, how did one go about doing so? The answer lay in a correct diet or regimen, understood here in the most expansive sense as the maintenance of a proper relationship of the body to its environment. The medieval reception of Galen systematized comments he had made in a number of his writings into a theory of the six non-naturals, which gives a clearer sense of the fuller meaning of regimen (see volume introduction). Essential to this physiological theory of disease is that while external factors influence the internal balance of the body's humours, a disease is not an external entity that penetrates the body and causes it to become ill so much as it is the result of an internal corruption of the body brought about by, for example, the inhalation of corrupted air or by eating too much of the wrong food. Put another way, diseases have no existence independent of the diseased body and because each body is the product of a different humoural configuration, no two bodies become diseased in exactly the same way or respond in the same fashion to the six non-naturals.[9] The theory sketched here in a brief fashion explains how epidemic disease, for example, could afflict a community by means of a common factor that all members would be exposed to – in the case of plague, physicians often identified corrupted air – while also explaining how certain individuals were able to survive it due to a more advantageous humoural composition (either inherent or fortified through the use of drugs).

Following the dissolution of the Western Roman Empire in the fourth century CE, Galenism remained dominant in the now-Christianized Mediterranean as a prevalent medical framework for understanding disease, although the Latinate world of the Western Mediterranean lost access to many of his works, some of which were recovered through later translations from the Arabic (see Glaze in this volume).[10] The emergence of an Islamic caliphate in the Eastern Mediterranean in the seventh century CE introduced scholars of a new Abrahamic faith to the philosophical corpus of Hellenism in which Galen played an important role, although systematic translation of his and other works related to medicine would wait until the ninth century and the concerted sponsorship of the 'Abbasid caliphate and its elites in Baghdad (Gutas 1998).[11] Once translated into Arabic, Galenism was quickly restructured and commented

DISEASE 67

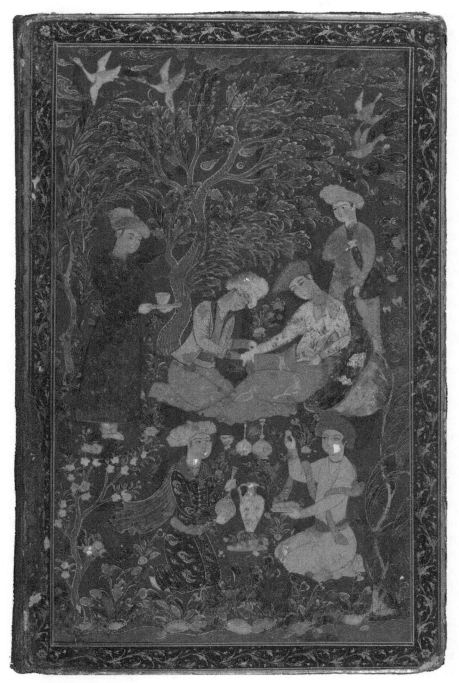

FIGURE 3.1: Taking the pulse, Avicenna, *al-Qānūn* (The Canon). Binding board of manuscript of 1632. Wellcome Library, London, Or Arabic MS 155. Credit: Wellcome Collection/Public Domain.

upon by such figures as Ibn Sahl b. Rabbān al-Ṭabarī (d. after 240/855), Muḥammad b. Zakariyyā al-Rāẓī (d. 311/923), and finally Ibn Sīnā (d. 428/1037), the Latin Avicenna, whose masterful synthesis and development of Galenism, *al-Qānūn* (The Canon), would prove influential in Gerard of Cremona's (d. 1187) twelfth-century translation.[12] In broad terms, the two translation movements and concerted appropriations of medical knowledge in ninth-century Baghdad and then in eleventh and twelfth-century Iberia led to scholars of medicine of the three Abrahamic faiths largely sharing the same framework for understanding disease.

DISEASE IN THE EYES OF GOD AND MAN

Abrahamic scripture seldom introduces the subject of disease without framing it in relationship to the Divine. In the Hebrew Bible, in Numbers 12, Moses' sister Mariam is punished with a disease, often translated as leprosy, for criticizing Moses for having married an Ethiopian woman and for having asserted her own prophet-hood.[13] Here, disease is a punishment for both human moral failing on the one hand and the rejection of God's authority on the other. As such, it can be situated in a broader genealogy of punishment of the body going back to Eve, who along with her descendants, is afflicted with the pains of childbirth when she was cast out from the Garden of Eden in Genesis 3. However, it is less than clear if disease always fits into God's punishment of humans, which is often visited upon the descendants of those who committed the sin (along with Eve, the example of Noah's son Ham comes immediately to mind) (compare with Shoham-Steiner 2014: 144–9). The book of Job includes arguably the most complex treatment of disease, for Job argues at length with his friends over both the reason he has been afflicted with disease and also the proper response to this affliction. The book conflates Job's being struck with a 'severe inflammation' (Job 2:7) by the enigmatic Adversary of God with the other calamities visited on him – setting the stage for the subsequent extended and largely unresolved contemplation of why innocents suffer. Yet Job is urged by his friend Eliphaz to understand his suffering as Divine instruction: 'See how happy is the man whom God reproves; Do not reject the discipline of the Almighty. He injures, but He binds up; He wounds, but His hands heal' (Job 5: 17–18; Berlin, Brettler, Fishbane 2014: 1511).

In his survey of Midrashic commentaries on the Bible, Brody has described how, as early as the second century CE, Jewish scholars were describing disease, in this case leprosy, as the direct result of specific types of sin (Brody 1974: 116–17; Stearns 2011: 169). More recently, Ephraim Shoham-Steiner, building on Brody's work, has surveyed both the continued linkage of leprosy with sin in medieval European Jewish writings and its use as a metaphor to refer to heretical beliefs, a use to which it would be widely put in medieval Christian writings as well (Shoham-Steiner 2014: 45–71). This does not mean, however, that Jewish authors in the Middle Ages saw disease merely as punishment or a metaphor for sin. Rather and as in Job, disease provided an opportunity to think through man's relationship to the divine. Considering deformity together with disease, Shoham-Steiner observes:

> The learned elite and the authors of ethical manuals sought to see physical deformity as an opportunity for soul searching, a call to inventory one's deeds in an attempt to identify a correspondence between a person's deformity and the actions for which he or she was presumably punished. Physical disability was addressed on the personal and communal level, and despite the ethos that views deformity as a sin or as a manifestation of God's will, the circumstances of each particular instance affected the extent to which the case at hand was viewed as an expression of this moral principle.[14]
>
> —Shoham-Steiner 2014: 149

The possibility of God using disease to either punish or test the pious continues into the Christian New Testament, where, however, it is supplemented by Jesus' ability to heal the sick. His own divinity is attested to by his repeated cures, particularly of leprosy (Luke 17), a power that extends to his raising of the dead.[15] As with the later Jewish scholars discussed by Shoham-Steiner, some early Christian commentators on the Bible saw disease not necessarily as internal sin made visible in the flesh, but as a trial or affliction of the pious. Origen (d. 253/54) and the fourth century Archbishop of Constantinople, Gregory of Nazianzos, described Job's skin disease first as elephantiasis and then as leprosy, especially striking considering the later popularity of leprosy among Christian authors as a metaphor for heresy (Stearns 2011: 41).

Christian commentators on the Bible in Late Antiquity often drew on disease in connection not with physical affliction, but metaphorically, in connection with heretical belief. These types of equivalences were facilitated by the New Testament itself engaging in a sustained close reading of the Hebrew Bible in a figurative manner, primarily to explain how Jesus fulfilled its prophecies and how Christianity was a universalization of the Abrahamic covenant of the Jewish people. Heresy became more prevalent in scholars' minds after Christianity became the Roman Empire's official religion in the fourth century. The Councils of Nicaea in 325 and Chalcedon in 451 were two in an ongoing series of attempts (including the Councils of Constantinople in 381 and Ephesus in 431) to define the limits of Christian orthodoxy. All of these were attempts to define the proper understanding of the Trinity and, in the process, they led to the labeling of groups such as the Arians and Nestorians as heretical.[16] Commentators such as Ambrosiaster in the fourth century, and St Jerome (d. 420) in the fifth, drew on Paul's first letters to the Corinthians (1 Corinthians

70   A CULTURAL HISTORY OF MEDICINE IN THE MIDDLE AGES

5:6–8) and the Galatians (Galatians 5:9) to warn of the dangers of associating with heretics, in the process equating heresy with disease and contagion (Stearns 2011: 170–2). During the Middle Ages the equivalence of false belief with disease, especially contagious disease, was not only directed towards Christian heresies, but, as we will see below with the sermons of Saint Vincent Ferrer, was also used in powerful and effective ways by Christian scholars to describe the dangers of associating with Jews and Muslims.

Like their later Muslim colleagues – such as al-Ghazālī (d. 505/1111), whom I will come to below – when faced with disease medieval Christian scholars struggled to reconcile the omnipotence of God – and his presumable power to cure any affliction – with human efforts to treat disease. The discussion found at the beginning of the early ninth century *Lorsch Book of Remedies* brings up many of these same concerns (Wallis 2010: 84–93, and see also Glaze in this volume).[17] The unknown author of what Fischer describes as 'the earliest, fairly certainly dateable medical book of the Western Middle Ages' prefaced his longer discussion of medical treatments with an apology for medicine itself and, in so doing, referred both to early medieval authorities such as Isidore of Seville (d. 636) as well as numerous quotations from both Old and New Testaments (Fischer 2010: 187). Disease, here, was defined both in relation to man's proclivity to sin and to humoural medicine:

> It is not for nothing that that which restores a man to the exercise of good works is called the gift of the Holy Spirit. For diseases happen to the body for three reasons; namely because of sin, because of a trial [of faith], and because of the intemperance of the passions. However, human medicine can be of help only for the last kind of illness, and for the others, only the compassion of the divine mercy. But in fact, even these will sometimes not be cured without human relief. We will demonstrate this better if we produce evidence. It was indeed because of sin that Saul [*that is, St Paul, prior to his conversion*] was smitten with the loss of his eyes, but nevertheless he was not cured without the laying on of a man's hands [Acts 9:8–18].
>
> —Wallis 2010: 86

While there is here no reason to doubt God's immanence, the text stresses the inevitability of human affliction and the fact that God works through terrestrial means to cure disease. Acknowledging that these means may not have been clear in the case of Job, the text offers us Jesus' example when the prostitute anointed his head with ointment in the house of a Pharisee. Noting that, by doing so, she had prepared his body for burial, Jesus rejects the criticisms of his disciples. The author of the *Lorsch Book of Remedies* observes, regarding this episode, that Jesus had shown that 'medicine and human means of relief ought not to be refused' (Wallis 2010: 88). Yet while the text gives

DISEASE 71

many examples of early Christian authorities who used medicine, it also stresses that God uses disease to cure believers of their vices and to teach them not to place too much importance on this world. One can rightfully describe both God and Christ as physicians come to heal the world of its sin and so, as long as one does not ask from God other than what He decreed, one should try to cure disease. The text recognizes that a proper understanding of disease is complex, however, for if medical treatments do not work, one should not doubt the doctor, but rather ascribe the power of the ailment to God's will or the sin of the afflicted. Thus, we see how God works through secondary causes but only when He wants to. The author of the text finishes his preface by stressing at some length the duty of the believer to visit the sick and to offer them comfort – this service being rendered to Christ himself (Wallis 2010: 92). Throughout the *Lorsch Book of Remedies*, disease plays an important role in the relationship between God and man, both as a reminder to man to focus on his own limited, sinful nature and the importance of the world to come and as an incentive to humble himself in service to the suffering of others.

In Islamic scripture, disease played a role similar to the two previous Abrahamic faiths, although it appears rarely in the Qur'an. Outside of one passage in which Abraham rebukes his father and community for not believing in a single all-powerful God who demonstrates His power by, among other ways, healing him when he is sick (Q26:80), disease appears figuratively as a sign of deficient faith (Abu Zayd 2002; Perho 2003). The sayings and witnessed actions of the Prophet Muḥammad (d. 632), the *ḥadīth*, however, provided a wealth of material on the nature, meaning and treatment of illness. Collected by the third/ninth century in a series of volumes that would subsequently become largely authoritative among Sunni Muslim scholars (Shi'a Muslims had a separate canon of collections that emerged in the fourth/tenth century), the Prophet appeared as medical authority, prescribing remedies, recommending forbearance in the face of suffering and denying contagion while describing the transmission of disease.[18] Drawing on this group of traditions, during the Middle Ages a group of Muslim scholars developed a genre that came to be called Prophetic Medicine or *al-ṭibb al-nabawī*. Current scholarship does not view this genre, as an earlier generation of scholars argued, so much as solely a recasting of Arab folk traditions with Prophetic authority as a creative and extended synthesis of Prophetic traditions with Galenism that at times positioned itself in explicit competition with Islamic Galenism.[19]

While there were times that Muslim authors used the metaphor of disease and contagion to warn their readers about associating with the wrong (spiritual) crowd, this seldom occurred when compared to Christian scholarship. The parallels with the previous Abrahamic faiths with regard to the types of discussion are more readily found when it comes to making sense of disease. An excellent example is offered here by al-Ghazālī (d. 505/1111), who, in his influential *Iḥyā 'ulūm al-dīn* (*Revival of the Religious Sciences*), brought together earlier writings by jurists, Sufis, theologians and philosophers to discuss, among other things, the proper attitude of the believer towards disease (al-Ghazali 2001: 106–40). The central problem regarding disease that al-Ghazālī faced in chapter thirty-five of the *Revival* concerned how a believer could maintain an internal reliance upon God while also believing in the effective powers of medicine (e.g. al-Ghazali 2001: 120–1). Disease was, in this context, both an affliction which warranted medical attention and an opportunity to display one's spiritual station and to measure one's own reliance against that of the pious ancestors. The ambivalence al-Ghazālī displayed when discussing disease and to what extent the believer should rely on God's habitual actions relates directly to the individual believer's spiritual station. Trusting in God means seeing God's immanent and constant presence behind everything that happens, including the transmission of disease and the affliction of disease itself. Like Job, whose example is not referenced here, the true believer is not distracted by the apparent causal relations that occur; instead he focuses on the foundational importance of God's causative power.[20] What al-Ghazālī means by this is clarified when he glosses the famous Prophetic tradition that one should hobble one's camel and trust in God (al-Ghazali 2001: 107):

> Now you may say: if one who trusts in God takes up weapons as protection against enemies, secures his door as protection against theft, and hobbles his camel to keep it from running away, what can trusting in God mean? I would respond: Such a one is trusting in God by knowledge and by state. With regard to *knowledge*, it is knowing that if the thief is repelled, securing the door did not suffice to repel him, but that he is only repelled by God Most High himself repelling him. For how many doors have been secured to no avail? How many camels have been hobbled and yet have died or escaped? . . . With regards to *state*, one is content with whatever God Most High decides for him as well as for his household, and says: O God, if you exercise Your authority overall what is in the house, then let whomever takes anything be on the way to You, and I shall be content with your judgment.
>
> —al-Ghazali 2001: 108–9

A few pages later, al-Ghazālī turns this insight on how to balance reliance on God with human agency to the matter of disease. The same basic point made above is repeated here, with God being described as a physician who prescribes for us what we need, even when we do not know it ourselves:

> This is like the sick person in the hands of a sympathetic doctor, content with what he does for him. Should he prepare nourishment for him, he is happy, saying: "Had he not known that the nourishment would help me and

DISEASE   73

that I would be able to take it, he would not have set it before me." And
when he kept food away from him after that, he would be happy and say:
"Were it not that the food would harm me and lead to my death, he would
not have kept me from it." Unless one has faith in the graciousness of God
Most High like the sick person has faith in the compassionate father versed
in the knowledge of medicine, trust in God will never be genuine in Him.

—al-Ghazālī 2001: 112

By giving al-Ghazālī's thought so much space here I do not mean to reduce
Muslim scholarship to his work, despite its admitted importance and influence
(Garden 2014). Nevertheless, al-Ghazālī's attentiveness to the complexity of
the meaning of disease is indicative of disease's broader significance in Islamic
scholarship in the Middle Ages. In *Revival*'s bringing together of a number of
religious discourses – theology, jurisprudence, Sufism among them – to offer a
new synthesis of Islamic thought to its readers, it also provides glimpses of the
diversity of meanings disease may have possessed for Muslims of its time.
Writing four centuries later in the early-fifteenth century, Ibn Ḥajar al-'Asqalānī,
by training and disposition a very different type of scholar than al-Ghazālī,
shared many of the earlier scholar's concerns when he devoted a long treatise
to the plague. Beyond being a terrifying disease that had been ravaging the
population of his native Egypt for over half a century in recurring waves, what
was its overarching significance?

JINN, MARTYRDOM AND RATIONALITY IN A MEDIEVAL EGYPTIAN PLAGUE TREATISE

Due to the author's stature in the field of Islamic scholarship and the later
influence of his writings, modern scholarship on the plague in the Muslim
world has devoted considerable attention to Ibn Ḥajar al-'Asqalānī's fifteenth-
century plague treatise. In his foundational *The Black Death in the Middle East*,
Michael Dols (1977: 110–21) referred to it as a quintessential example of its
kind – as representative of 'orthodox Islam' – and relied on it extensively when
discussing intellectual responses to the plague.[21] While I have taken issue with
Dols' characterization of the representativeness of Ibn Ḥajar's treatise, there is
no doubt that it was influential for later generations and that it continues to
offer a valuable window onto the broader significance of disease in the Muslim
Mediterranean (Stearns 2011: 85–89).

Ibn Ḥajar's *An Offering of Kindness on the Virtue of the Plague* is comprehensive
in scope and while its author is first and foremost a Shāfi'ī legal scholar and
specialist on Prophetic Tradition (his commentary on Bukhārī is still popular
today), he draws extensively on a broad number of genres, including the Arabic
reception of Galenic medicine.[22] The first of the book's five chapters takes up the

question of the nature of the plague, its origins and nature. Ibn Ḥajar demonstrates here the methodology that he will use throughout his book, relying first and foremost on adducing relevant Prophetic traditions and including other sources when necessary. What quickly becomes clear is that, unlike most other diseases, plague has a long history, having originally been sent down by God as a punishment on the Jews in the time of either Moses or David and then having been first experienced by the Muslim community between 638–40 at 'Amwās (Emmaus) during its expansion into the Levant.[23] It is a specific sub-category of epidemic, the symptoms of which are varied, and here Ibn Ḥajar cites earlier religious scholars, with Ibn al-Athīr (d. 630/1232) describing it as 'an epidemic that corrupted the air' and al-Nawawī (d. 676/1277) enumerating its symptoms as follows:

> a very painful pustule [*bathar*] and swelling [*waram*] involving inflammation [*lahīb*]. It renders the surrounding area black, green or a purplish red like flowing blood [*durra*], and brings about heart palpitations [*khafaqān al-qalb*] and vomiting. It often appears in the groin and the armpits, as well as on the hands and fingers and the rest of the body.
>
> —al-'Asqalānī 1990: 97

Lest it be thought that Ibn Ḥajar was drawing only on exegetical literature, he follows these descriptions immediately with a longer section on how Ibn Sīnā and other expert doctors have understood the plague:

> [They said] The plague is a poisonous substance that causes a deadly swelling in soft tissues and the joints of the body, and it usually occurs under the armpits, behind the ears or next to the nose. It is caused by spoiled blood prone to decay and corruption that becomes a poisonous substance and corrupts the organ and the surrounding area. It affects the heart negatively and causes vomiting, nausea, fainting and heart palpitations. Due to its vileness it afflicts those parts of the body that are naturally weak, and its worst effects are on the chief organs. Few survive the kind of plague that is black, while the red followed by the yellow is less dangerous. Ibn Sīna said: Plagues are plentiful during a time of epidemics and in epidemic countries. Because of this, the term 'epidemic' was applied to 'plague' and vice-versa. Ibn Sīna said also: Concerning the epidemics, it is a corruption of the essence of the air, which is the substance of the spirit and upon which it depends. Humans and animals cannot, therefore, live without breathing it, to the point that when an animal is deprived of inhaling it, it dies.[24]
>
> —al-'Asqalānī 1990: 98–9

Having laid out a wide set of definitions of the plague and taken care to differentiate the plague from other epidemic diseases, Ibn Ḥajar now presents

DISEASE 75

his argument for why the plague is unlike other diseases in both aetiology and significance. In doing so, he stresses the importance of both personal experience and of the proper interpretation of empirical evidence.[25]

Drawing on a well-known Prophetic tradition that stated that plague was the result of the jinn piercing humans, Ibn Ḥajar argues against the belief of Ibn Sīnā and other doctors that it was caused by a corruption of the air or miasma. It was precisely the involvement of jinn that differentiated plague from other epidemic diseases and which, again in accordance with a Prophetic tradition, separated it from all other diseases for which God had created cures. Nevertheless, Ibn Ḥajar hastened to explain that the jinn's agency took place within a Galenic framework, for the symptoms of the plague were precisely the result of jinn piercing the humans internally. His rejection of plague being caused by a corruption of the air was entirely empirical and in conversation with humoural medicine:

> If the plague were caused by the air, then it would affect humans and animals alike. We find that the plague strikes many people and animals, and next to them are those of their kind whose temperament is similar who are not struck. It has been witnessed that it takes all the people of a house in a village, and does not in any fashion enter their neighbors' house, or that it enters a given house and only strikes down some people. It has also been witnessed to be less prominent when the air is corrupt than when it is well balanced. Finally, the corruption of the air necessitates a change of the humors that causes a multitude of sicknesses and illnesses, while this kills without sickness or with a mild sickness.
>
> —al-ʿAsqalānī 1990: 105

Ibn Ḥajar continues his argument for the singular nature of the plague by drawing on a Prophetic tradition that states that the Muslim community will die either by being pierced (ṭ'an) or because of the plague (ṭāʿūn), both of which will result in the martyrdom of the believer (al-ʿAsqalānī 1990: 109).[26] To be sure, dying of the plague did not guarantee the status of a martyr: as with engaging in *jihād*, intention is everything. Similar to the Muslim who dies as a hypocrite while fighting the enemies of God and only achieves the status of martyr in this world and not the next, so the believer who dies of the plague while fleeing it will not be rewarded by God in the world to come (compare al-ʿAsqalānī 1990: 189 and 194 with 196 and 200). The importance of proper intention in remaining to face the plague with forbearance is so great that if one remains in a plague-struck land knowing that God has determined both one's health and death and trusting entirely in Him, then even if one dies of something other than the plague, one will still be rewarded with the status of martyrdom (al-ʿAsqalānī 1990: 200).[27] Not surprisingly, Ibn Ḥajar strongly advises against fleeing the plague, although he seems open to the rather curious possibility of leaving a plague-struck country if one does so with the belief that leaving would not change what God has decreed.[28] What he means by this is clarified when he turns to the famous episode of the second Caliph 'Umar, who, having arrived at Sargh in southern Syria, was told that the plague (of 'Amwās) had broken out, and after deliberating with companions, decided to return to Medina. In doing so, 'Umar had been acting correctly, like someone who chooses not to enter into a house on fire. Yet the matter is confusing enough for Ibn Ḥajar to have to spend some time discussing it, especially in light of the troubling report that 'Umar had repented on his deathbed of returning and not advancing toward the plague (al-'Asqalānī 1990: 283–7).

In the context of the above, it should come as no surprise that Ibn Ḥajar uses the debate on the question of whether disease can be transmitted to focus on the importance of believing in God as the source of all things, including disease. The plague is clearly not contagious, as he has already shown with his explanation of jinn being the causative factor, but what about other diseases? Leprosy demands attention, as the Prophet had known and interacted with lepers and had said a great deal about them, including some things that could seem contradictory (Stearns 2011: 31–5). Ibn Ḥajar explains that it was possible that God had made interaction with lepers a cause for disease transmission, but that it was preferable to understand those Prophetic traditions that warned against proximity to lepers to have been intended to protect Muslims whose trust in God might be weakened by mistakenly coming to believe that diseases could transmit themselves (al-'Asqalānī 1990: 296–7).

Ibn Ḥajar's discussion of the plague is particularly useful here because, while he spends a great deal of time arguing that the plague is not like other diseases, his overall discussion illuminates the nature of disease itself as a category and its significance for his community. It is first and foremost an opportunity to rededicate oneself to a proper relationship with the Divine. But it is also a social problem, one that demands an answer both regarding a Muslim's duty to others and the medical opportunities open to him as an individual (al-'Asqalānī 1990: 303). Here, Ibn Ḥajar draws explicitly on earlier medical authorities and praises Ibn Sīnā's advice to bleed the patient, to use cupping glasses if needed and to use various cold substances to strengthen the heart. The medical authorities of his own time, he complains, are ignorant of Ibn Sīnā's writings and reject bloodletting as treatment for the plague. Considering that the plague was caused by jinn piercing humans internally, inflaming their tissues until it reached the heart, killing them, bloodletting was the necessary treatment. Ibn Ḥajar continues his attack on the authority of the doctors of his day by disagreeing with the famed Tāj al-Dīn al-Subkī (d. 771/1370) that if two trustworthy doctors testified to the plague being transmittable, their testimony should be accepted. Instead, Ibn Ḥajar stressed that the same empirical evidence that had shown that air could not be the causative factor in the case of plague had proven that it was not transmitted from one person to another (al-'Asqalānī 1990: 340–2).

Ibn Ḥajar's view of the plague, while influential, was not the only one, or even the only prevalent view in the Muslim world. Much has been written about the Andalusī plague treatises, written in the decades after the Black Death, that supported the concept of contagion and which, significantly, chose to ignore the Prophetic traditions on the plague being a martyrdom for believers.[29] Similar opinions were set out by the Kurdish scholar Idrīs al-Bidlīsī (d. 1520) in a plague treatise written in the Ottoman Empire roughly two generations after Ibn Ḥajar.[30] So while Ibn Ḥajar's specific views on the plague should not be taken as representative of all Muslim views on disease in the medieval Mediterranean, how he chose to make disease meaningful is indicative of broader cultural

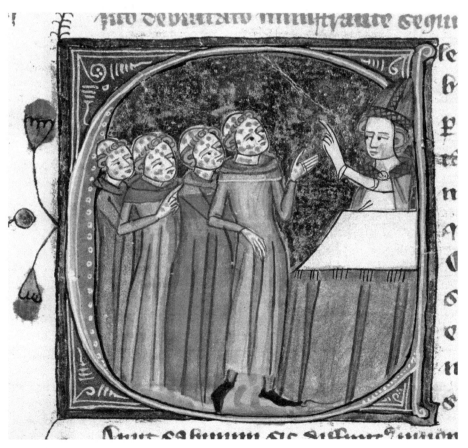

FIGURE 3.2: Bishop instructing clergymen with leprosy, James le Palmer, *Omne bonum* (late-fourteenth century). London, British Library, MS Royal 6.E.VI, vol 2, fol. 301 (detail). Credit: British Library/Public Domain.

considerations shared by his fellow scholars. Muslim jurists, doctors, theologians and mystics constructed disease as an affliction of the body, a challenge to the social fabric of the Muslim community and a test of proper belief as well as an opportunity to demonstrate one's reliance on God. In so doing, they drew on scriptural and empirical evidence, depending on their own beliefs and inclinations. In this they were largely similar to their Christian neighbours, although their responses were shaped by distinct, if related, scriptural and theological texts.[31] I stress this similarity here because, as I turn to Vincent Ferrer's deployment of leprosy in his sermons in fifteenth-century Valencia, I do not wish to imply that his discussion of disease is so much a counterpoint to Ibn Ḥajar's as yet another example of a shared Mediterranean meditation on the significance of disease.

HERETICS, CORRUPTED FAITH AND THE MEDICINE OF CHRIST

Vincent Ferrer (1350–1419), a Dominican priest from Valencia who played an important role in the Great Schism that split the Latin Christian Church in the late-fourteenth and early-fifteenth centuries, was the most influential preacher of his day and famously held strong feelings regarding Jews and the importance of protecting Christians from them (Daileader 2016: 101–36). Ferrer's preaching was so famous and the number of miracles associated with him so well attested that he was canonized surprisingly quickly as Saint Vincent Ferrer in 1455 (Smoller 2014). I have previously considered Ferrer's sermons in light of his description of Jewish and Muslim bodies as diseased and contagious, dangerous to those Christians in their proximity. Here I would like to focus on how he frames disease more generally within a broader metaphor of Jesus Christ as doctor being sent to cure the Christian community of their sins. Parsing disease through a metaphorical lens is perhaps all too obvious in light of the Christian exegetical imperative to explain the Hebrew Bible as foretelling the coming of Christ and thus to read it figuratively, a tendency only strengthened by Jesus' own fondness for parables in the Gospels and the love for metaphor shown by Paul in his letters. Similarly, it is certainly nothing new to draw attention to the central attraction that metaphor held in medieval Christian writings.[32] As Augustine (d. 430), who himself often described sin metaphorically as disease, had famously noted in a striking phrase: 'I find more delight in considering the saints when I regard them as the teeth of the Church. They bite off men from their heresies and carry them over to the body of the Church, when their hardness of heart has been softened as if by being bitten and chewed' (Augustine of Hippo 1996: 63; Stearns 2011: 65). Yet it would distort the full range of cultural significance of disease in the Middle Ages to omit the figurative work to which disease was put, particularly when one considers that Ferrer's sermons were heard by thousands in Valencia and Castile as well as beyond the

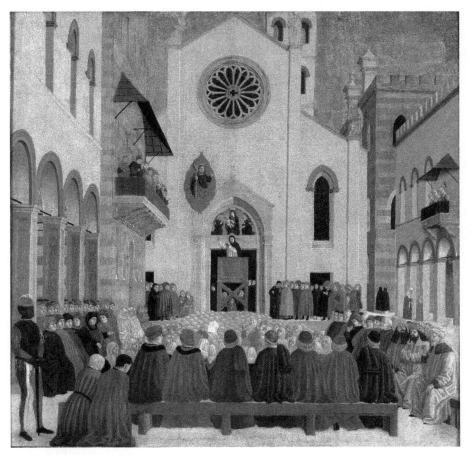

FIGURE 3.3: St Vincent Ferrer preaching, part of an altar piece originally in S. Domenico, Modena, by Bartolomeo degli Erri and his brother Agnolo (late-fifteenth century), now Ashmolean Museum, Oxford. Credit: Getty Images.

Pyrenees. Including the role played by metaphor gives us an impression of what conceptions of disease were held by the broader non-literate public.

For Ferrer, disease was both affliction and medicine. In a series of sermons given in Castile in 1411 or 1412 we find him touching on many of the ways in which he framed disease. He assured his audience that God does not enjoy visiting illnesses or suffering upon them: He does so to lead them out of sin. Similar to the author of the *Lorsch Book of Remedies* and al-Ghazālī, Ferrer argues that the believer should see disease as an opportunity to turn to God: 'In this fashion, if you stray from the path to paradise, God prods you with his goad so that you turn towards Him' (Cátedra García 1994: 380). To be sure, not all paid attention to God's efforts: Ferrer argued that the Jews, for example, required ceaseless affliction 'as they never desired to do anything good', ignored the efforts of Moses and had to be forced out of Egypt by the Egyptians. Moses, himself, in the case of leprosy, had mixed the blood of a bird with water and applied this to the skin of a leper, healing him.[33] Ferrer sees in this moment a prefiguring of the healing power of the sacrament of the baptism – a theme to which he returns repeatedly in his sermons – as in 1 John 5:6 Jesus had been foretold to come with water and blood (Cátedra García 1994: 383). The remedy for the world afflicted with the infection of sin lies in the preaching of the monastic orders of the Dominicans and the Franciscans, preaching that had been prefigured in that of Paul, who had cured all diseases with the name of Jesus Christ. Similarly, Jesus had referred to the preaching of the monastic orders in the Sermon on the Mount with the words: 'You are the salt of the earth' (Matthew 5:13).[34]

Ferrer is, to be sure, not interested in presenting a coherent metaphorical discussion of disease. His primary focus in these sermons lies in exhorting his audience to pious belief and action and the avoidance of sin, warning them of the dangers of associating with Muslims and Jews and contemplating the coming of the anti-Christ and the end of days. He uses disease within this framework, developing leprosy extensively as a disease of the soul in one of his Valencian sermons (Ferrer 1932–88: vol. 3, 210–17): as the leper is cured by God in the one manner through the washing of his body, so Jews, Turks and Muslims are purified of their sins through baptism; as Jesus cured lepers in Matthew 8 by extending his hand, so true contrition purifies the heart; as Jesus sent ten lepers who approached him to the priests, so the soul is purified through confession; as Moses turned his own hand leprous by placing it next to his body, so do all sins come from the flesh; as Moses' sister Mariam was cast out from the community for plotting against her brother and was afflicted with leprosy, so one should distance oneself from the company of sinners if one does not wish to become leprous oneself.[35]

Ferrer generally differentiates spiritual from physical affliction, although in his extended use of metaphor the difference can at times become blurred. In a sermon on Matthew 8:2 ('There was a leper who came to him') he notes that if a person wishes to be cured of his or her illness he or she needs to admit their sin and receive the medicine of penitence (Ferrer 1932–88: vol. 5, 16–20). As leprosy creates tumours within the body, pride inflates the sinner and requires remorse; as lust drives the sinner to spread his sin to others, leprosy is infectious and is transmitted from one person to the next (the reason for their being cast outside the city); as the sinner's sense of charity has been lost – a foundational characteristic of any Christian – so a person becomes a leper through the corruption of one's radical humour.[36] Treatment of this type of spiritual leprosy consists of contrition, confession and good works, possibly supplemented through self-discipline, devotion to Christ and the sacraments of baptism and the taking of the Eucharist.[37]

Similar to the example of Ibn Ḥajar above, we should not understand Ferrer's largely figurative discussions of disease as representative of all medieval European scholarship, which was just as rich as the Islamicate scholarship on the southern and eastern shores of the Mediterranean. Yet it illuminates another dimension of disease in the broader Abrahamic Mediterranean and reminds us of the evocative uses to which disease was put even when it was not actually present, of the importance of the role it played within elite and popular discourses beyond the clear role that it occupied in the worlds of the doctors and those that visited them.

CONCLUSION

There is something hopelessly quixotic about making any statement regarding the cultural history of the Middle Ages and the Mediterranean and it is impossible to do this without being convinced that, by doing so, one is flattening the period or leaving out something vital. In this chapter, I have argued for understanding medieval scholarship on disease through the shared framework of the Christian and Muslim scholarship around the Mediterranean. Familiar absences appear immediately: What about India? Africa? China? The significance of disease on Jewish or pagan thought? The evidence provided to us by archaeology, architecture and art history? The sins of omission are numerous and yet, admitting them even if only ritually, allows me to return to the chapter's central argument.

In the Middle Ages, disease represented a physical and spiritual challenge to both Muslims and Christians. It was both an absence of health that needed to be addressed and a dilemma for the believer who was forced to reconsider both his relationship to God and his fellow man. In making sense of disease, Christian and Muslim scholars drew on a shared, interwoven heritage with roots in both Galenism and the broader body of texts associated with the Abrahamic revelations. They differed, naturally, in how they did so, which texts, metaphors or theories they emphasized at different times and contexts, but these various attempts were mutually intelligible in their internal logic and coherence. Thus, while Ferrer's depiction of Muslims needing to recognize the healing power of the host as well as the miracle of Jesus' resurrection after his crucifixion would have been deeply offensive to Ibn Ḥajar had he had the opportunity to read it, Ibn Ḥajar shared with Ferrer the need in times of illness to entrust oneself to God and to view the importance of disease diachronically within a Sacred History of God using disease to both punish and instruct humanity. They were both descendants of Abraham wrestling with the problem of the suffering of diseased bodies and the responsibility to provide a broader community with guidance and reassurance.

ACKNOWLEDGEMENTS

I would like to thank both Louisa Burnham and Nahyan Fancy for their comments on a first draft of this chapter and only wish I had been able to fully address all their suggestions. I am additionally grateful to Iona McCleery for her close reading of a later draft and her editorial work throughout the process of assembling this volume.

NOTES

1. For a discussion of the usefulness of the Middle Ages to describe Europe up until the nineteenth century, see Le Goff (2015).
2. For one sustained attempt to write the history of the early Muslim community into Roman Late Antiquity, see Fowden (1993) and Fowden (2014). The general point had been previously made by Brown ([1971] 1989: 189–203). The influence of the Roman Empire and presence of Christianity in the Mediterranean was, of course, varied. For one example of this regional variation, see Shaw (2003).
3. Like all categories, the Mediterranean is naturally problematic in its own ways. When preparing this chapter, I came upon the introduction to Langermann and Morrison (2016), in which the editors, while acknowledging the problems involved in defining the Mediterranean rigidly, also stress the region's productive character in breaking down established binaries.
4. For a recent comprehensive account of the extent of the influence of Latin translations from the Arabic and the humanistic debates during the Renaissance about the original contributions of Arabic texts, see Hasse (2016). The older work of Felix Klein-Franke (1980) on the same subject remains valuable.
5. In the field of the history of science, this tendency can be seen most explicitly in the scholarship of figures such as Toby Huff, whose two books champion Europe's exceptionality: see Huff (2003 and 2010). For his understanding of medieval science and medicine in Europe, Huff drew significantly on the work of the medievalist Edward Grant, who shared his views on the exceptional nature of Europe and its institutions. In a curious fashion, the teleological view of Huff and Grant is paralleled in the influential exhibition *1001 Inventions*, which champions the influence of Arabic works on European scholars to the extent that it draws a direct line between medieval Muslim thinkers and twentieth-century technology, eliding in the process all intellectual and cultural production of the Muslim world following Latin authors' appropriation of Arabic and Greek thought. For a critical evaluation of the exhibition see Brentjes, Edis, Richter-Bernburg, eds. (2016).
6. On the reception of Galen in the Middle Ages and beyond see Nutton (2008). For one compelling argument against reducing medicine in the medieval Mediterranean to Galenism, see Fancy (2013: 71).
7. On the editing of Galen's work down to a manageable size, see Nutton (2008: 362). For the work of Galen eclipsing that of his predecessors in Late Antiquity and providing the authoritative means by which they were interpreted, see the narrative provided in Nutton (2013).

DISEASE 83

8. For an overview of Galen's understanding of the body, see Nutton (2013: 236–52).
9. For the emergence of the aetiological standpoint that characterizes our modern understanding of disease, see Stearns (2011: 3–4).
10. The extent to which Galen's works were unavailable to scholars working in Latin can be measured by the attention the twelfth-century translator Gerard of Cremona paid to them when he came to Toledo to translate philosophical texts from the Arabic to Latin: see Burnett (2001: 279–80).
11. On the importance of and context for Ḥunayn b. Isḥāq's translations of Galen into Syriac, see Watt (2014).
12. On this reception, see also Forcada (2011: 121–61), where the author traces the close relationship of medicine to philosophy in the Islamic reception of Galenism.
13. Moses' brother Aaron, who criticized Moses in the same fashion, goes unpunished. For a brief overview of the role of leprosy in the Hebrew Bible, including how most contemporary scholars believe that the Hebrew term *sara'at* refers to a distinct skin disease, see Stearns (2011: 169–70).
14. Space has not permitted me a sufficient discussion of the recent literature on disability in the Middle Ages, but on the medieval Muslim world see Richardson (2012).
15. For Jesus and his followers considering the leprosy of the Hebrew Bible to be the same disease that they witnessed during their lifetime, see Miller and Nesbitt (2014: 20–21). The rather enthusiastic larger argument of this book that medieval Christian thinkers overwhelmingly saw leprosy as a blessing and that negative views of leprosy were the result of Germanic influence should be approached with caution as this is hardly borne out by Luke Demaitre's excellent study of leprosy in Late Medieval Europe (Demaitre 2007). See also Demaitre (2015) for his critical review of Miller and Nesbitt's book.
16. Christological debates continued in Western Christianity until the ninth century: see Cavadini (1993).
17. On the vexed nature of the authorship and precise date of this work, which was preserved in the Lorsch monastery in Germany, see Fischer (2010). I find Fischer's (2010: 180–84) argument against previous proposals for the authorship of the text convincing.
18. On the canonization of Prophetic Tradition, see Brown (2007). For the Prophet's statements on contagion, see Stearns (2011), where I discuss how Muslim scholars negotiated the tensions in the Prophet's various statements on contagion and disease transmission. For an example of a Shi'ī work of Prophetic medicine, see Ispahany and Newman (2000), and for a general survey of the importance of traditionism in early Imamī Shi'a thought, see Haider (2014: 150–3).
19. For the now outdated characterization of Prophetic medicine, see Ullman (1978: 22) and Bürgel ([1968] 2016). Ullman and Bürgel relied for this characterization on Ibn Khaldun (1958, vol 3: 150–1). This seems to be one of many occasions on which scholars have taken Ibn Khaldun's views as indicative of an entire scholarly canon. Compare with Perho (1995), Pormann and Savage-Smith (2007: 71–750), and Stearns (2011: 73–9). On Prophetic medicine as explicit competitor with Galenism, see Bürgel ([1968] 2016: 423–32).

84   A CULTURAL HISTORY OF MEDICINE IN THE MIDDLE AGES

20. Al-Ghazālī's argument is, therefore, distinct from that of the author of the *Lorsch Book of Remedies* in that (here at least) he rejects secondary causality for an occasionalist understanding of reality in which God creates everything at each moment and any apparent causal relations exist only in the human mind.

21. The repeated use of the term 'orthodox Islam' on Dols' part – which seems to imply that Ibn Ḥajar's views represented the consensus of the majority of Sunni Muslim scholars – is regrettable due both to its being inaccurate and due to its distorting the dynamics of Islamic scholarship which was premised on a broad diversity of opinion. For my critique of Dols' depiction of Muslim scholars' stance on plague, see Stearns (2011: 160–7), and for a cogent critique of the term orthodoxy in Islamic Studies, see Wilson (2007). For a recent thoughtful and extended discussion of how to define Islam, see Ahmed (2016), especially 270–8 on the issue of orthodoxy.

22. The editor's introduction and overview of earlier Muslim writings on plague is particularly useful: see al-ʿAsqalānī (1990).

23. Ibn Ḥajar discusses various possibilities and reasons why God would have punished the Jews with plague at different times, as well as the possibility that with reference to Q7:134, that the plague was that which had been sent against the Pharaoh: see al-ʿAsqalānī (1990: 82–88). For a brief overview of the plague of ʿAmwās, see Stearns (2016).

24. The last quotation of this section is not taken from Ibn Sīnā, who in his section on 'plagues' in the *Qānūn* does not refer to the corruption of the air as a general cause of the plague, although this view is well attested in the writings of scholars both before and after him such as al-Rāzī (d. 311/923), Ibn Lūqā (d. 308/920) and Ibn al-Nafīs' (d. 687/1288). In the following pages, Ibn Ḥajar discusses a variety of taxonomies of plague, including a comparison of plague to leprosy and, following Ibn al-Nafīs' *Mūjaz fī-l-ṭibb*, the terrestrial and heavenly causes of epidemics (al-ʿAsqalānī 1990: 100–1). For a strong argument against Ibn al-Nafīs being the author of the *Mūjaz*, see Fancy (2013: 117–20). This and all further translations of Ibn Ḥajar's text are my own.

25. See al-ʿAsqalānī (1990: 101), where the author notes that: 'In all of this, one should rely on experience (*al-tajārib*)'.

26. As always, Ibn Ḥajar discusses the various versions of the tradition and then turns to how it can be properly understood when clearly not all Muslims have died in these two ways. For the historical and theological environment of the Muslim community in the first/seventh century that would explain how dying of the plague could be linked to martyrdom, see van Ess (2001).

27. To be sure, there are numerous other problems to deal with, such as how the plague can be both a punishment for the unbelievers and a blessing for the believers. Ibn Ḥajar addresses all of these. On this specific case, see al-ʿAsqalānī (1990: 213–18).

28. Ibn Ḥajar later quotes al-Ghazālī to give an additional humoural justification for how leaving a plague-struck land would not help in any case: 'Air does not damage at the point of its encounter with the body's exterior, but through uninterrupted inhalation that reaches the lungs and the heart and affects them. It does not appear

DISEASE 85

on the exterior until it has affected the interior. And the one who leaves the country in which it occurs, usually does not get rid of the affair that had previously been prevalent, although he may imagine that he has' (al-'Asqalānī 1990: 303).

29. See Stearns (2011: 79–85) and relevant footnotes, where I cite prior discussions of Ibn Khātimah (d. 770/1369) and Ibn al-Khaṭīb's (776/1374) treatises.

30. I discuss this treatise in Stearns (2017). Al-Bidlīsī's most original contribution to the genre may lie in his including of the *barzakh*, the intermediary world of images between the physical and spiritual worlds, in his discussion of plague.

31. I have previously compared Christian and Muslim responses to the plague in Stearns (2009).

32. For an overview of how late medieval European Christian scholars read the Bible, see Ocker (2002) and for an extended consideration of the role of metaphor in medical writings see Ziegler (1998).

33. A reference to Leviticus 14: 2–7. Ferrer has changed the meaning of the passage somewhat, as in these verses God had instructed Moses how to ritually reintegrate an already healed leper into the community, not heal him.

34. Combining references from Cátedra García, ed. (1994: 382, 582), and the extended discussion of the history of the world after the coming of Christianity (Ibid: 638–9). See the last two pages cited here on how the Virgin Mary interceded with Christ not to destroy the world and to give the monastic orders an opportunity to save it from sin. The reference to Saint Dominic being the salt of the earth is given in Ferrer (1932–88: vol 3, 23). On the spiritual value of preaching, see his discussion of Luke 16:21 (misidentified by the editor as Psalms 67:24) where preachers are described as the dogs of Christ, who heal with their tongues (Ferrer 1932–88: vol 1, 159).

35. In another sermon Ferrer gives an overview of the art of medicine, enumerating ten different types of cures recommended by doctors, all of which he then proceeds to explain metaphorically (Ferrer 1932–82: vol 4, 116–20). Compare with the various ways Ferrer describes Jesus functioning as a doctor (Ferrer 1973: vol 1, 72).

36. It is unclear what exactly he is referring to here in a medical sense. For an overview of leprosy aetiology in medieval European medicine, see Demaitre (2007: 184–95).

37. For the power of the host to heal, see Ferrer (1932–88: vol 2, 163–5) and Ferrer (1973: vol 2, 163).

CHAPTER FOUR

Animals: Their Use and Meaning in Medieval Medicine

KATHLEEN WALKER-MEIKLE

INTRODUCTION

This chapter will examine the cultural history of medicine through animals. Historical scholarship on animals has grown exponentially in the last decades. Described as the 'animal turn', it offers new perspectives on human culture by examining the roles animals have played in human society, although it often still remains at the margins or between disciplines (Ritvo 2007: 118–22). It includes cultural history (Resl 2009), archaeology (O'Connor 2013), environmental history, intellectual history and the study of animals as commodities, encompassing fields as disparate from zoo studies to evolutionary history.

In the field of medieval studies, animals have remained at the periphery of medical history and are rarely the focus of scholarship. Although they are accorded due attention in veterinary history, there has been little work on their place in medical history.[1] This chapter hopes to inspire the reader with a brief survey of the multiple ways in which animals and humans intersect in medieval medical history, looking at animals as medical metaphors; animals as a source of ill health and injury; animals used for nourishment and healing; and the parallels between the treatment of animals and humans.

ANIMALS AS MEDICAL METAPHORS

Animals frequently appear as metaphors for disease, body parts or signs of disease. From the resemblance between the swollen lymph nodes of scrofula to a pregnant sow through to the retina resembling a spider's web or skin lesions resembling the swarming of ants or the scales of fish, analogies abound. Verbs of biting, gnawing or devouring were frequently used in medical literature to describe the destructive nature of a sign of disease. For example, the Latin verb *corrodere* (to gnaw to pieces) can be used to describe the effect of tissues being eaten away; the destruction of humours, ulcers, and wounds; or the corrosive or destructive effects of medicines, poisons or caustics. In John Trevisa's late fourteenth-century Middle English translation of Bartholomaeus Anglicus' early thirteenth-century *De proprietatibus* (*On the Properties of Things*), he translates *corrodere* using the verbs *gnauen* and *frēten* to describe this biting action on the body, so that, for example, a 'posteme [swelling] cometh of pure colera, and gnawith and fretith the membre that hit is inne, and hatte among phisicians *herpes* and *estiomemus*, as it were gnawinge and fretinge itself' (Trevisa 1975: 416).

Cancer and lupus

Cancer, the Latin word for crab, was applied to the disease by the Roman physician Celsus as a translation from the Hippocratic term *karkinos*. By the late medieval period, the analogy of cancer as a hungry beast was well established. Roland of Parma (fl. early-thirteenth century, author of the *Rolandina*, a commentary on Rogerius, referred to below), commented on how the cancer, like a crab itself, would 'crawl backwards while eating the flesh' (Demaitre 1998: 621–24). For the French surgeon, Henry de Mondeville (d. 1316), cancer had all the characteristics of the crustacean. It was round, clung on fiercely, and was surrounded with long bent veins like a crab. It would gnaw and move in all directions, paralleling the movements of a crab. The crab metaphor could even be extended for treatment, as when Guillaume Boucher suggested to a female patient suffering from breast cancer in *c.*1400 to boil crayfish, soak a cloth in the infusion and place it on the afflicted breast (Pouchelle 1990: 176). Its hungry animal-like nature was attested by the surgeon Guy de Chauliac (*c.* 1300–1368) who described the 'wolfish fury' of ulcerated cancers and the need to feed the beast-like disease. The tumour must be 'fed' with food to avoid it eating the patient's flesh:

> Some people appease its treachery and wolfish fury with a piece of scarlet cloth, or with hen's flesh. And for that reason, the people say that it is called 'wolf' because it eats a chicken every day, and if it did not get it, it would eat the person.
>
> —Pouchelle 1990: 168

ANIMALS

Lupus is a disease that was not categorized as such in Antiquity. The first reference of the disease called 'the wolf' appears in a tenth-century affidavit by Eraclius, Bishop of Liège, who attested that he had been healed at the shrine of St Martin of Tours from an affliction called *lupus*. A later thirteenth-century chronicler claimed that the same bishop had been cured of an affliction 'which people call the wolf' which consumed the bishop's flesh in a 'wolfish manner'. Physicians were at a loss and although chickens were regularly split open and applied to the afflicted region of the body, he was not cured until he visited the shrine. For the twelfth-century Salernitan surgeon, Rogerius Frugardi, who wrote a *Practica Chirurgiae* (*Practice of Surgery*) the term *lupus* was used to describe corrosive facial lesions and lesions on the lower limbs. On the face it was *noli me tangere* (touch me not), and on the thighs, it was a type of cancer. His student, Roland of Parma, called the lesions on the lower body *lupula* (little she-wolf) (Benedek 2007: 2). The twelfth-century theologian, Peter of Blois, mentioned how an archbishop of Palermo had died of a disease that people called 'the wolf' and that it was *herpes estiomenus* (a Classical term for a corrosive skin disease, *herpes* from the Greek term to 'slither like a serpent', as the disease appeared to creep across skin and *estiomenus*, for 'eating'). In the mid-thirteenth century, Gilbertus Anglicus in his *Compendium* likewise claimed that *lupus* was *herpes estiomenus*. The term *herpes* gradually became preferred in medical texts, with the snake analogy replacing the wolf (Demaitre 2013: 92–4).

Leprosy

Different forms of leprosy could be distinguished by an excess of one of the humours and each one was given an animal metaphor which best characterized the signs of the disease. Constantine the African's late eleventh-century *Pantegni* (his adaptation of the tenth-century medical encyclopaedia of 'Alī ibn al-'Abbās al-Majūsī, known as Haly Abbas in Latin) established the basic scheme of four types of leprosy with their animal metaphors (Rawcliffe 2006: 75). By the time of the Montpellier professor of medicine Bernard de Gordon (fl. 1270–1330), the four sub-types of *elephantia*, *leonine*, *tyria* and *alopecia* were fully developed (Demaitre 2007: 176–8).

Elephantia was ascribed to the elephant and was caused by an excess of black bile. The skin would be blackish and thick, accompanied by nodes. The term *elephantia* itself was contentious, as it had a long history from Ancient Greek medicine and, confusingly, could be used as a synonym for leprosy or as a separate disease that caused extremities to swell (which is still called elephantiasis). In the Canon of Medicine of Avicenna (Ibn Sīnā, d. 1037), elephantiasis was a leg affliction and one of the stages of the manifestation of leprosy. In Constantine the African's late eleventh-century *Viaticum* (an adaptation of Ibn al-Jazzar's *Kitab Zād al-musāfir wa-qūt al-ḥāḍir*), *elephancia* was one of the four forms of *lepra* (Demaitre 2007: 86–9). For the early thirteenth-century physician Gilbertus Anglicus, in his *Compendium medicinae*, what he termed *elephantia* was due to melancholic blood:

> It takes its name from the elephant, just as the elephant surpasses other animals in size and strength and ugliness, so this variety is greater and stronger than the others, as regards both its cause and cure. Likewise, as the elephant is a spotted animal (*maculosum*), so in elephantia (but this is common to all forms of leprosy).
>
> —Grant 1974: 753; Gilbertus Anglicus 1510: fols 339–40

Leonina was ascribed to the lion and yellow bile was given as its cause. The signs of leonina were the loss of eyebrows and a bulging forehead, accompanied by yellow skin and urine. The symbolic terminology of two of these sub-types, elephantia and leonina, had a very long history. The Ancient Greek physician Aretaeus discussed in detail the rough skin of the elephant when detailing the former, and how the wrinkles on the forehead of the latter resembled a lion or an angry person. Avicenna would similarly remark that *leonina* made the patient's face look terrifying (and added that this form was mostly commonly seen in lions themselves). For Gilles de Corbeil in the late-twelfth century, the ferocity of the lion was itself a metaphor for this terrible disease (Demaitre 2007: 91–3).

The third form was *tyria* which had the characteristics of a snake. It was named for the highly venomous tyrus snake, which lived in the region around Jericho (Rubin 2014: 234–53). A patient suffering with *tyria* (caused by an excess of phlegm) would have a very pale face, with white scaly skin and pale urine. Descriptions of this form often emphasized the snake-like shedding of skin. In his thirteenth-century *Practica*, surgeon Roger de Baron characterized the disease as a serpent that 'gets rid of its filth by rubbing, thus those afflicted by this sort of leprosy are always wanting to scratch themselves' (Pouchelle 1990: 174).

Finally, *alopecia*, caused by an excess of blood, was ascribed to the fox. It was the least harmful of the sub-types and sufferers would be burdened by hair loss and a red face and eyes.

These animal metaphors probably explain why eating the flesh of certain animals was alleged to be one of the causes of leprosy. Lion meat, according to one Salernitan author, might cause the leonine form of leprosy. Avicenna and other authors blamed the meat of donkeys (along with other 'bad foods' such as lentils) as a probable cause. Donkey meat was considered to be a melancholic meat (i.e. possessing the qualities of being cold and dry like the humour of black bile). Similarly, slugs were considered to be probable causes of the disease due to producing 'melancholic blood'. For the second-century Greek physician

ANIMALS

Galen, phlegmatic meat was to blame (caused by the animal in question eating reptiles). Medieval authors were not consistent in identifying the meat to be avoided, as a variety of animals were suspected. This included eating fish and milk together, hare, the excessive consumption of beef, along with less commonly eaten animals such as foxes or bears (Demaitre 2007: 164–6).

Senses and humours

Animal analogy could also extend to the senses and humours. For the thirteenth-century Dominican writer Thomas de Cantimpré, certain animals surpassed man in each of the five senses: the eagle and the lynx in their sharp sight, the vulture in its sense of smell, the ape in its sense of taste, the spider in the sense of touch, and both the mole or the wild boar were man's superior when it came to hearing (Thomas de Cantimpré 1973: 106). These analogies were not definitive; for some, touch was most perfect in man in comparison to animals. The scheme laid out by Pliny the Elder in the first century gave taste and touch to man, with the eagle having vision, the vulture smell and the mole hearing (Woolgar 2006: 27).

In addition, animals and man could perceive sensations in different ways. For sight, animals had their eyes turned to the ground, while man had eyes high in the head so that he might look towards heaven. The sight of the basilisk, one of the most feared venomous serpents, could cause death merely by looking upon its victim. The sound of its hiss was similarly deadly (although its enemy the weasel was immune from its actions). Man could not compete with the night vision of creatures such as owls and vultures, while cats could see in the dark thanks to light shining from their eyes. The uncertain and transitory light of twilight was known as *inter canem et lupum* (between dog and wolf), when clear identification of beasts was difficult. For smell, apart from the vulture, other animals like the bear, elephant and the fox, were also considered to have an excellent sense of smell. In the bestiary tradition the panther has a marvellous odour, which attracts all the other animals and symbolizes Christ (Woolgar 2006: 148–150).[2]

By the end of the Middle Ages, four animals were linked with each one of the four humours. This appears to have originated in the fourteenth-century *Gesta Romanorum* (Deeds of the Romans) which recounts that after the Flood, in an attempt to cultivate the wild grapevine, Noah takes the blood of four animals (a lion, a lamb, a pig, and an ape) and pours it on the roots of the plant. The resulting wine, which makes Noah drunk, is sweetened by the blood of the animals. The origins of the story are very nebulous. A similar tale appears in the *Midrash Tanhuma*, a Late Antique collection of rabbinical material with the same animals, although the source that the *Gesta Romanorum* used is unclear. The *Libellus de imaginibus deorum* (*Little Book on the Images of the Gods*, *c*.1400) notes that the god Bacchus was depicted by the Ancients with a pig,

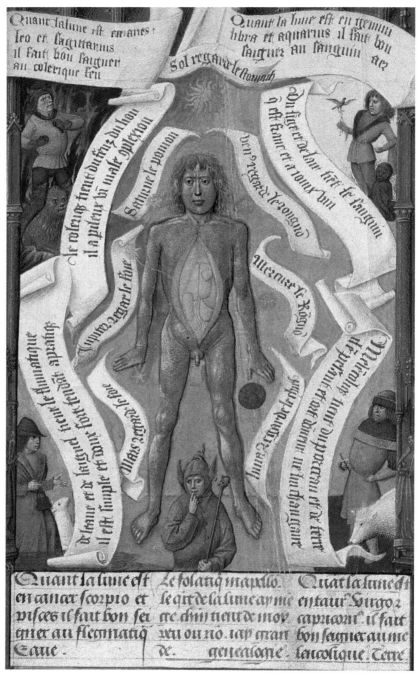

FIGURE 4.1: Planet man, Book of Hours (late-fifteenth century). Oxford, Bodleian Library, MS Douce 311, fol. 1v. Credit: Bodleian Library.

lion and an ape at the foot of a vine, stressing the connection of these animals to drunkenness. The *Calendrier des Bergers* (published by Guyot Marchand in 1493 and, ten years later, translated into English as the *Kalender of Shepherdes* – see Figure 0.3) connects a humoural complexion to a type of drunkenness associated with each animal. Thus, the choleric has 'lion wine' and 'when he is drunk he wants to dance, make noise and fight'. The sanguine has 'ape wine, the more he drinks the more cheerful he becomes and pursues the ladies'. The phlegmatic has 'sheep wine ... when he is drunk he seems wise and more intent on his business than before'. The melancholic has 'swine wine' and 'when he is drunk he wants only to sleep or to dream' (Janson 1952: 239–50).

In a late-fifteenth-century manuscript now in the Bodleian Library (and in early printed Books of Hours from Paris in the 1490s), there is a depiction of Planet Man with personifications of the four humours in each corner (see figure 4.1). The humours' respective animals follow the same scheme as that laid out in Marchand's text; however, these books predate his work by a few years, thus their source must be elsewhere. Notably, drunkenness is not mentioned at all. The relevant labels for each complexion and their corresponding animal in this iconographic scheme are the following (there are also labels that connect the zodiac signs and elements to each complexion, and each of the planets to an inner organ):

The choleric has fire and the lion, he has a perilous bad complexion
The sanguine has the monkey and the air, he is frank and joyful
The phlegmatic has water and the sheep, he is simple and sweet with a strong tendency for the practical
The melancholic has the pig and the earth, he is heavy and does not care for honour.

ANIMALS AS A SOURCE OF ILL HEALTH AND DISEASE

Urban health and animals

Animals, both alive and dead, abounded in medieval urban landscapes and had to be controlled by the authorities to ensure public health. Towns abounded with animals for a variety of reasons. To ensure a supply of fresh meat, animals had to be herded into towns and slaughtered in situ, so that the purchased meat would be fresh. Animals used for transportation and for moving goods would be stabled and moved along the lanes and roads. Small-scale animal husbandry was practised profusely by urban inhabitants, many animals roamed around the towns, and some might be kept to serve as guards or pets. Zoo-archaeological remains abound in excavations of medieval urban environments and are a valuable source in understanding how animals and humans lived in a shared space (Sykes 2009: 347–61; Choyke and Jaritz, eds. 2017; O'Connor 2013).

The idea that foul air (miasma) could adversely affect human health played a major role in the attempts to lessen the impact of noxious animal smells on the urban population. As also pointed out earlier in this volume by Jørgensen, animal manure on the streets was recognized as an issue that had to be addressed, both as a cause of ill health and because it impeded the passage of people in the streets (Ciecieznski, 2013: 91–104). A fourteenth-century ordinance from Oxford remarked that, along with the smells from the butchering trade, manure could affect the population's health as:

> so much filth, dung and other offal is in the streets, ways and lanes within the walls, that the air is so infected by abominable smells that certain of the magnates and others who come to the town and the scholars and burgesses there are often detained by severe sickness and some die.
>
> —Ciecieznski, 2013: 95

Animals were butchered within the boundaries of medieval towns and cities. Ordinances and other regulations, like those discussed earlier by Jørgensen, sought to control where animals could be slaughtered and the proper disposal of hides, offal, blood and other waste products. The location of animal markets and butchers might be established by ordinance. For example, in an example already mentioned briefly by Jørgensen above, the butchers of St Nicholas Shambles in London were the object of complaints concerning the pernicious smells and their practice of throwing entrails on the pavement. In 1342–1343 they were given a small section of land by the Fleet River to encourage them to go to a pier and dispose of the animal entrails there. However, a few years later, the Prior of the Hospital of St John of Jerusalem complained that the pier belonged to the hospital and that the practice of disposing animal remains caused 'stench arising therefrom . . . so bad as to be injurious to the health'. Complaints about butchers abound in urban regulations and the authorities attempted to regulate the practice in diverse ways, from legislating how the waste was to be disposed to ordering that animals not be butchered on the street but behind it (Carr 2008: 450–61).

Many urban centres attempted to control the presence of live animals meandering inside their walls. Swine, in particular, were considered to pose a danger to material goods, property and people. Some regulations banned roaming swine on the streets, some allowed them loose on a certain day of the week when they were allowed out of their sties so that their owners could clean their enclosures. The disposal of the pig manure during the cleaning of their sties could also be regulated. Urban pigs belonging to multiple households might also be taken en masse out to pasture by a swineherd. Some towns banned

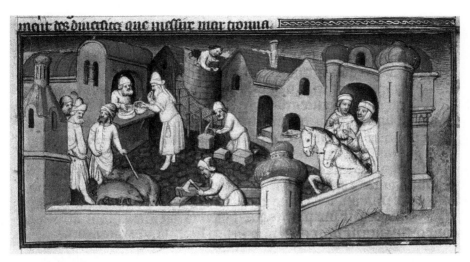

FIGURE 4.2: Urban pigs, Marco Polo, *Le livre des merveilles* (early-fifteenth century). Paris, Bibliothèque Nationale, MS français 2810, fol. 7. Credit: Getty Images.

the keeping of pigs inside their walls altogether, only allowing pigs destined for slaughter to enter. An exception to the common ban on swine roaming at will was usually made for the pigs belonging to the Hospital Brothers of St Anthony. The pig was long associated with St Antony; a combination of various traditions, including the use of pig fat in treating St Antony's fire (*Ignis sacer*) and the saint's association with swineherds and the healing of pigs. Late medieval iconography of the saint depicts him with a pig, often with a bell around its neck. Pigs considered unsuitable for slaughter would have a bell attached to their necks by the order's proctor. The Hospital Brothers of St Antony's swine were allowed to roam free in the streets, with their identifying bells. Inhabitants considered it meritorious to feed these animals, and they served as income for the house. However, this privilege could be abused; in 1311 the City of London demanded that the house's tenant, Roger de Wynchester, stop putting bells on any pigs that he found, as only those that had been given formally to the house should be belled (Jørgensen 2013b: 429–51).

Animals attacking the body: venom and poison

Bites by venomous animals, notably snakes, scorpions, spiders and rabid dogs were considered to be distinct from wounds inflicted by other means and could cause severe physical and mental symptoms for the patient, including derangement and hallucinations. In medical literature on animal bites, venomous animals receive the larger share of attention (Walker-Meikle, 2017: 151–8). Nearly all the sources concentrate on the idea of the animal biting or puncturing the skin's surface. The bites of non-venomous animals receive little attention in the literature, which might briefly discuss the bites of animals such as apes, cats, non-rabid dogs, crocodiles and weasels, but the symptoms were almost always considered mild (pain at the site of the bite). Birds almost never appear among the categories of biting animals, which is limited to quadrupeds, aquatic animals and the crawling beasts.

On the subject of venomous snakes, Avicenna's *Canon of Medicine* was a major source for the Latin tradition, along with Classical antecedents (Avicenna 1556: 911–40). In Albertus Magnus' monumental thirteenth-century commentary on Aristotle, *De animalibus* (*On Animals*), nearly all the information on the bites of serpents derives from Avicenna. After dividing them into three classes – from the most deadly to least venomous – and listing conditions which could change the toxicity of the snake's venom (sex, age, geographical location, emotional state and the weather) and the hot nature of snake venom, he detailed sixty-one venomous 'crawling creatures'. Analogies abound in the descriptions of the animals and the signs of their bites. For example, the teeth of an asp extending out of its mouth are compared to those of a boar. The bite of the horned asp was like being pricked by pins or having nails driven into the site of the bite. A patient bitten by the *falitusus* or the *prester* was compared to someone suffering with dropsy. The *serps* consumes the flesh and bones akin to a 'voracious flame' while

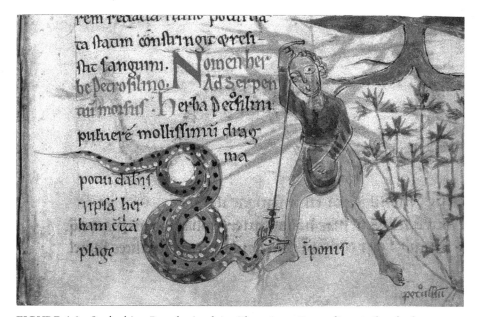

FIGURE 4.3: Snake bite, Pseudo-Apuleius Platonicus, *De medicaminibus herbarum* (late-twelfth century). London, British Library, MS Harley 5294, fol. 42 (detail). Credit: British Library/Public Domain.

the flesh of one bitten by the *spectaficus* liquefied like oil (Albertus Magnus 1999: 1708–38).

In the next chapter, Albertus discusses vermin (bees, mosquitoes, toads, flies, etc.), some of which were also considered venomous. The patient bitten by the rutela spider would urinate a watery material that resembled a spider's web (and at times, something that resembled a spider could be found in the urine). A firefly was so cold that it could put out a fire like ice. The scorpion's venom was considered to be cold (as opposed to the hot venom of the viper) and the pain of the bite was compared to being pricked by a needle. A patient stung by a scorpion might believe that they were being crushed 'in the pestles used to crush salt'. If the scorpion had a 'strong malice', the patient will feel as if it the spot had been cauterized by fire (Albertus Magnus 1999: 1739–64).

Despite these highly alarming signs, many authors stressed that most venomous snakes, spiders and scorpions did not reside in their own geographical locations. Bernard de Gordon, professor of medicine, remarked that the tyrus, dragon, asp and basilisk did not reside around Montpellier and that most local snakes were not very venomous (although one had to keep an eye on scorpions, which were common in regions such as Avignon). Similarly, the French surgeon Henri de Mondeville notes that many of the most venomous serpents were never seen in France, the local spiders were quite harmless, a few non-venomous lizards might bite and the major cause of snake bite was due to people dragging grass snakes out of their burrows and shoving them in sacks or harassing them in other ways (Walker-Meikle 2013–2014: 85–104).

A curious connection can be found between melancholy and spider-bite in the case of the tarantula. Tarantulism is addressed by the physician William of Marra, who wrote an extensive treatise on poisons for Pope Urban V entitled *Sertum papale* (The Papal Garland, *c*.1362). A tarantula bite could be treated by playing music, as its venom caused melancholy (an excess of black bile) and music could produce joy and prevent the venom from penetrating the patient's vital organs. William of Marra dismissed the explanation of the 'vulgar' who claimed that it was due to the tarantula itself singing as it bit the victim, who himself could be treated by hearing similar music. This narrative is likely one of the earliest sources on Southern Italian tarantism, a form of hysteria resulting in uncontrollable dancing believed to be caused by the bite of a tarantula.[3]

Animals could also be a font of poison, whether by eating or touching them. For William of Marra, following other authors, a variety of animals are poisonous (in contrast to venomous animals that bite). Animals could be poisonous in themselves (such as the Spanish fly or the sea hare), could have poisonous body parts (eating cat brain could drive a person witless), or an animal by-product could have gone off, such as coagulated milk or cold fish that was three or four days old (for more on fish as a problematic food, see Iona McCleery's chapter in this volume). Marra even listed as poisonous the act of choking on roast meats (for which the first recommendation was to make the patient vomit). If a live green frog had crawled into a patient's mouth, warm water was to be shaken near the mouth, to encourage the animal to depart.[4]

Rabies and the imagination

The rabid dog, with its poisonous saliva, was considered to be one of the mostly deadly of venomous beasts. In Antiquity, hydrophobia was the most famous symptom. Other symptoms, mostly derived from the patient's own imagination, start to make an appearance in late antiquity but were developed and expanded on by medical writers in Arabic and became hugely influential in the later Western medical tradition.

The seventh-century medical author, Paul of Aegina, who was a great influence on Avicenna and other writers in Arabic, considered the disease to be a form of melancholia, the poison taking on the nature of black bile and thus, like many melancholics, the rabid patient would fear things. Patients may say that they see an image of the dog that bit them in the water (Paul of Aegina 1846: 163).

The rabid patient adopting canine behaviour and barking is remarked on by Rhazes (Muhammad ibn Zakariyyā al-Rāzī, 841–926) who, apart from suggesting therapeutics for rabies, described the behaviour of his afflicted patients. One of his patients barked like a dog at night and soon died. Another patient saw water and was seized by trembling, which ceased once the water was removed. Another refused to drink water, despite having the desire, as he claimed that it contained the entrails of dogs and cats (Rhazes 1544: 194–6).

Avicenna was hugely influential on medieval scholarship of the disease. Psychological symptoms included melancholic ideas, nightmares and a fear of light and open spaces. In the final stages of the disease, the patient would have visions of dogs, see the entrails of dogs in water, and believe that their urine was full of pieces of flesh in the shape of little dogs (Avicenna 1556: 923).

On the influence of these authors in medieval medical tradition, the Montpellier medical author, Bernard de Gordon, in his *Lilium medicinae* (*Lily of Medicine*) would adapt what he had read in Rhazes and Avicenna. Following Avicenna, the patient suffers nightmares, has hiccups, and feels stings all over their body; once they refuse water and lose their mind, they are almost certain to die. The explanation of why patients abhor water, claiming to see dog entrails and dung in it, following Rhazes, is because naturally and rationally a man would abhor those things, even though the only reason the patient believes that they see those things is due to their imagination being corrupted. And finally, concerning the peculiar sight of others observing the flesh of puppies in their urine, Bernard de Gordon explains that it is due to the poison (of the rabid dog) being cold, which congeals blood in such a way that what look like pieces of flesh is actually congealed blood (Bernard de Gordon 1486: 14r).

ANIMALS

A similar approach was taken by the early fourteenth-century French surgeon Henri de Mondeville in his *Chirugia*, who wrote extensively on animal bites. His major source was Moses Maimonides' influential late twelfth-century treatise on poisons and their remedies, which had been recently translated into Latin in the early-fourteenth century.[5] De Mondeville stated that it is only the patient who sees things, and they are the product of his imagination. Thus, the victim of a rabid dog-bite should not examine his own urine, because he may see what seem to be tissue shreds in the form of little dogs. When bled, he should not look at his blood, because he would imagine that he saw bits of the dog's entrails. For Mondeville, the fear of water is due to internal corruption of the patient's imagination. He claimed that when rabid patients see water their imaginations stray; they believe that they see the water inside themselves. When asked why they fear water, the patients reply that it is full of the dog's intestines and feces and thus what little reason remains in their minds is enough to be horrified by the products of their own deranged imaginations (Henri de Mondeville 1893: 456–7).

The great commentator of Avicenna, Gentile da Foligno (d. 1348), questioned the possibility of the imagination of the bitten patient producing these forms, arguing:

> Against the appearance of minute forms or particles like dogs in the urine of one suffering from hydrophobia it is argued that serpents do not so appear when one is stung by a scorpion, and that neither the matter, agent, nor place is favourable for generation. On the other hand, it is pointed out the dog's nature is more like ours than is that of the serpent or scorpion, and that the slower action of the canine poison gives more opportunity for such an effect. The counter question is then raised whether if such a man bit another man, human or canine forms would appear in the second case.[6]

However, other authors maintained that the imaginative powers of the deranged patient could produce these canine substances. The Paduan Pietro d'Abano (*c.* 1257–1316) reading the same Arabic sources, described how the moment the patient saw water, they would imagine dogs to be in that water and, even though dying of thirst, they would run away for fear of the dogs they imagined they saw (once this happened, there was no hope for the patient). As the disease takes its course, the patient becomes crazed (*rabidus*) and emits sperm and phlegm in the shape of little dogs (*in modum catulorum*). This is due to the imagination of the patient, which seals the shape of dogs onto damp substances (Pietro d'Abano 1476: ch. 65: 9).

In the mid-fourteenth century, William of Marra wrote extensively on rabies when discussing all types of poisons. Dogs are more prone to rabies, even though there are more melancholic animals (colder and drier) such as wolves and bears, due to the changeable nature of a dog's lifestyle: eating different things, sometimes sleeping by the fire indoors, at other times sitting outside in the cold. In addition, a dog can become very sad or angry due to the actions of its master, whether due to unkind words or beatings and may thus become more melancholic and more prone to rabies. Rabid humans attack others with their teeth as they have become canine in their nature. William claimed that the afflicted patient often dislikes water as it reminds them of the dog that bit them. This was due to vapours from the patient's eyes that are reflected from the water, and as the vapours are infected with rabies, the patient believes he sees the dog in it. He explains that seeing little bits of flesh or fat in the patient's urine is due to both the *spiritus* of the dog and the imagination of the patient. William uses as an example to back this up the maternal imagination of a pregnant woman, whose foetus can be affected by what her mind concentrates on.[7]

Parasites

Many human parasites, such as lice and intestinal worms, were believed to be spontaneously generated, be that by an excessively hot head producing hair lice or worms generating in ulcers. Many authors claimed these parasites were born by putrefaction, often caused by a combination of heat and humidity. Worms and flies were believed to be born from the earth, a completely accepted natural phenomena, like the fleas that Albertus Magnus described as being 'born from dust that has been warmed and moistened, especially if animal hair and the spirit exhaled from animals' bodies are mixed.' Similarly, 'the *seta* is a vermin about one cubit long . . . it is born by chance, from the hairs of horses' or 'the woodborer . . . is born out of a corrupt humor in the wood' (Albertus Magnus 1999: 1752, 1759, 1763). Their parasitical equivalents were born in the putrefying dead or living body. They had a strong association with sin and the concept of the body after death of being 'food for worms' as remarked by Alan of Lille in the twelfth century:

> O man, remember that thou were a liquid of semen, and that as thou art receptacle of filth, though shalt also be food for worms. For after death, a worm is born from the tongue, which represents the sin of the tongue; thread-worms are born of the stomach to signify the sin of gluttony; a scorpion is born of the spine to mark the sin of lust; a toad is born of the brain to show the sin of pride.
>
> —Pouchelle 1990: 169–71

ANIMALS NOURISHING OR HEALING THE BODY

Regimens of health

This genre of dietetic texts was extremely popular in the late medieval period, as pointed out in this volume by Iona McCleery. Readers could attempt to bring

ANIMALS

their health into balance by regulating the non-naturals (see volume introduction). Each food had two qualities (hot, cold, dry or moist), and could be connected to the respective humour. Thus, there could be 'good' animals to eat and 'bad' animals whose consumption should be avoided. The late thirteenth-century *Regimen Sanitatis Salernitanum* (Salernitan Regimen of Health) is a metric poem that counsels the reader with mainly dietetic recommendations to maintain the body in balance and its recommendations are similar to other regimens of health. Good food included testicles, pig intestines (other animal intestines were to be avoided), pork (with wine, without wine it was worse than mutton), brains (that of chickens was the best), marrow, veal, fowls of all kinds (e.g. quail, partridge, pigeon) were considered nourishing. Animals to avoid included venison, goat, beef and rabbit as these were viewed as melancholic and thus detrimental. Eels were bad for the voice. The milk of assorted animals was praised, from goats to camels, although asses' milk was considered the best. Cheese had a cold quality and could cause constipation; it could be eaten with bread by a healthy person, but without if the person was in ill health (cheese was good to serve after meat, as were nuts after fish). Offal, the heart and stomach of animals, was viewed as hard to digest. Milk was to be avoided directly after blood letting (Wallis 2010: 485–510).

Animals as materia medica

Animal products played their part in medieval pharmacology. Both imported and freshly obtained animal products were used in medical recipes. Eggs, milk, blood, flesh, bile and grease from a variety of animals were regularly used. Animal excrement was used as an ingredient but overwhelmingly was used topically. Two of the most notable imported ingredients were castoreum and ambergris. Castoreum is the secretion from a beaver's castor sacs (not its testicles, despite the popular medieval tradition) and a major ingredient in many compound recipes. Beavers were hunted for their meat, fur and precious castor sacs. Ambergris, a substance formed in the intestines of sperm whales was another prized product and was found washed up on beaches. The use of the animal in particular recipes might have a theoretical background based on its qualities (a mixture of hot, cold, moist or dry) or experimental (based on practice) (Ventura 2010: 303–62). In the experimental vein, the late thirteenth-century medical practitioner and Dominican Friar, Nicholas of Poland, praised greatly the virtues of serpents, lizards and frogs, which he recommended that his patients eat (Eamon and Keil 1987: 180–96).

One of the most popular compound medicines was theriac, which had an animal connection in both its ingredients and what it treated and was widely manufactured and supplied by medieval apothecaries. The drug was prized as a panacea for a variety of ailments from snake and reptile bites to expelling dead foetuses and nephritic and intestinal conditions. The list of ingredients was very long, including mumia, castoreum, pitch, poppy and the ground-up flesh of either vipers or the tyrus snake. The latter was the venomous serpent from Jericho, which also gave its name to the 'snake-like' type of leprosy, as seen above.

Living animals could also be used to assuage ailments. A long tradition, dating back to Pliny the Elder, maintained that a small dog, pressed to the stomach could alleviate pains due to its animal heat. Pets were noted for their ability to assuage cares. The thirteenth-century chronicler Richard of Durham describes a bishop of that diocese keeping pet monkeys 'to ease the burden of his worries'. In the thirteenth-century Tristan Romance, Tristan gives his beloved a magical lapdog with a bell which banishes loneliness (Isolde is quick to remove the bell so that she does not forget her love, although she keeps the dog) (Walker-Meikle 2012: 90–1).

PARALLELS BETWEEN ANIMAL AND HUMAN MEDICINE

Veterinary medicine

Veterinary medicine in the period overwhelmingly focused on the horse, although there were also texts on care for hounds and hawks. Medieval hippiatric medicine had many parallels to human medicine, particularly when many authors of the former adopted Galenic humoural theory. Thus blood letting was a fundamental therapy when treating horses. In a similar way, medical astrology, where planets and stars were believed to influence the body, was adapted in hippiatric texts. The author Laurentius Rusius (1288–1347) in his *Hippiatrica sive marescalia* was likely the first to apply to horses the medical theory of 'zodiac man'. The sky was divided into twelve sections, each ruled by one of the twelve signs of the zodiac. When the moon was in a particular sign, no surgery or any medical treatment was to be attempted on the part of the horse's body ruled by that zodiac sign. For example, if blood-letting the horse was planned, if the moon was in Aries, the horse's head should not be bled; if the moon was in Virgo, the shoulders should not be bled; and similarly, if the moon was in Cancer, the area around the shoulders should not be bled. It was a direct parallel to the zodiac correspondences for human patients, with hooves instead of feet for Pisces or the rump instead of thighs for Libra (Laurentius Rusius 1867: 432–4).

There were two iconographic traditions of the 'zodiac horse.' The first appears in vernacular manuscripts of Laurentius Rusius' work and depicted the horse under a prominent sun, with lines from twelve moons going to the zodiac signs which were placed by the body part they influenced. The second iconographic scheme, seen in Manuel Díes' early fifteenth-century *Libre de cavalls* (Book of the Horse), had the horse placed in a circle. Apart from a prominent moon and sun and indications of the corresponding zodiac for each body part, all the

ANIMALS

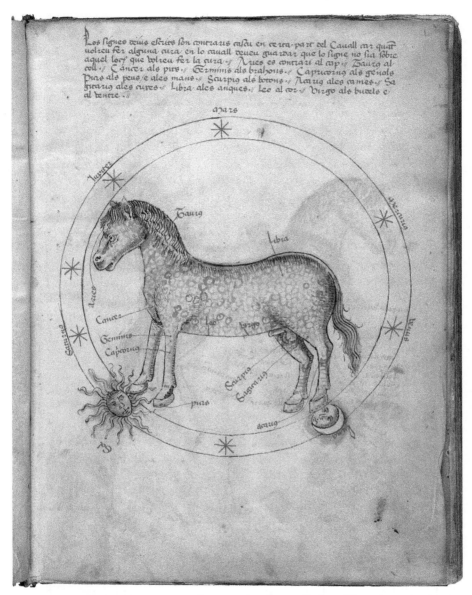

FIGURE 4.4: Zodiac horse, Manuel Díes, *Libre de cavalls* (late-fifteenth century). Beinecke Rare Book and Manuscript Library, Yale University, Beinecke MS 454 fol. 1. Credit: Beinecke Rare Book and Manuscript Library, Yale University.

planets, which similarly influence the horse's health, are depicted in the circle (Plancas 2012).[8]

Saintly healing

There are also parallels between animal and human cures in hagiographical literature and in studies of saints' cults. For example, the miracles of William of Norwich (compiled in the 1170s), include the healing of a horse, a sow, a sparrow-hawk and the oxen of one Goscelin le Gros. Many of the animals in the sources are horses and hawks, belonging to the elite, but there were also livestock like sheep, cattle and swine, and some more unusual animals, such as a woman who asked St Thomas Cantilupe (d. 1282) to cure her pet dormouse that had been stood upon. The exact ailment is often not mentioned, just that the animal was ill, but occasionally there are references to swellings, broken limbs and other afflictions. The saint might be invoked by prayer or by a written or verbal charm, but a visit to the shrine by the owner might be in order. Surviving wax *ex votos* placed at the tomb of the fifteenth-century Bishop Edmund Lacy of Exeter include both human and animal parts (such as a horse leg). The animal itself might even be sent to the shrine for healing or even for prophylactic purposes. Louis Duke of Orléans (1372–1407) sent his entire pack of hounds to Saint-Mesmer so that they might be protected from rabies. When the dogs arrived at the shrine itself, a mass was sung and wax and money were presented to the saint (Aitchison 2009: 875–92).

Animals for anatomical study and experimentation

Anatomical texts of animals for didactic purposes were studied for parallels to human anatomy. One text was notable for its inclusion and influence. The *Anatomia porci* (*Anatomy of the Pig*) or *Anatomia Cophonis* (*Anatomy of Copho*) was written in Southern Italy (most likely at Salerno) at the end of the eleventh or beginning of the twelfth century. It was at times included in the *Articella*, the collection of medical texts that was a core part of the university curriculum. It is a short text detailing the dissection of a pig and maintains that the internal structure of this animal most resembles human anatomy. It instructs readers on how to conduct their own porcine dissection and thus understand the human body using the body of the pig (O'Neill 1970: 115–24).

Human medical treatment could even be preceded by experimentation on animals, to assure success in the former. The early twelfth-century chronicle of Guibert of Nogent recounts how King Baldwin I of Jerusalem (d. 1118) was suffering from a lance wound. His doctor was sceptical at the idea of covering the area in poultices and planned to operate on a Saracen prisoner with a similar wound to determine the best course of action. Baldwin refused so the physician suggested instead the use of a bear, saying to the king:

ANIMALS 105

If you have decided that no man's life can be spent on your own well-being then at least give the order to bring forward a bear, an animal useless except for show, and have it hung up by its front paws, then struck with an iron blade that I may examine its entrails and I shall be able to measure how far it went in and therefore determine the depth of your own wound.

—Mitchell 2004: 161–2

A bear was delivered to the doctor, who performed his experiment, which confirmed his suspicions that it would be harmful to cover the wound without removing the pus first.

CONCLUSION

From rampaging pigs, delirious rabid patients, and beaver body parts to metaphors of disease and its pernicious attack on the human body, this chapter has attempted to present an overview of some of the multiple aspects in which animals had a meaning and a place in medieval medicine. It is clear that there are strong future directions for the development of animal studies in medical history. Significant work has already developed regarding animals and urban health and in zoo-archaeology, but further work could be done on animals in medical iconography and the symbolic use of animals in medical literature (briefly touched on here when discussing medical metaphors). Pharmacology is a particularly rich vein, as animals abound in the sources. Current scholarship (e.g. Ventura 2005, 2010; Buquet 2016) could be expanded by further research into the myriad sources and the animal products themselves, in both compounds and simples. A comparative approach, observing the huge influence of Galenism on equine medicine, would help broach the disciplinary divisions between 'human' and 'animal' medicine. Animals as nourishment are addressed in scholarship on food but perhaps the subject could be approached through a detailed examination of categories of animals. All in all, the field is vast, with interdisciplinarity at its centre, thus there is much still to write on animals in medicine.

ACKNOWLEDGEMENTS

Part of this work was supported by the Wellcome Trust (grant number WT090591MA).

NOTES

1. For example, see Pouchelle (1990: 160–78), who discusses animal metaphors in Henri de Mondeville or Ventura (2005) on animal ingredients in recipes. For a

selection of recent scholarship on veterinary medicine see Shehada (2012), Curth (2013) and McCabe (2007).

2. For example, see Aberdeen University Library, MS 24 fol 9r. Originally available online: www.abdn.ac.uk/ bestiary/ms24/f9r (accessed 1 October 2017).

3. Bibliotheca Apostolica Vaticana, MS Barbarini Lat. 306, pp. 145–7.

4. Animals crawling into the body, particularly snakes, is a long-standing motif: see Ermacora (2015) and also Bibliotheca Apostolica Vaticana, MS Barbarini Lat. 306 p. 97.

5. De Mondeville used Giovanni da Capua's translation of 1305: see Bos (2009: xv).

6. Bibliotheca Apostolica Vaticana, MS Vat Lat 2418, fols 210v–211: *Gentilis Commentarium super Tractatu Mesues de Venenis, qui est VIa IIIIti*. Question: *Utrum in urina morsi a cane, possint apparere canes.*

7. Bibliotheca Apostolica Vaticana, MS Barbarini Lat 306, pp. 124–35.

8. The first iconographic tradition can be found in Pierpont Morgan Library, MS M735; London, British Library, MS Add 15097; and Naples, Bib Gerolamini, MS Cf.2.7. For the second scheme, see Figure 4.4 as one example. For an incomplete list of manuscripts, see Cifuentes and Ferragud (1999: 93–127, n. 18).

CHAPTER FIVE

Objects: The Archaeology of Medieval Healing

GEMMA L. WATSON AND ROBERTA GILCHRIST

INTRODUCTION

Medieval healing encompassed a broad range of approaches informed by science, religion and folklore, performed by an equally diverse group of practitioners – physicians (often monks and priests), surgeons, apothecaries, herbalists, lay-sisters, bone-setters, tooth-drawers, astrologers, wise-women, midwives, druggists and leeches. Historians of medicine previously focused on practices that conform to our understanding of Western medicine today, while frequently dismissing other approaches to healing as 'magic gibberish'. This has resulted in traditional, folk-based practices becoming invisible in both historical and archaeological studies of medicine. (Rawcliffe 2011: 391; Shaw and Sykes 2018). A narrow definition of medieval medicine is compounded by the fact that many aspects of healing are hard to reach through documentary sources alone. For instance, texts on the various learned medical traditions have survived, but in most cases, we do not know how they were used or by whom. The methods of the common healer are unclear as they would have learned their craft orally and through practice; and the methods of sorcerers and other magic healers are even more obscure (Horden 2008: 418). The objects used by medieval healers represent an important source with potential both to address some of the gaps in historical knowledge and to explore the agency of healers and their tools (Hartnell 2017a, 2017b). This chapter discusses the contribution that artefactual analyses make to a cultural history of medieval medicine and, more specifically, what the study of archaeological sources can offer, drawing principally on evidence from medieval Britain.

Archaeological approaches reveal a broad range of healing practices that were employed by medieval healers. Through contextual analyses of material culture, burial evidence, buildings, and environmental data, archaeology can make a significant contribution to the cultural history of medicine, providing insight into the agency of practitioners and the embodied experience of the patient. This is especially significant for the study of social and spatial contexts that texts are unable to reach, such as healing practices employed in the home, but archaeology also challenges prevailing ideas about institutionalized care and medieval understandings of the body and soul (Gilchrist 2020).

ARCHAEOLOGY AND THE CULTURAL HISTORY OF MEDICINE

Cultural history seeks to understand how people in the past made sense of their lives, of the natural world, of social relations and of their bodies. Mary Fissell defines it as 'making meaning from the margins', although she cautions us not to fetishize the marginal – cultural history must look beyond the bizarre and weird (Fissell 2008: 364–5). It is also about how categories are made and remade; about understanding and analysing how cultural categories work as ongoing sets of negotiations. Cultural history is about meaning – what it meant to be a patient, a healer, a physician or a surgeon. But how can we begin to reconstruct the medieval experience of healing? What was it like to be sick in the medieval period? How was illness understood by medieval people? What was it like to be a healer? Historians look for meaning through analysing contemporary thinking written down in documentary sources. To gain a better picture of the actual *experiences* of people in the past and their understanding of the world in which they lived, the cultural history of medicine would benefit from analyses of a wider range of sources and by working collaboratively with other disciplines, such as archaeology (McCleery 2013: 86).

There is no sub-discipline of 'cultural archaeology' that mirrors cultural history or cultural geography. This is partly a reaction among archaeologists against the 'culture history' approach that dominated archaeology before the theorization of the discipline from the 1970s onwards, which divided past societies into distinct ethnic and cultural groupings according to types of material culture. Instead, 'social archaeology' developed from the 1980s onwards, which holds similarities with the cultural turn in other disciplines, addressing themes such as power relations, ethnicity, gender and identity, age and the life course, religion and belief systems. The history of the body is one area where cultural history and archaeology are complementary and collaboration between the two fields would be beneficial, especially for those studying medieval healing and medicine.

Cultural historians have critiqued prevailing approaches to the history of the body and called for deeper considerations of the body as a cultural site (Fissell

2008: 371; Hartnell 2018). Archaeological theorizing of the body was initially influenced by phenomenological approaches: an archaeology of the body assumes that social understandings of the body were created and reproduced through associations with material culture. The body is seen as a site of lived experience, a social body and a site of embodied agency (Joyce 2005). More recent approaches have developed the concept of 'body worlds' as a tool for thinking about the centrality of bodies in human lives. A body world encompasses the totality of bodily experiences, practices, and representations in a specific place and time that are at the heart of how we understand the world (Robb and Harris 2013). Medieval archaeologists have been influenced by these approaches in their analyses of burial evidence and material culture. Medieval conceptions and understandings of the body have been explored in relation to gender, personhood, magic and the life course (e.g. Gilchrist 2008; 2012; Graves 2008; Standley 2013; Gowland and Penny-Mason 2018). An archaeological perspective provides a direct link to the practices performed on the body and therefore offers rich potential for understanding the embodied experience of healing.

Archaeology can contribute significantly to the cultural history of medicine through analyses of material culture connected with healing. One of the dominant themes in the cultural history of medicine is the attention given to rhetorical form. Cultural historians study textual narrative, analysing the meanings behind how and why texts were constructed, the language used, in addition to their content (Fissell 2008). But medieval healing had a practical as well as a narrative component that used tools and materials alongside words (Jones and Olsan 2019). A more practice-based approach is therefore needed to balance this focus on narrative, which can be developed through the study of material culture. Archaeology's concern with materiality is especially relevant to the study of medieval healing and the belief in the efficacy of plants, stones and animals, be they scientific or magical, to ease various afflictions (Gilchrist 2020). In many cases, archaeology is the only means by which we have access to this type of healing. Indeed, practice-based healing that was learned and transmitted orally would probably have made up the main body of medical knowledge, since the majority were illiterate in the Middle Ages.

Spatial context is vital when analysing archaeological sources as this will give potential information on the type of healing being evidenced, who was being treated, and by whom. There are no distinct archaeological typologies to discern healing objects: many objects were multi-purpose and recognition of their healing function relies largely on archaeological context. For instance, many objects used for bodily grooming had multiple applications; surgical instruments had a whole host of other practical purposes and, unless they are excavated from secure 'medical' contexts such as hospitals or monastic infirmaries, are unlikely to be identified as such; devotional objects were utilized in 'folk medicine',[1] but are only recognized in this respect if found in burials or in the home. The most common archaeological contexts for studying healing are burials, hospitals, monasteries and domestic buildings (Huggon 2018). These different contexts give insight into the agency of healing practitioners: healing in the home would have been performed predominantly by women, whereas learned male practitioners would have treated residents of religious institutions. For the most part, archaeologists study refuse rather than the use-context of material culture, but occasionally, a unique archaeological find will offer the chance to study healing where it was practiced, such as the surgeon's chest found aboard the sunken Tudor warship, the *Mary Rose* (1545), on which see more below. Burials also offer the opportunity to study the embodied experience of healing through objects found in direct contact with the corpse. It should be noted that it was not common to place objects with the Christian dead – the great majority of burials were simple interments in shrouds. However, archaeological evidence confirms that objects were placed with a small minority of people buried in medieval churches and monasteries (2–3 per cent of excavated burials from medieval England: Gilchrist and Sloane 2005). It has been suggested that many of these objects were connected to the healing and transformation of the body (Gilchrist 2008; Gilchrist 2012).

INSTITUTIONAL CONTEXTS: HOSPITALS AND MONASTERIES

Religious institutions are the most common archaeological context for identifying medieval medical practice. These institutions are believed to have focused on treating the soul rather than the body – the cure of the soul, through the medicine of the sacraments, was more important than the relief of bodily infirmity (Horden 2007). There were two main types of religious institution that cared for the infirm. First, there were hospitals founded to care for the poor and elderly who suffered from physical, spiritual and occasionally mental affliction. Physical treatment was largely limited to bedrest and an adequate diet, administered in a clean warm environment. This was in keeping with the medical concept of the *Regimen Sanitatis,* the proper management of the body through diet and moderation to achieve equilibrium. It would have also provided the sick poor with access to food, medicine and comfort not widely available to them outside these institutions (Gilchrist 1992: 101; Gilchrist 1995: 32; Rawcliffe 2002b: 58; Horden 2007). Secondly, there were monasteries that provided specialist care for monks and nuns in their infirmaries and separate provision was sometimes made for the sick poor and for pilgrims. The monastic infirmary formed a self-contained community, with buildings mirroring the functions of the main claustral complex, with its own hall, chapel and ancillary buildings; larger monastic infirmaries were sometimes arranged around a cloister, resembling a small hospital (e.g. the infirmary cloister of Thetford Cluniac Priory, Norfolk) (Miller and Saxby 2007: 122–9).

The infirmarer's duty was first and foremost to care for the soul of his patients, although he would have also been medically trained, usually in-house, having an understanding of humoural theory. The Barnwell Observances outline three kinds of sick persons allowed within the infirmary: those suffering exhaustion and weakness from overwork or overindulgence; those suffering fevers, bodily pains or spasms; and those struck with sudden illness such as strokes and heart attacks. The first were prescribed rest in the infirmary for a short time; the second needed a physician, baths and medicine; and the third needed only care for their departing soul (Clark 1897). Monks would have also visited the infirmary on a rotating basis to be phlebotomized, resting there for three days to recuperate. Periodic bloodletting was practised in medieval religious communities, where healthy men and women were bled at regular intervals as a prophylactic measure (Yearl 2007: 176). Some elderly monks would have retired permanently to the infirmary once they were no longer able to fully partake in the monastic regime. They would have benefited from bedrest in the warmer and cleaner environment that characterized medieval hospital care (Gilchrist 2005: 165–6).

New archaeological evidence is challenging previous assumptions about the treatment and care provided in medieval hospitals and monastic infirmaries. The archaeology of healing at these institutions is diverse and includes buildings, burials, objects and environmental data. Study of the buildings of religious institutions where care was provided can reveal much about the organization and development of treatment over time, something that is difficult to establish from documentary sources alone (e.g. Cardwell 1995; Durham 1992; Price and Ponsford 1998; Roffey 2012; Smith 1979; Thomas et al 1997; Harward et al 2019). However, it is the study of the associated cemetery populations that has provided the greatest archaeological source for medieval healing (e.g. Cessford 2015; Connell et al 2012; Magilton et al 2008; Roffey and Tucker 2012; Willows 2017). Bioarchaeology can provide much information on the health of individuals, the types of diseases and infirmities that they suffered from and, occasionally, the care that was provided to them.

The health of an individual can be ascertained by looking for certain indicators on their skeleton. Some chronic diseases, such as tuberculosis, leprosy and arthritis, are visible on the human skeleton in the form of changes in bone structure (Roberts and Manchester 2005; Roberts 2009). Poor diet can be revealed through looking at the teeth; for instance, enamel defects reflect stress brought on by dietary problems during growth in childhood (Hillson 1996). Stature is also a good reflection of the quality and quantity of diet during the growth period (Roberts 2009). Dental caries and diffuse idiopathic skeletal hyperostosis (DISH – a condition that causes ligaments of the spine to calcify and vertebrae to fuse) may indicate an excess in diet leading to poor oral health and obesity (Hillson 1996; Rogers and Waldron 2001; Patrick 2014).

Stable isotope analysis also enables archaeologists to reconstruct diet from the skeleton by looking at the chemical composition of bone collagen (Müldner 2009). Living and working conditions can sometimes be ascertained from studying the human skeleton. For instance, sinusitis – which can be caused by a number of factors including allergies, air pollution, and smoke inhalation – can be recognized on the skeleton as bone formation; while lesions on ribs are indications of lung disease, which can be caused by poor air quality (Roberts 2007; 2009). The mass burial pits excavated at the hospital of St Mary Spital (London) provide poignant evidence for the devastating impact of recurrent famines and epidemics on medieval London. Phases of mass burial at St Mary Spital correspond with major outbreaks of famine thought to have been caused by climatic fluctuations resulting from a massive volcanic eruption in Indonesia in 1257. Osteological analysis revealed that the cemetery population underwent a period of prolonged stress, reflecting repeated incidences of famine and associated infectious disease (Connell et al 2012).

Access to specialist medical treatment in the form of surgery has been observed on a small number of skeletons buried in hospital cemeteries. For instance, three individuals from the cemetery of the hospital of St Mary Spital had trepanation preformed on them, including a man (estimated 36–45 years old) who also displayed a number of pathological changes to the skeleton indicating a chronic pulmonary condition, traumatic lesions to his arms, a fractured rib, and a number of injuries to the skull. The individual had suffered an assault to the top of his head by a bladed instrument or weapon used with extreme force. This had left a sub-triangular hole that appeared to have been deliberately enlarged in an attempt to open up the area of the wound for inspection and/or cleaning. This suggests that surgical treatment was available at St Mary Spital and of sufficient standard to enable the individual to survive the trauma (Connell et al 2012). Archaeologists excavating at the hospital site of St Mary Magdalen (Winchester) discovered one individual who suffered from leprosy who had his lower left leg amputated sometime before death. There was very little evidence of infection associated with the amputation, suggesting that the individual received some degree of medical care (Roffey and Tucker 2012: 175). Evidence for amputation of the lower leg has also been found on the skeleton of an individual excavated from the hospital of St James and St Mary Magdalene (Chichester) and at St Mary Spital (Magilton et al 2008: 258–9; Connell et al 2012). These examples of surgery performed at medieval hospitals challenge previous assumptions regarding the care available to residents: despite ecclesiastical opposition to the spilling of blood and the fragmentation of the body, specialist surgical intervention was sometimes provided at medieval hospitals when required. This would have been from visiting physicians and surgeons, such as those recorded at Norwich Cathedral, Westminster Abbey and Ely Cathedral (Gilchrist 2005: 166; Rawcliffe 2002b, 46; Harvey 1993; Holton-Krayenbuhl 1997, 168).

Specialist medicines were also provided for hospital and infirmary residents, some of which would have required expert skill and knowledge in their preparation. Evidence for distilling has been found at a number of monastic and hospital sites in Britain (Booth 2017; Moorhouse 1972; 1993; Tyson 2000; Gilchrist 2020). Alembics and other distillation vessels, urinals and vessels intended for chemical and medicinal purposes, were identified amongst the objects found in a small area at the end of the dormitory range during excavations at St John's Priory (Pontefract) (Moorhouse 1972). This equipment could have been used for distilling wine into *aqua vitae*, which had a wide range of medicinal uses including relieving toothache, expelling poison and treating cancer (Moorhouse 1972; Prioreschi 2003: 353). More recently, a small building at St Mary Spital has been identified as a distillery based on the peat-burning hearths covering its floor, a common industrial method employed by distillers. Residual evidence of arsenic, lead, copper and iron was found in the building, and glass and ceramic distilling vessels were excavated from a nearby pit. Tests on residues within the vessels revealed the presence of mercury, lead, iron, arsenic and copper; one deposit also contained calcium and phosphorus, possibly from a crushed bone (Harward et al 2019). In the medieval period,

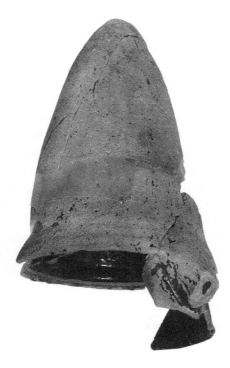

FIGURE 5.1: Distillation vessel (ceramic alembic, fourteenth century, height 290mm) from St Mary Spital, London. Credit: Museum of London Archaeology.

mercury was used in a large number of medicines and lead carbonate was employed in the treatment of conjunctivitis (Connell et al 2012).

Environmental data also provide evidence for some of the remedies prepared and employed to treat the sick body at religious institutions. For example, a fifteenth-century drain excavated at Paisley Abbey (Renfrewshire) yielded plant remains for medicinal plants which may have grown in the abbey's physic garden (Dickson 1996). These plant-based remedies were used to help relieve the sick body rather than treat the soul. The pollen of tormentil was found at Jedburgh Observantine Friary (in the Scottish Borders) and could have been used to treat whipworm. The pollen of ivy and viola were also found; ivy berries were used as a powerful purgative in the Middle Ages and the leaves were sometimes crushed to make poultices for wounds and sores. Violets were used as emollients, expectorants and laxatives (Dixon 2000). The artefactual and environmental evidence for the production and consumption of specialist medical remedies challenges previous assumptions that medieval hospitals primarily treated the soul. Archaeological evidence confirms that the medieval hospital also treated the sick body through the provision of remedies employing specialist knowledge and skill.

MEDICAL OBJECTS

Hospital and monastic sites have provided large assemblages of artefacts, but it is difficult to identify objects with an exclusively medical purpose. A good example is the assemblages of knives and scissors that are commonly found at medieval hospital sites: for instance, thirty-four knives and blade fragments were excavated from the hospital of St Giles by Brompton Bridge, Yorkshire (Cardwell 1995: 194–6). These could have been used for medical purposes, such as in phlebotomy, preparing medicinal ingredients and cutting up dressings. However, it is difficult to assign a specialist function to these multi-purpose tools as they could also have been used for domestic and craft-working activities. In fact, no specialist medical tool has been identified definitively from medieval England (Egan 2007: 65).

However, a unique archaeological find from British waters, a barber-surgeon's chest from the Tudor warship the *Mary Rose*, has provided a rare opportunity to study specialist medical care in situ. A significant number of specialist medical objects were found within the wooden chest and were also recovered from around the barber-surgeon's cabin. These include surgical equipment, drug jars, bandages and syringes. Most of the surgical instruments were made from iron and steel, therefore only a few have survived in a recognizable state. However, a wide range of artefacts made from non-ferrous materials such as ceramic and wood have survived, as well as two pewter syringes. A large number of containers also survived from the Tudor warship.

Samples were taken of the residues still adhering to containers, flasks, syringes and bandages, as well as from a possible spillage identified lying loose within the chest. These include inorganic powders and concretions, mixtures of organic and inorganic material and various organic resins and lipids. One canister contained peppercorns and in others there were residues of beeswax, butter or tallow, pine or spruce resin and frankincense. Scientific analysis demonstrated the use of a wide range of metallic compounds – mercury, tin, zinc, lead, and copper – dispersed in organic matrices. These ingredients are known from Renaissance surgical texts to have been used in a wide variety of therapeutic drugs, ointments and dressings; for instance, pine resin is a natural antiseptic and haemostatic (aiding the coagulation of blood), and lead plasters were used to treat severe bruising and contusions from Classical Greece to the early twentieth century (Derham 2002; Castle et al 2005).

Surgical equipment is rarely found archaeologically, which makes the *Mary Rose* discovery even more significant. Documentary evidence can provide

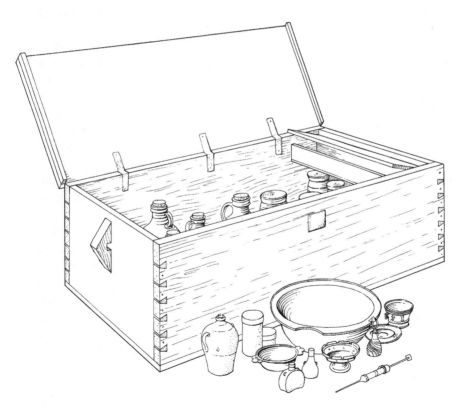

FIGURE 5.2: Reconstruction of the Barber-surgeon's chest and contents as found on the Tudor warship the *Mary Rose*, with other equipment from the cabin. Credit: Mary Rose Trust.

information on the types of surgical tools that could be found in the archaeological record. According to Guy de Chauliac (c. 1300–1368), a surgeon's essential equipment consisted of knives, razors, and lancets for making incisions, cautery irons, grasping tools, probes, needles, cannulas and a tool for trepanation (Siraisi 1990: 155). The wooden handles from surgical instruments were found among the contents of the barber-surgeon's chest on the *Mary Rose*, including the handles for specialist needles, dental instruments, probes, hooks, an amputation knife and bow saw, a cautery iron, and a chisel. Parts of a metal object found concreted to the handles in the chest has been interpreted as a trepan head. The object is tubular and originally had teeth around its edge (Castle et al 2005: 208–12).

Another rare archaeological discovery is that of the skeleton of a possible barber-surgeon found with his kit, perhaps the victim of an accidental death. The remains of a male were found beneath a toppled sarsen stone at Avebury (Wiltshire) and were interpreted as a medieval barber-surgeon due to the objects found associated with his body: coins date the burial to c. 1320–50, and a pair of scissors and a possible lancet or probe suggest his craft (Gilchrist and Sloane 2005: 73).

Northern European monastic hospital sites have yielded rich assemblages of specialist medical material culture, including surgical instruments. For instance, objects excavated from Alvastra Abbey (Östergötland, Sweden) include scalpels, a cautery and a surgical hook, as well as glass and ceramic medicine vessels, spatulas, probes and forceps, and curettes for cleaning fistulae and wounds (Bergqvist 2014). At the Augustinian monastery and hospital of Skriðuklaustur in Iceland, eighteen lancets, scalpels and pins (possibly used for surgical purposes) were excavated. A vial and a ceramic bottle were also found, interpreted as being used for medication (Kristjánsdóttir 2010: 52). Similar rich assemblages have yet to be identified in Britain, perhaps indicating regional differences in attitudes towards healing between the two areas.

The urinal, or jordan, is the best-known medical instrument of the Middle Ages and became the symbol of the medieval physician. It is, perhaps, the most direct evidence we have for specialist medical objects in the archaeological record. Physicians used urinals, made from glass, to examine urine samples for consistency, colour, clarity and odour, which signified particular diseases or states of health and was one of the mainstays of a medieval physician's diagnostic and prognostic repertoire. The technique was closely associated with astrology, which influenced the diagnosis and the recommended cure (Rawcliffe 2006). Usually the rounded bases and necks of green-glass urinals are the only parts of the container that survive in the archaeological record. This is because they are thicker and sturdier than the body of the walls, which are blown very thin so that the contents could be easily observed (Charleston 1975: 213). Fragments of just two glass urinals, possibly dating to the fourteenth century, have been

OBJECTS 117

excavated from the hospital at St Mary Spital (London). They have been interpreted as being of the piriform type: pear-shaped with sloping sides that run up to a wide rim (Gilchrist 1995: 36; Thomas et al 1997: 111). Urinals are not only found at hospital and monastic sites, but also in domestic settings, suggesting that trained physicians also operated in wealthy mercantile contexts. For example, fragments of three green-glass urinals were excavated from the High Street C excavation in Southampton, dating to the fourteenth and sixteenth centuries (Platt and Coleman-Smith 1975: 216–26); and many fragments of urinals were among a large glass assemblage excavated at Upper Bugle Street III, also in Southampton, from a garderobe and cellar tunnel dated to the later fifteenth century (Watson 2013).

Vessels used for storing and preparing medicines are even more challenging to identify in the archaeological record than specialist medical objects because many vessels had multiple functions, making context vital for interpretation. Ceramic vessels were used in the preparation and storage of basic medicines, such as laxatives, diuretics, sedatives and stimulants (Gilchrist 1995: 34). Albarellos, or drug jars, are the easiest vessel type to identify for use in medical contexts. These were specialist vessels imported from the Mediterranean containing exotic drugs for the dispensary. Examples have been identified at a number of monastic and hospital sites in the UK including a possible example in Spanish tin-glaze ware excavated from the infirmary at St Mary Merton Priory (Surrey) suggesting that medicines were kept there (Miller and Saxby 2007). Other examples have been reported from the Carmelite friary in Linlithgow (West Lothian) (Stones 1989), the nunnery of St Mary Clerkenwell (London) (Sloane 2012: 238) and the hospital of St Mary of Ospringe (Kent) (Smith 1979). A fragment of a fifteenth-century drug jar from Glastonbury Abbey (Somerset) was confirmed, by chemical analysis, to be from Tuscany (Blake 2015: 270).

At the hospital of St Mary Spital, 5.5 per cent of the ceramic assemblage from the first phase, dating from 1235–80, comprised ladles and small pipkins (a type of vessel with three feet and a handle placed over direct heat to warm its contents), an unusual vessel form for medieval London. Some of the pipkins show evidence of sooting and may have been used in the preparation of medicines. Those without burning could have been used for mixing (Thomas et al 1997: 111). At St Nicholas' (Fife) jugs are predominant amongst the pottery assemblage in contrast to cooking pots which characterize burgh sites. Could this represent a specialized function for hospital pottery in contrast to the contemporary urban pottery? Special forms, unique to the hospital assemblage, are present within the local ware (Scottish East Coast White Gritty Ware) which may have fulfilled a particular need within the hospital. These include a flat-based open bowl, glazed green internally and externally smoke-blackened, and a small squat jug, possibly with a glazed tubular spout (Gilchrist 1992: 110;

Gilchrist 1995: 36). Medical vessels can sometimes be identified by the residues still clinging to them, like a jar excavated from Soutra Hospital (Scottish Borders) reported as having an organic residue still adhering to it comprising hemp, opium poppy, rose, cedar and pine, all plants known to have been used in healing remedies (Moffat et al 1986–9: 79).

There are candidates for specialist and personalized vessels that may have been used to care for the sick: for instance, a reversible, ash-wood double bowl from St Mary Spital (see Figure 5.3). This could be turned over and used again from the other side and may have been designed specifically for a second person to hold steady by the foot while an infirm person was fed (Egan 2007: 68). During excavations at St Mary Magdalen (Winchester), fragments of two pottery vessels were found in the grave of an individual with leprosy who exhibited severe facial deformities. These have been interpreted as personal food bowls, perhaps indicating assisted feeding or dedicated utensils (Roffey and Tucker 2012: 176). A maple wood feeding bottle, measuring 145 x 66mm, found within the *Mary Rose* barber-surgeon's chest, would have been used to feed the very sick and those with facial injuries. Other vessels that could have had a specialist medical function are bowls used to catch blood during bloodletting, such as the twelve earthenware dishes for bloodletting purchased for the Durham infirmarer in 1397–98 (Gilchrist 1992: 110). A possible pewter bleeding bowl was found in the *Mary Rose* barber-surgeon's chest. It is a small, shallow bowl with a domed centre and two opposed trefoil handles. Two pewter saucers, also found in the chest, may have also been used during bleeding (Castle et al 2005: 200–3).

Stone mortars have been recovered from hospital sites which may have been used to grind up medicinal plants. The rim of a mortar made from sandstone was excavated from a fourteenth-century context at St Bartholomew's (Bristol) and fragments of four mortars were found at St Mary of Ospringe, including one of Purbeck marble and another that had been reused in a nineteenth-

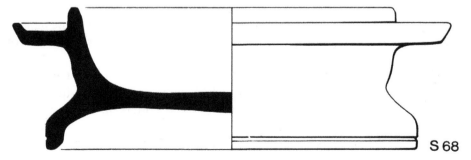

FIGURE 5.3: Drawing of a reversible, ash-wood double bowl excavated from St Mary Spital, London (diameter 170mm, height 56mm). Credit: Museum of London Archaeology.

century wall (Price and Ponsford 1998: 166–7; Smith 1979: 153–4). A limestone apothecary's mortar, dating to the fifteenth century, was excavated from the Dominican friary in Arundel (West Sussex) (formerly thought to have been the hospital of the Holy Trinity). It has been suggested that limestone may have been preferred because it eliminated the risk of particles of quartz entering mixtures of medical compounds, in contrast with mortars made from sandstone (Dunning 1969). A copper-alloy mortar and chafing dish were among the *Mary Rose* barber-surgeon's belongings. The mortar has four external rings or handles, two round and two square, one of which had another ring through it, indicating that it could be suspended over the chafing dish if required to heat the ingredients being prepared (Castle et al 2005: 202–5).

MATERIALS

Certain materials were believed to possess therapeutic or occult properties in the Middle Ages. How these materials were used by medieval healers can sometimes be ascertained by looking at the archaeological context for their use. Mercury, also known as quick silver, was thought to have a cold, wet, complexion; it was valued for its regenerative and purgative qualities and for its capacity to destroy

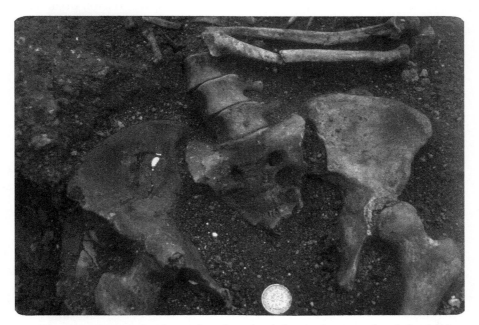

FIGURE 5.4: Mercury droplets as found on the skeleton of a young female buried in Exeter Cathedral Green. Credit: Royal Albert Memorial Museum and Art Gallery, Exeter.

infected flesh and remove unsightly blemishes (Rawcliffe 2006: 224). High levels of mercury were found in the bones of skeletons excavated from Danish medieval cemeteries: mercury was present in the bones of 79 per cent of leprosy cases and 40 per cent of syphilis cases examined, which was attributed to the treatment of these diseases with mercury-containing medicines. In addition, a substantial number of the skeletons of monks interred at the Cistercian abbey of Øm, Denmark, also exhibited increased levels of mercury, which could have occurred from preparing and administering mercury-containing medicine in the hospital there (Rasmussen et al 2008). Mercury droplets have also been found on the skeleton of a young female in her early to mid-twenties buried in Exeter's Cathedral Green (Devon) in the late medieval period. Her skeleton reveals that she suffered from scoliosis and, possibly, miliary tuberculosis. The droplets were found on her right hip bone, and had caused the bone to blacken (see Figure 5.4). It is possible that the droplets came from a medicinal vial hung from her waist that has since disintegrated (Kingdom 2019).

Copper was believed to reduce acute pain, swelling and infection – even today magnetic copper bracelets are used to treat arthritis. Furthermore, modern medical science has shown that copper is toxic to certain bacteria (Gordon 2014: 66). Therapeutic objects made from copper alloy have been found on the skeletons of individuals buried in medieval cemeteries. For example, copper-alloy support plates were found on the skeleton of an adult male from St Andrew's Gilbertine Priory, Fishergate, in York. The man had suffered a severe rotary fracture to the right knee, which was supported by two copper-alloy plates on either side of the joint. The plates were horse-shoe-shaped and measured approximately 100mm in length; they were pierced by rows of perforations, probably intended to carry some form of binding or stitching. Leather was found adhering to the corrosion products of the plates. The plates had stained the man's tibia green, showing that they had been bound to the damaged joint. Similar examples are known from other religious houses in Britain and northern Europe. Two copper-alloy plates were found associated with a badly necrosed and osteomyelitic right humerus from an adult woman (see Figure 5.5), excavated from the leper hospital of St Mary Magdalene (Reading). Remains of dock leaves were found lining the plates, indicating that the plates held some form of poultice or treatment used to treat skin conditions (Gilchrist and Sloane 2005: 103–4). Copper ligatures have also been identified on medieval skeletons. Excavations from the churchyard of St Mark's in Lincoln revealed a late eleventh-century skeleton, the upper arm of which was wrapped in a spool of copper alloy wire (Gilmour and Stocker 1986: 41).

Copper may have been considered efficacious against bubonic plague and it has been suggested that copper-alloy scourges were used as protection against the Black Death. Several examples are known from England: Rufford Abbey (Nottinghamshire), Rievaulx Abbey (North Yorkshire), Roche Abbey (South

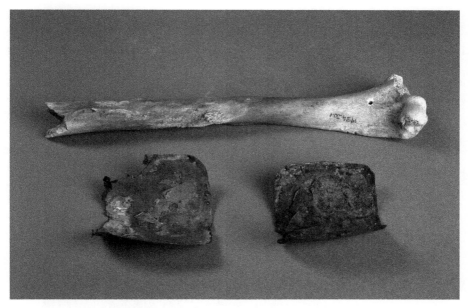

FIGURE 5.5: Copper-alloy plate associated with the humerus of a woman from the cemetery of St Mary Magdalene leper hospital, Reading. Credit: Reading Museum Service.

Yorkshire), Grovebury Priory (Bedfordshire), St Mary Spital, Bordesley Abbey (Worcestershire) and the London Charterhouse (*British Archaeology* news item 2016; Livius 2016; Egan 2019). In addition, the Black Death cemetery at East Smithfield (London) contained the body of an adult male with a copper link wrapped around the base of the tibia (Grainger et al 2008: 16). Could this have been intended as an amulet against the spread of the plague?

Mainstream medicine also used gems, linking them to the theory of the humours (Harris 2016). For instance, sapphires were a cold stone used to treat excessive body heat, ulcers and other ailments. Sapphire rings are a relatively common occurrence in the graves of high-ranking ecclesiastics (Gilchrist 2008: 138). Red coral was believed to hold occult, apotropaic properties and was used during childbirth, as well as being a popular material used to protect infants. Coral pendants are recorded as birth gifts from the fourteenth century and are widely depicted in Italian paintings of the Christ-child and other infants. The close connection between coral and infants also led to the popularity of coral charms as baptismal and wedding gifts, the latter to promote conception and safe birth (Musacchio 1999: 137; Gilchrist 2012: 143). The Peterborough lapidary specifically attributes coral with the power to bring love and aid fertility (McSheffrey 2006: 62). Archaeological evidence of coral is relatively rare in England but includes a pendant from a fifteenth-century house in Brook

Street (Winchester) and two pins from London. Waste from coral bead production was also recovered from Trig Lane (London) confirming that the raw material was imported and worked there (Egan and Pritchard 2002: 304; Gilchrist 2012: 143).

Jet is another material regarded as possessing occult powers. According to medieval lapidaries, jet could ease childbirth and heal dropsy and epilepsy (Egan 1998: 299; Egan 2007: 69–70; Gilchrist 2012: 141, 166). It has been suggested that a jet bowl recovered from fifteenth-century deposits at Trig Lane (London) may have been used within the medieval birthing chamber to ease the pains of childbirth. The unusual selection of jet for the bowl suggests that liquid was intended to be consumed directly from the bowl, being a similar action to the ingestion of holy relics and occult materials that is known from medieval pharmacopoeia (Rawcliffe 2002a: 122; Gilchrist 2012: 141).

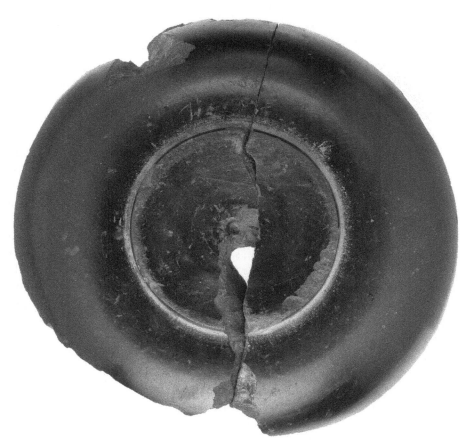

FIGURE 5.6: Jet bowl from Trig Lane, London (diameter 130mm, height 27mm). Credit: Museum of London Archaeology.

BODY AND SOUL

The study of material culture from religious institutions suggests that care of the body was not exclusively curative but that preventative measures were also undertaken to prevent ill health, evidenced by objects associated with personal grooming (such as toothpicks). Bodily hygiene may have taken on deeper spiritual significance, given the close connection that medieval people perceived between the health of the body and the soul. Johanna Bergqvist has argued that care of the body was a means of demonstrating pious religiosity and that gender differences can be discerned. She has studied the material culture of healing at four Cistercian monastic sites in Sweden: the male houses of Alvastra and Varnhem and the female houses of Vreta and Gudhem. Bergqvist identified a gendered correlation in the material culture used in bodily maintenance from male and female monastic sites. Depilation tweezers were found at female institutions, whilst completely absent from the male monasteries. Female hair was a potent symbol of female sexuality and, consequently, medieval nuns would cut and conceal their cephalic hair. Plucking facial hairs may have also been practised amongst pious nuns as a means of domesticating their body. It is a practice also observed in medieval court fashions and was criticized in guides on female behaviour; for example, in the late fourteenth-century tales by Geoffrey de la Tour Landry, *The Book of the Knight of the Tower* (Offord 1971: 76–8). Cosmetics were closely related to female health as beautification was a crucial precursor to procreation (McCleery 2013: 94). Bergqvist also observed that objects of a more specialized medical nature, such as probes, forceps and curettes, predominate at the male institutions, but are absent from the female institutions. Personal hygiene also appeared to be less important among the nuns than among the monks: ear scoops and toothpicks are totally absent from Vreta, but are abundant at Alvastra; and depilation seems to have been a solely female practice (Bergqvist 2014).

The contrast between the male and female communities may have resulted from gendered attitudes to the body and to differing levels of access to medical knowledge. Bergqvist concludes that the abundance of equipment for surgery, medicine, wound treatment and personal hygiene at the male institutions of Alvastra and Varnhem suggests that a well-tended body was consistent with the prevailing view of the male body being more cultured and civilized. She interprets the absence of material culture for hygienic purposes and for surgery at the Cistercian nunneries of Vreta and Gudhem as an expression of female pious religiosity. She links the negative evidence for bodily grooming with the female religious tradition of voluntary asceticism: she argues that the nuns were willing to suffer sickness and infirmity and to forsake personal hygiene as a pious embodiment of disease (Bergqvist 2014: 102).

Other preventive practices included devotional objects worn on the body to protect it from various afflictions and common hazards, such as mass-produced souvenirs purchased from shrines. Many women undertook pilgrimages to help them conceive or to prepare them for safe childbirth, invoking the saints' protection for the unborn foetus and a safe delivery for the mother and child. A souvenir from a shrine or relic renowned for obstetric miracles served as a surrogate relic, attributed with the same protective and curative properties that were possessed by the original. This was achieved by the object coming into direct physical contact with the relic or shrine, transferring healing or apotropaic power to the souvenir. Souvenirs included badges, bells, whistles and candleholders, all cheaply cast from lead/tin alloy, in addition to pictures, votive figurines and candles (Spencer 1998: 5; Gilchrist 2012: 135). These souvenirs, along with relics, textual amulets on parchment, precious stones, herbal remedies, and the recital of verbal charms, were used by the attending midwife to assist and promote a safe delivery (Jones and Olsan 2015).

Textual birthing amulets comprised benedictional formulae written on parchment scrolls and applied to the abdomen, right knee, back or side (Skemer 2006: 237; Rawcliffe 2003). There is an extant example in the Wellcome Collection, Wellcome W MS 632, which depicts the instruments of Christ's passion on one side of the scroll and a promise of safe delivery written on the other (Gilchrist 2012: 140). Amulets were sometimes collected as heirlooms for family use, the best surviving of which is from the French town of Aurillac in Auvergne (Aymer 1926). It comprises handwritten and printed amulets kept together in a linen sack as a 'birthing kit' that was used for centuries by the same family (Skemer 2006: 242).

Parchment rarely survives in archaeological contexts, but there are two possible examples of birthing amulets known to the authors. A mature adult female excavated from the eastern cemetery at the Benedictine priory of St James (Bristol) was buried with a small parcel on her abdomen, formed from a sheet of lead. The lead was carefully folded into a rectangular package that contained a granular material thought to be parchment. The second example is from the cemetery of the hospital of St Mary Spital where a wrapped textile bundle containing a granular material, possibly parchment, was found between the legs of an adult female (Gilchrist 2008; Gilchrist 2012: 140–1). Textual amulets were also folded and placed on open wounds to staunch blood (Gilchrist 2008: 125).

Archaeological evidence confirms that the written word was inscribed on a diverse range of objects in the Middle Ages. Devotional words were inscribed on jewellery, armour, and household objects, particularly from the thirteenth to fifteenth centuries. The inscription of holy words transformed these objects into charms, which were worn on the body and kept in the home to confer protection, good fortune and healing (Skemer 2006: 10; Gilchrist 2012: 163). For instance, the names of the Three Magi served as a verbal charm to protect against epilepsy, falling sickness, sudden death and from all forms of sorcery and witchcraft (Hildburgh 1908: 85). It is one of the most famous charms of the Middle Ages and is found on a plethora of medieval objects including finger rings, brooches, and drinking cups. Examples include two fifteenth-century finger rings, one made from gold from Castle Hill (Edinburgh) and one of silver from Stoke Trister (Somerset). They are both simply inscribed on their exterior with the names Caspar, Melchior and Balthazar (Standley 2013: 79–80).

Koen De Groote has highlighted the occurrence of scratched-mark pottery at nunneries in north-western Europe (De Groote 2016). For example, a large ceramic assemblage from the St Claire monastery of Petegem (Belgium) is inscribed with letters and other marks (see Figure 5.7). One hundred and four examples exist, mainly on redware, representing 12 per cent of the total ceramic assemblage. These appear on bowls, dishes, pipkins, skillets, chafing dishes and a flowerpot. Most are probably linked with the identity of their users, but a large number of them seem to represent an abbreviation of a religious kind; for instance 'MA' for Maria, 'I' for Jesus, 'IC' for Jesus Christ, 'IM' for Jesus and Maria and 'F' for Saint Francis (De Groote 2005: 33–4). Food and drink ingested from these vessels may have been perceived to acquire curative properties transferred from the inscribed vessel.

It was not only the bodies of the living that needed to be treated, cared for, and protected, but also the bodies of the dead. Healing charms were sometimes included in the graves of the deceased (Gilchrist 2008). Archaeologists have found possible examples placed with individuals whose affliction left a pathological

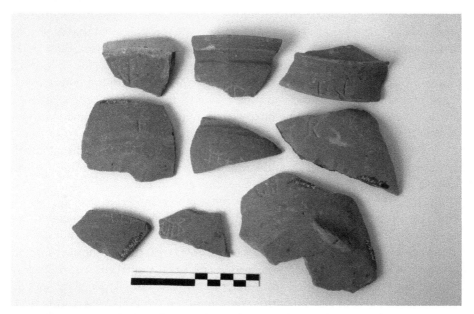

FIGURE 5.7: Scratched marks on redware from St Claire monastery of Petegem, Belgium. Credit: Flanders Heritage Agency.

signature on the skeleton. For instance, a middle-aged woman at St Nicholas' (Aberdeen) and two others from St Giles' Cathedral (Edinburgh) suffered from adult rickets and were interred with a religious badge, a timber rod, and coin, respectively. A woman buried at Holyrood Abbey (Edinburgh) with a silver penny near her hip, suffered from osteochondritis dissecans, a condition that would have affected the circulation and mobility in her legs and feet; and an adult male at Raunds (Northants) buried with a pebble in his mouth, had suffered from poliomyelitis in his youth and later developed tuberculosis (Boddington 1996: 42). The Anglo-Saxon penitentials and later hagiographic and theological writings indicate a belief that a dead body might heal. Lives of saints include details of their holy bodies remaining incorrupt after burial, and their injuries and infirmities healing miraculously after death. For instance, a twelfth-century account of the exhumation and translation of the body of St Etheldreda states that a tumour on her neck had healed after burial (Gilchrist 2008: 149).

The placing of items on the corpse would have occurred during the preparation of the body for burial, when it was washed and dressed, or wrapped in a shroud. In a secular context, women of the family, or perhaps a midwife,[2] prepared the body in the home, while the monastic dead would have been prepared in the infirmary (Gilchrist and Sloane 2005). Healing charms were part of the popular tradition of folk magic, routinely performed by women in the care of their families, by herbalists and midwives and, occasionally, by male practitioners such as surgeons, physicians and mendicant friars (Jones and Olsan 2015; Olsan 2003). There is a long tradition of women using charms and sympathetic magic in caring for their families, and it is suggested that their roles as healers extended to include nurturing the dead (Gilchrist 2008: 152). Outside the family, the destitute, sick and dying were cared for by nursing sisters in hospitals, who had taken religious vows. The hospital sisters would have prepared the corpses of hospital residents for burial and archaeological evidence confirms that healing charms and amulets were sometimes included within their burials (Gilchrist 2012: 154–5).

Caroline Walker Bynum argues that souls were regarded by medieval people as disembodied spirits that could suffer bodily tortures: the condition of the corpse in the grave reflected the fate of the soul in purgatory (Bynum 1995: 206, 296). Archaeological evidence for medical items interred still adhering to the corpse may confirm a popular belief in the sustained connection between the soul and the body (Gilchrist and Sloane 2005: 103–5). It has been argued that these objects were therapeutic devices intended to treat or heal the corpse while it was in the grave, in preparation for the corporeal resurrection at the day of judgement (Gilchrist 2008: 150). Examples include the copper alloy support plates discussed above and a hernia truss found on the body of a mature adult male excavated from St Mary Merton (See Figure 5.8; Gilchrist and Sloane 2005: 103–5).

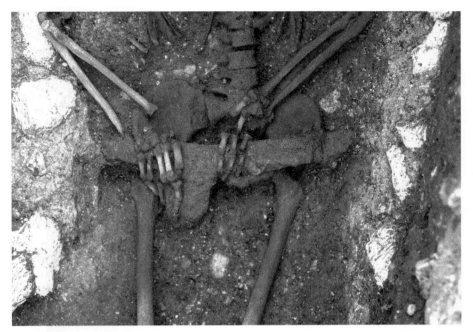

FIGURE 5.8: Hernia truss as found in the grave of a mature-adult male in the north transept of the church of St Mary Merton, Surrey. Credit: Museum of London Archaeology.

In contrast, Stephen Gordon offers an alternative interpretation for copper ligatures found on the body: he proposes that these were used to 'bind' the flesh of a swollen and potentially restless corpse. The *Lacnunga,* an Anglo-Saxon medical miscellany dating to the eleventh century, contains numerous charms which illustrate how ligatures were seen as powerful devices for curing, or 'binding', physical and spiritual ailments and Gordon conjectures that this practice continued into the later medieval period. Gordon compares the medieval evidence for binding with interpretations in anthropological literature, specifically Alfred Gell's study of contemporary Polynesia and conceptions of magic. The power of magical substances resides in the ability of the viewer to comprehend the ambiguous properties of an object or thing's creation (Gell 1998). Abstract forms such as ligatures, knots, woven patterns, and difficult incantations, bewilder the senses. Such patterns are difficult to process because they are ambiguous with no readily understandable form. Consequently, the object of the bind, or the agent of disease, becomes trapped in the pattern (Gell 1998: 85–90). Gordon notes that some medieval physicians, such as John of Gaddesden (*c.* 1280–1360), were aware of the popular belief in the power of knots, specifically the use of ligatures to cure ailments such as toothache and gout (Gordon 2014: 65).

Gordon argues that the act of tying ligatures to curtail disease can be extended to include bodily and spiritual disorders afflicting the deceased (Gordon 2014: 65). Dangerously swollen bodies needed to be contained to prevent them from returning to the world of the living as revenants, people who had died a 'bad death', unable to confess their sins. A revenant was believed to spread disease, such as the story of the Ghost of Anantis,[3] who would emerge from his tomb each night, accompanied by a pack of howling dogs and a terrible, pestilent stench, causing many people to die of plague (Gordon 2014: 57–9). Gordon argues that copper ligatures may have served as amulets on the corpse, preventing decay and restlessness and, consequently, the spread of disease (Gordon 2014: 66).

CONCLUSION

Through its focus on contextual analysis, archaeology reveals undocumented practices and expands and challenges existing models of medieval medical practice. Archaeology provides evidence for specialist medical care of the body in medieval religious institutions, previously thought to have provided only palliative care and being primarily concerned with caring for the soul. Excavations at hospitals have provided possible evidence for surgery on residents, as well as the manufacture of specialist pharmaceuticals on site. Archaeology also provides new insight to the experience of health and healing beyond the confines of elite texts that represent the mainstay of medical history. The excavation of hospital cemeteries provides source material for study of the sick poor in medieval society and the osteological study of their remains reveals much about their health and the care they received at these institutions (Roberts 2017).

Archaeology offers insight into the experience of patients and the roles of undocumented healers, such as lay sisters in hospitals, women and midwives in the home, and the barber-surgeon at sea. Archaeology also provides a new source for medieval understandings of the body and soul through the practices employed in healing the dead, previously unknown from documentary sources.

The archaeological study of medieval healing is still at a formative stage. Future research might explore regional differences in healing, as highlighted by the difference in material culture found at hospitals and monastic sites in Britain compared with continental northern Europe. Why have specialist medical objects rarely been found in Britain? Does this reflect a regional distinction in medieval understandings of the body and its care? The study of women's health also needs to broaden beyond issues of fertility and childbirth. Most historical sources are written by men, making it very difficult to find female perspectives on female health issues. Archaeology can help to address this imbalance through analyses of female skeletons to consider health, diet and longevity and living conditions in the archaeological record. For example, a recent osteological study of young women from England has provided insight into health issues connected to living conditions and employment (Shapland et al 2015). Archaeology brings a practice-based approach to the study of medieval healing, highlighting the importance of context, materiality and embodied experience, to bring new insights to the cultural history of medicine.

NOTES

1. Folk medicine today is also termed 'traditional' or 'indigenous' medicine. The World Health Organization (WHO) defines traditional medicine as 'the sum total of the knowledge, skills, and practices based on the theories, beliefs, and experiences indigenous to different cultures, whether explicable or not, used in the maintenance of health as well as in the prevention, diagnosis, improvement or treatment of physical and mental illness' (World Health Organization 2000: 1). As such, folk medicine may also be regarded as inherited traditions, knowledge and practices defined as 'intangible heritage' by UNESCO. Folk medicine is often interpreted as a body of belief and practice separate to the social and cultural mainstream. It thus tends to be conceptualized within a hierarchical model which places official, scientific medicine at the top and folk medicine below (O'Connor and Hufford 2001). The term 'folk medicine' did not exist in the medieval period but is sometimes defined as popular medicine based on received tradition of herbal lore (e.g. Hunt 1990). For the purposes of this chapter, folk medicine relates to healing practices that were performed in the home outside of institutional care and was circulated via oral tradition rather than through learned medical texts.
2. Midwives were part of a larger community of women healers practising in the medieval period (Green 1989). The term midwife means 'with-woman'. There is some debate over the professionalization of midwives in the Middle Ages, but generally they are not well documented until the thirteenth or fourteenth centuries. There is documentary evidence, however, for local women assisting in this role prior to this date. Midwives are likely to have been married women or widows who were able to draw upon their experience to assist with childbirth (Green 2005: 15; Harris-Stoertz 2014). For further discussion on the role of medieval midwives see the work by Monica Green (2005; 1989) and Fiona Harris-Stoertz (2014).
3. The Ghost of Anantis is one of twenty-five supernatural stories in the late twelfth-century *Historia Rerum Anglicarum* of William, canon of Newburgh Priory, North Yorkshire.

CHAPTER SIX

Experiences: Feeling Unhealthy in the Middle Ages

NAAMA COHEN-HANEGBI

INTRODUCTION

Identified only by his name and provenance, some intimate detail is known to us about the life of a certain nobleman named Martin of Germany. A medical *consilium*, issued by the Perugian physician Mattiolo de Mattioli (aka Mattheolus de Perusio d. 1480), discloses that Martin sought the physician's advice because he feared he might have inherited his parents' gout. Martin's noble birth contributed further to the danger that he might succumb to the disease. Mattiolo goes on to mention a few of the symptoms described by his patient, most probably in writing, perhaps through a mediator: his organs had a lax composition and were not very stable and he would tire and suffer pain easily. He was also fearful and his sight had deteriorated (Munich, Bayerische Staatsbibliothek, MS CLM 363, fol. 188). This list of Martin's symptoms offers a glimpse into a personal experience of failing health and its all-encompassing influence. It also allows us to try to piece together what it meant to be healthy or ill in medieval times, how such concepts were defined and what the criteria were for either designation.

Health, illness and disease are elusive terms. What they describe and how their boundaries are identified varies according to point of view (professional or lay), discipline (medical, linguistic, literary) and ethical positions (Boyd

2000). In contemporary bioethics and the philosophy of medicine, these notions have been dissected thoroughly, providing definitions which range from scientific-based naturalism to normative positions. Stark naturalists regard health as the absence of disease and disease as a state of internal impairment or limitation of functional ability. Normativists consider health and disease as value judgements dictated by social codes (Ereshefsky 2009; Wakefield 1992; Murphy 2015). In between the two polarized (and much criticized) views there is an ongoing effort to explain, or rather ascertain, what these words encapsulate. In twenty-first-century societies this deconstruction of seemingly self-evident concepts has been instrumental for numerous actors, including institutions of health services, policy makers, insurance companies, patients' advocate groups and for more personal individual needs. The multiplicity of ideas and definitions at hand validates the constant role of social and cultural positions constructing the meaning of health and illness. The important contribution of historical studies to this debate is therefore in demonstrating just how profound the influence of culture is, not only with regard to changing values, but also in shifting perceptions of 'nature' and of what is 'natural'.

In turn, bringing this awareness to the study of medieval texts reminds us that, although words translate to modern English seemingly easily from medieval Latin, or other vernacular languages, the cultural meanings imbued in terms needs to be addressed as well. More importantly, this awareness demands that we return to the sources which discuss health and illness and recover their attributed meanings. Looking at sources such as letters, medical consultations, miracle inquests and medical contracts, which provide a range of experiential information about illness, this chapter will consider how illness/health was discerned, the function and forms of communicating illness and the relationship between physical, mental and spiritual health. Above all, espousing the viewpoint of narrative medicine, this study will examine the use and meaning of categories of illness in late medieval culture and how this matches the documentation of personal experiences of health and illness.

METHODOLOGY

The necessity of tending to the narratives of patients to ascertain the meaning of health and illness has been a central argument in health studies for three decades. Motivated by social movements dedicated to human rights and multi-culturalism, this branch of scholarship was written with a commitment to enacting change in public health care and in health practices. Such was the mission of Arthur Kleinman in *The Illness Narratives: Suffering, Healing, and the Human Condition*, which sought to raise awareness of the importance of listening to patients' accounts of their illness, and of becoming more attentive to the cultural embeddedness of experiences (Kleinman 1988). For Kleinman, a primary goal

EXPERIENCES

of this awareness was to assist patients' recovery by allowing sufferers a voice and by encouraging the sensitivity of care-givers. However, the message has no less potential for scholars eager to fathom concepts of health in present or past societies. Anthropologists, psychologists, scholars of literature and history all gain new insights into the feelings of the sick and suffering when they concentrate on patients' own words and vocabularies.[1] Historian Roy Porter has further nuanced this critique by arguing that the physician-patient prism is bound to be restricted and non-representative of the life of the sufferer. Based on early-modern findings, he proposed that much of the daily interaction surrounding ill health occurred among family, community and with other methods of healing. A more complete historical account of experiences of health and illness must rely on sources that go beyond the viewpoint of the medical profession (Porter 1985).

Studies in early-modern European history that espoused the narrative approach to the history of medicine have discovered, for example, that sufferers were active in producing narratives of their own illnesses for various purposes. Narratives often reviewed one's lifespan rather than just current episodes of illness, intimating a sense of continuity and ongoing fragility. Such texts also show that patients repeatedly sought reasons for their ill-health, often resorting to self-blame for having a predestined poor constitution, or describing themselves as sinners (usually of a sexual nature) whose sins weakened their bodies and rendered them prone to illness (Stolberg 2011: 46–7). These and other models of reasoning disclose that experiences of illness which are usually associated with modernity, such as lay engagement with professional medical discourse or an inherent link between health and moral behaviour, have a longer history. The few studies that assumed this approach in studying medieval healthcare demonstrate that these themes recur in narratives of this period as well, although the task of finding and interpreting them is perhaps less straightforward (McVaugh 1993: 18–28; McCleery 2009; 2011).

Medieval intimations of illness are often as daunting as they are revealing. Reports of illness from the period are seldom narratives in the sense referred to by contemporary anthropologists or literary critics. Apart from a few single texts, autobiographical writing is generally rare until late in the fifteenth century, leaving us with limited first-person reports of illness. Among existing materials, comprehensive accounts of one's own infirmities, appended by a narrative of self-formation through illness, are singular examples (Frohne 2015). To fill this gap, it is necessary to examine available accounts of illness and disease, and to assemble narratives from them. Nonetheless, even when such reports are available, making sense of the feelings that underpin them is a task fraught with methodological difficulties. As scholars who studied illness narratives inform us, such texts, as personal as they are, are nevertheless manufactured and their use of language habitually employs literary schemes such as metaphors, symbols and allusions which respond to common notions.[2] This is particularly true for medieval texts. Marion Turner (2016), for example, has shown that Middle English narratives of illness are replete with literary mechanisms, but concomitantly less fabricated texts also subscribe to language norms in recounting histories of illness. In addition, as will be discussed below, the conundrum of deciphering the private and personal meanings attributed to illness is even more intricate since medieval narratives often serve as didactic treatises for moral emendation. It is therefore necessary to identify conventions, undertake close reading and consider how these conventions assist and inform the act of making sense of health and illness.

Martin's story is a case in point. In this document produced by the physician, our insight into the patient's motives is skewed. The narrative suggests that Martin interpreted his failing health as an early sign of gout. His fears were understandably grave as gout was considered (then as now) a chronic disease and his hopes for recovery might have been low. What, then, did he expect to gain from the physician? Presumably, he was after a regimen of palliative treatment. But, as the case is told, it seems that Martin was also in need of some assurance or knowledge of his condition. Naming the disease was valuable for the patient no less than for the physician. In some way, it appears, it was different from soliciting the physician for general weakness and anxiety. Did naming his condition allow him to better plan for the future? Did it provide credence to his otherwise inexplicable suffering? Unfortunately, such questions must remain unanswered. However, it is noteworthy that we find that both patient and physician shared a conceptual framework regarding the feared disease. The patient's self-diagnosis was confirmed by the physician, who then added further professional information about the specific manifestation of the disease in this specific patient.

At the same time, it is through the intervention of professional language that another model of approaching the patient's ailments is proposed. Introducing the notion of *complexio*, the physician moves from considering the specific symptoms and the disease in a narrow sense – gout – to discussing the patient's overall condition. Thus, the physician broadens the patient's point of view and connects his localized aches and pains to a holistic perspective. The notion of *complexio* also highlights another salient feature of Galenic medicine, namely the emphasis on individual health rather than implying a strict dichotomy between health and disease. Though this corresponds to the tone of the patient's complaint, the professional terminology sets the experience of disease within a comprehensive system of thought which lends sense and meaning to the processes of the body.

Thus, we have two voices in this medical *consilium*. The first is the retrieved voice of the patient, the sufferer; the second is of the medical man. The two voices express notions and concepts of health and disease as discussed above, but

EXPERIENCES

also provide us with a personal – if fragmented – narrative of illness. Further points of view regarding the nature of health and disease emerge in medieval sources that deal with the body and its ailments; these include miracle stories and inquests, letters and sermons, contracts and court-cases. Their diversity foretells the plurality of definitions and approaches to illness found in the period, which range from the functional to the spiritual. Though these texts often bow under the heavy weight of generic conventions and cultural expectations, they do not obliterate first-person narratives. Exploring these fragments of personal experiences of health allows us to further deepen our understanding of how ideas about health and illness resonated among individual people.

Recent research in the history of emotions and sensibilities opens new and helpful avenues for this pursuit. Assembling diverse responses to pain in varied disciplines, Esther Cohen's *The Modulated Scream* (2010), for example, pointed out the necessary task of identifying the stage at which a certain pain has been uttered to uncover the meaning it assumed. For although pain could be understood as salvific punishment for sins, it could still be an unwelcome symptom of a wound requiring surgery. The plurality of medieval points of view is even more revealing when they coincide. Thus, recognizing the overlapping meanings and the interplay between registers has been shown to be a profitable hermeneutic method for the study of pain in devotional literature (Yoshikawa 2009). Paying close attention to disciplines, genres and registers helps, therefore, to open a gap through which narratives – in our case, illness narratives – may come to light. In drawing attention to the ways authors make use of conventions of speaking about health, we may overcome the problematics of veracity and adequacy of capturing the experience of illness, a difficulty to which even medieval authors allude (Turner 2016: 67).

DEFINING SICKNESS

Categories of illness and health are shaped by cultural settings to which environmental and social circumstances contribute. The medieval European context with its high mortality rates among the young, famines, plague and – as perceived by modern popular culture – the dubious effects of its medicine, is often considered to be apathetic and indifferent to illness and death. Monty Python's 'bring out the dead' scene certainly assisted in imprinting this portrayal on recent generations. Scholars, too, contributed to a stereotype of medieval illness as a fatally extreme state. This may have been catastrophic, echoing Boccaccio's description of the plague in the introduction to the *Decameron* as severing all cultural and social ties, or trivial, as seen in some discussions of parental love and child mortality (Wray 2004; Oosterwijk 2008). It was also proposed that in the medieval period people excluded the sick from their communities, mostly in cases of leprosy, because they were thought to have incurred divine punishment for their sins (Turner 1995: 84; van Dam 1985: 259–61). In recent years, the bleakness of this narrative has been moderated as more attention has been paid to the social practices formulated in the face of disease and imminent death. These studies show that the ill – women after childbirth can also be included in this category – were an important part of the living community (Rieder 2006: 60–80, 123–45). Although most evidence derives from records of the wealthy and powerful, there is sufficient indication that, among most layers of society, sickness invited reliance on near-kin and further strengthened networks among the broader local community (Pilsworth 2011; Wray 2009: 170–4). It is, therefore, important to state that it is now

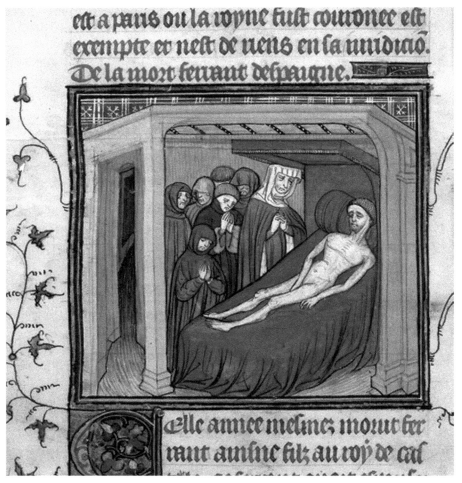

FIGURE 6.1: Death of Fernando of Castile in 1252, *Chroniques de France* (late-fourteenth century). London, British Library, MS Royal 20 C VII, fol. 11 (detail). Credit: British Library/Public Domain.

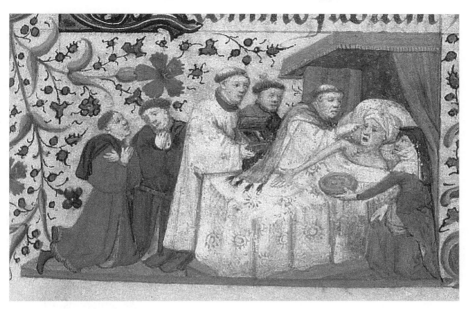

FIGURE 6.2: Administering the Last Rites, Matins of the Office of the Dead, *The Dunois Hours* (mid-fifteenth century). London, British Library, MS Yates Thompson 3, fol. 211 (detail). Credit: British Library/Public Domain.

commonly recognized that medieval society maintained an ongoing preoccupation with illness. In the same way that death called upon rituals involving spiritual, bodily and communal practices, illness was an axis around which congregated a host of social and cultural anxieties (see Figures 6.1 and 6.2). It inspired concern among the living whose hopes, worries, funds and daily routine were invested in their own health and that of their kin.

Substantial evidence indicates that illness was not conceived of in the period in binary terms as the opposite of health and that, in certain circumstances, a more complex understanding prevailed. A rather technical perspective on how medieval people regarded illness can be learned from agreements drawn up between patients and healers, such as those found in the archives of late-medieval Bologna. A repeated condition of the contract is the restoration of the patient's ability to perform certain tasks, such as dressing and feeding himself or cutting bread (Pomata 1998: 27–9; Shatzmiller 1989: 137). In such cases, health was associated with regaining functioning ability and the alleviation of symptoms. These agreements suggest that it was the patient who determined whether the treatment was successful, yet the focus on abilities and actions delineates this visibly. Malpractice suits also relied on visible means to settle claims. In contested cases, as well as in litigations regarding bodily harm, testimonies of external medical experts were necessary to determine the plaintiffs' state (Shatzmiller

1989: 150–1; Ferragud 2014; Carraway Vitiello 2014; Cosman 1973). This method for assessing health indicates that, at least in the legal sphere, it was seen as a state that could be recognized beyond the personal experience.

From the late-thirteenth century on, there is evidence that physicians and surgeons assessed wounds of the victims of violence in court to determine the degree of harm. In cases surviving from the fourteenth-century Italian town Reggio Emilia, for example, these professional witnesses evaluated the victims, some badly hurt, according to their chances of dying from the injury. Their verdicts ultimately attest to a binary view between health and death. A recurrent statement in these documents considers the shedding of blood and the amount of bleeding. Blood serves as an externally visible marker of degree, which assists in conveying to the court the expert's analysis of the patient's state in non-professional terms (Carraway Vitello 2014: 143–5). This need to summon professional witnesses demonstrates the frailty of the objective stance. In addition to an underlying awareness of the personal experience of impairment and disease, lawsuits and legal action demanded definitive categories.

Furthermore, it is not by chance that this judicial evidence largely concerns ailments of a particular bodily organ or symptom. These situations are more susceptible to clear-cut judgement. A greyer area, between health and illness, was nevertheless observed and discussed within the more abstract discourse of academic medicine. Galenic medicine maintained two models for defining states and degrees of health. The primary model rested on the concept of complexions and mixtures, suggesting that health and disease existed on a continuum and that they were subject to inevitable movement. Health was defined not as perfect balance, for such a state was almost impossible to maintain, but as the normative equilibrium of each individual. Infraction of this balance resulted in loss of health and required restoration through medicine and regimen (Isidore of Seville 1911: Book IV; Kaye 2014: 205–40). Such infractions were nevertheless unavoidable, being part of everyday living and being part of everyday living conditions. The language of balance imagines health as a fluid, ever-changing mode of being in which health or illness was hardly ever an absolute term. In tandem with this approach, healthcare was not for the sick alone; it was rather a necessity of everyday life.

A more methodological view is, nevertheless, apparent in the scholarly medical literature from the twelfth century onwards; but it is also not binary. Following Galenic ideas, some physicians considered another intermediate state (*neutrum* or *neutralitas*) between health and disease. The category was developed among physicians for their own use as a term helpful for diagnosis and for formulating accurate practice (van der Lugt 2011). It was not discussed more broadly, nor was it conceived with the intention of capturing or reflecting on patients' experience. However, these theoretical discussions reveal physicians' engagement with the reality that, for example, the health of a person with a permanent disability should be judged differently from the health of a young girl. In this respect, the aspiration to provide medical care for diverse circumstances not only demanded calculation of age, seasons, gender, geography and the vocation of the patient in prescribing the correct dosage, but also envisaging different goals for each patient.

Although elaborate distinction and terminology (such as *neutrum*) belonged primarily to the discourse of learned physicians, other medical ideas – such as the theory of mixtures/qualities and the four temperaments – circulated among the wider public, shaping terminology regarding the body and its health. These helped to express the intuitive idea that different bodies were healthy in different ways, and that one person's natural state could be another's malady. Authors of penitential manuals, for instance, advised confessors to pay attention to penitents' complexions, because they may have influenced the inclination to certain sins and actions (e.g. Alain of Lille 1965: vol. 2, 31; Thomas of Chobham 1968: 418).[3] Coroners and judges considered humoural changes and individual temperaments to determine the mental state of the accused, or to ascertain cause of death (Butler 2015: 225–7). Literary works also mention humoural dispositions as salient attributes of their characters. Geoffrey Chaucer, John Lydgate and Fernando de Roja did so explicitly, particularly with regard to melancholic types. Others, such as Dante or Chrétien de Troyes, reference this scheme more subtly (Whitney 2011; Langum 2016: 125, Amasuno 2004; Boyde 2006: 159–60; Saunders 2015: 36–7). Defined wholly by their bodily complexions, both in physical terms and demeanour, such characters are never seen as completely healthy even if they do not suffer particular ailments.

Pastoral theology is perhaps the most binary among medieval perceptions of health. Employing a vocabulary of disease and illness, authors of devotional or didactic texts speak of sins as wounds and diseases that are a negation of health and righteousness. The repeated metaphor of the priest as physician gained in prominence in the later Middle Ages following its appearance in canon 21 of the Fourth Lateran Council of 1215 (Tanner 1990: 245). Reiterated in confessors' manuals and sermons, it taught that the confessor's role is to discern and diagnose the illness of the penitent; that diverse spiritual remedies extract sin by performing medical-like procedures; and that full health also offers the prospect of salvation (Ziegler 1998: 181–7; Smith 1998; Yearl 2014). This metaphorical trope was wedded to the idea that sin/illness is an antonym of salvation/health. However, theologians from the twelfth century onwards engaged in discerning varying states of sin and formulated a detailed analysis of venial and deadly sins. This precision in identifying sins was a development deeply rooted in the desire to adapt to a growing community of penitents. This effort to discern degrees and severity mirrors physicians' concern with the ineptitude of binary categories of health and illness (Cohen-Hanegbi 2017). This movement between establishing clear-cut categories and acknowledging

140   A CULTURAL HISTORY OF MEDICINE IN THE MIDDLE AGES

the many in-between experiences was thus central to the discourse of health and illness in the period.

CORRESPONDING ILLNESS

Epistolary exchange is an important window onto how health was discussed among families, friends, patrons or professionals. Letters, private and public, ordinarily contained at least a short mention of how the author or recipient was faring. Nevertheless, it is a highly problematic source, as the written exchange was always situated within generic conventions due to the public nature of correspondence in the period. Scholars of letters and epistolary collections remind us that the diversity of the genre and its process of composition and compilation demand particular care in deciphering the contexts and conventions guiding each letter (Ysebaert 2015). Thus, it is essential to consider how writing about health and illness was specifically prescribed in correspondence with family, physicians or other persons of authority. Still, it is through this formal and formulaic address, that we learn how different contexts shaped ideals and norms of conversing about experiences of health and illness (Cohen 2010: 115–20). We further learn how the telling of such experiences served to facilitate certain kinds of communication.

High medieval correspondence by nobility and ecclesiastics to their kin or peers of similar social standing shows the casual mingling of private health concerns with political calculations, sometimes as a means of softening one's agenda. In 1263, Marguerite of Provence (1221–1295) Queen of France, wrote a short letter to her brother-in-law King Henry III of England (1207–1272) mixing covert diplomacy with an overt expression of interest in the king's health (Champollion-Figeac, ed. 1839: 1. 148, letter 120). In another example, Lanfranc of Bec (1005–1089), in a letter to Pope Alexander II, mentioned the old age and chronic illness of a bishop under his jurisdiction to urge his release from duty; although it is clear from the letter that many other motives were at stake (Clover and Gibson, eds. 1979: 34–8). In another letter from 1076–1077, Lanfranc wrote that he had provided extensive health care for a sick monk out of reverence for the Archbishop of Rouen (Clover and Gibson, eds. 1979: 136). Fulbert of Chartres (d. 1028) fostered his close friendships and alliances through letters, which included personal advice of both a spiritual and a medical nature (Fulbert of Chartres 1976: 82–4, 118–28; McGuire 2010: 163–72). A similar, yet even more medically orientated approach, is seen in Anselm of Canterbury's (1033–1109) correspondence with his monastic circle of friends. Anselm's enquiries and advice which, as Giles Gasper noted, are not unlike those of a medical practitioner, emphasize his own patriarchal responsibilities as abbot, and reaffirm his learning and his role in the community (Schmitt, ed. 1984: vol. 4, 3–6, 61–2; Gasper 2004).

Despite the unavoidable burden of style and convention which might raise doubts about the authenticity of sentiment that letters express, we nevertheless learn from them about the common expectations of social and personal behaviour in times of sickness. Bernard of Clairvaux's (1090–1153) letter to his benefactor Beatrice of Villa, in which he complained (clearly to flatter) that no one else ever asks him about his health (*Quis umquam de nostra salute interrogat?*), elegantly captures the conjoined aims of care and political advancement (LeClerq and Rochais, eds. 1979: vol. 8, 298–9). Anselm of Canterbury's letters to Matilda of Scotland, Queen of England (1080–1118), similarly exhibit how loyalty is expressed through enquiries about health (Schmitt, ed. 1984: vol. 5, 344, 351). Looking ahead to the consolation letters of Italian humanists, such as Petrarch (1304–74) and Coluccio Salutati (1331–1406), we see that corresponding about one's pains continued to confirm and constitute friendships, even after modes of expression had changed (McClure 1991: 75–6). Moreover, the culture of consolatory letters also existed outside learned circles, especially from the

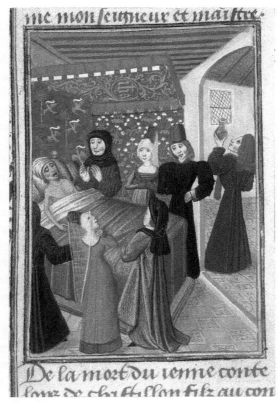

FIGURE 6.3: Sick man's bedside, Jean Froissart, *Chroniques* (late-fifteenth century). London, British Library, MS Harley 4379, fol. 125v (detail). Credit: British Library/Public Domain.

fifteenth century onwards, as private vernacular correspondence expanded among noble women, merchants and urban circles. One such example is the letter written in 1468 by the recently enthroned Duchess of Milan, Bonne of Savoy (1449–1503), to her mother-in-law, the former Duchess of Milan, Bianca Maria Visconti (1425–68). Bonne mentioned that she herself was sick at the time of writing the letter, implying perhaps a bond based on their shared experience of ill health. Although the relationship between the two seems to have had its challenges, the expression of filial care and Bonne's note about her constant prayers for Bianca's health can be considered a sincere, yet political, confirmation of their mutual bond (Nicoud 2000: 377). Similarly, in a letter from 1495, Isabella d'Este (1474–1539) conveyed to her sister-in-law, Chiara Gonzaga, her desire that her loving letters 'written with blood' would heal Chiara's illness (Isabella d'Este 2017: 68). Forging and extending kinship and friendship through informing each other about illness and poor health (one's own, and no less that of friends and neighbours) is also apparent in the prolific correspondence of the Paston family of Norfolk gentry, the noble Florentine Strozzis and the lesser-known Fernando Díaz de Toledo, Archbishop of Niebla (d. 1452), all active in the fifteenth century (e.g. Strozzi 1997: 87–91; Davis, ed. 1971: 216–7, 230–2, 246–7; Round 1980).[4] Finally, further evidence as to the social role that conversing about sickness had in the period can be gleaned from artworks depicting the sick surrounded by figures who appear to be partaking in a communal interaction that is not strictly that of providing medical care (see Figure 6.3).

A rather different testimony to the norms and degree of communal involvement in states of physical pain appears in Peter Abelard's (1079–1142) letter, known as the *Historia calamitatum*. In one of the first passages of the letter, Abelard tells of the time he returned to his family's home due to sickness to be cared for by his kin (Peter Abelard 2013: 8). Later on, following his castration by the avenging uncle of Heloise with whom he had had an illicit relationship, he is again surrounded by people, his neighbours, who come to his bed upon hearing of the attack. Abelard describes his deep shame and annoyance at the lamentation surrounding him, not wishing the embarrassing affair to be so publicly known. Though this is an unusual case of suffering, which is particularly awkward to share, the retelling of the affair in a letter to a friend (at least it is presented as such) charts the boundaries of sharing pain (Peter Abelard 2013: 46–50).

The intimate side of letters is also invaluable as a source for learning about experiences of illness during the period. Correspondence often provides first-hand information about sickness and daily routines of diet and medicine (Gasper 2004: 250–1; Whitaker 1993). Yet, when addressed to a member of the laity, complaints in these letters usually refrain from naming specific diseases or from giving a full account of their unfolding. Instead, they mention diverse pains – headaches, back pain – and chronic problems such as deteriorating

EXPERIENCES

eyesight and episodes of fever. Anselm, in a letter to Gilbert Abbot of St Étienne, complained about a sickness with harsh fever, symptoms of weakness, insomnia and loss of appetite that persisted even after the fever had subsided (Gasper 2004: 250; Schmitt, ed. 1984: vol. 3, 284–5). Alessandra Strozzi (1406–71) describes her failing health in more general terms of weakness and old age (Strozzi 1997: 213). Both Bonne of Savoy and Bianca Maria mention in their letters the inability to write because of illness (Nicoud 2000: 410).

Letters discussing the illness of a mutual acquaintance further demonstrate how incidents of poor health were recorded among the sick person's immediate community. In many letters, the symptomatic approach is again prominent. In 1487–95, John Paston urged Margery Paston to send a plaster to James Hobart who had an ache in his knee (Davis ed. 1971: 628). Blanche of Brittany wrote to King Henry III of England in the 1260s that his daughter Beatrice was sick with fever (Shirley ed. 1862: 334). Fever also appears as the sign of sickness in a letter Brother Edmund sent Sir Edmund Stonor in 1380 concerning his son (Carpenter and Kingsford ed. 1996: 109). Other letters tell of being confined to bed, of being weak, or rather active, recalling the language of the contracts discussed above, and identifying health with functionality (e.g. Klassen ed. 2001: 86). That the focus on functionality stretches the boundaries of the sick/healthy binary is also apparent in the letters. Sir Edmund Stonor's son is said to be with fever only in the mornings, while later in the day he is out and about; Benedetto Strozzi is said to have been feeling ill but 'not in a bad way' (Strozzi 1997: 73). Although both died not long after, they were reported to have been in an intermediate state for a while, neither healthy nor ill.

HEALTHY BODY/HEALTHY SOUL

Emotional or mental pain is another topic which appears in letters. Agony and grief tend to be expressed and emphasized through detailed descriptions of physical pain. Eleanor of Aquitaine (1122–1204) complained to Pope Celestine III (1106–1198) that incarceration of her son Richard left her in great misery and that she was growing thin and losing her eyesight. She adds that her grief is so harsh that she would rather her hand be cut off (Celestine III 1853: 1268–1272). The Dominican Riccoldo of Monte Croce (1243–1320), writing about the fall of Acre in 1291, described his great sorrow and anguish over the loss of the city. He writes about being consumed in thought, his aching heart and flowing tears – a sorrowful state which led him to a deep spiritual crisis; it is clear that the distress debilitated him (Röhricht 1884: 264, 272; Shagrir 2012).

These very evocative descriptions of a mental all-consuming pain have a literary feel to them. Indeed, similarly stylized descriptions of emotional states can be found in the more fictional genre of miracle tales. Caesarius of Heisterbach's stories include a number of acedia-stricken monks whose desperation and sorrow, often prompted by demonic intervention, made them blind, lethargic, pale and weak in body and soul (Caesarius of Heisterbach 1851: 1: 203–10). It can also be witnessed in other literary self-documentations, such as the mystical writings of Margaret Ebner, which open with the pre-devotional pains that afflict her body, mind and soul (Ebner 1993: 85); and, in a more professional manner, in the melancholy of religious and financial despair described by the physician Juan of Aviñón (fl. 1320–1381) (Cohen-Hanegbi and Melammed 2013; Cohen-Hanegbi 2016). The affinity between the language of correspondence and other modes of writing, which are seemingly less immediate and less committed to a factual account, reminds us of the need to be aware of the gap between actual experience and its verbal expression. Here we see that the underlying holistic point of view that associated physical ailments and pains with mental states relied on the physical evidence that bodily pains provided. These pains gave a material language to describe the intangible feeling and turned the abstract emotion into a somatic symptom.

The pain of crucifixion, too, particularly in its late-medieval evolution as a pain that could be transferred to the deeply devout in the form of *stigmata*, performs a similar act of localizing a *passio*. Its expression in letters may be seen as another aspect of the contemporary practice of correspondence about illness as a means of forming amicable relations, as well as gaining political recognition (e.g. Wiethaus 1993: 185). Bodily pains are also seen to be salvific and therapeutic to the troubles of the soul. This is a predominant feature of consolatory letters (or messages of reproach) to the sick. Lanfranc sent the sick Gilbert Crispin (between 1070 and 1089) a purgative together with a letter urging him to think of his illness as penance and therefore to thank God for his mercy (Clover and Gibson, eds. 1979: 103). Ivo of Chartres (1040–1115), entreating the assistance of Adela of Blois (1067–1137), expressed his hope that her illness would be a remedy to the *interior homo* and that the scourges of the body would wash away her sins (Ivo of Chartres 1854: 112). Petrarch (1304–1374) encouraged Niccolo, Bishop of Viterbo, to see the occasion of his bodily sickness as an opportunity to extend his spiritual fortitude (Petrarch 1863: 378–84). The friar Antonio de Verceil suggested to Bianca Maria, Duchess of Milan, that her illness was sent by God to cleanse her sins and increase her love of His glory (Nicoud 2000: 411).

As we have seen, this form of consolation was anchored in a very popular analogy between physical pain/illness and spiritual sin/penance. Sermons and devotional treatises expanded at length on this trope. Henry of Grosmont, Duke of Lancaster, (*c.* 1310–1361), for example, in *Le Livre de Seyntz Medicines* (Book of Holy Medicines) of 1354, pored over his sins, likening them to wounds which required the medicine of divine healing (Henry of Grosmont 2014). Yet, it was also much more than a metaphor. In 1438, King Duarte of Portugal (r. 1433–1438) composed the *Leal Conselheiro* (Loyal Counsellor), a treatise influenced by the vice and virtue devotional framework (Duarte, King

EXPERIENCES 145

of Portugal 2011). In several chapters dealing with *tristeza* (sadness) (chs. 18–25), he adopted a more private tone: reflecting on his fluency in medical discourse on melancholy, the king recalled his own history with the illness, listing the spiritual remedies he took upon himself to bring about his healing (McCleery 2009). Turning to one's own medical problems within the devotional setting of meditation on sin demonstrates more than the common invocation of God for healing; it illustrates the belief in an inherent linkage between the health of the body, the mind and soul. Margery Kempe's exposition of her devotional narrative describes a state of madness followed by a combined deterioration of her physical, mental and spiritual states (Staley, ed. 1996). A more casual example of this deeply intertwined view of health is recurrent in the letters of Fernando Díaz de Toledo, who repeatedly draws connections between joy, his physical health and spiritual well-being as an overall account of his state of health (Round 1980: 223, 234).

Naturally, this association – at times a conflation – of the physical, emotional and spiritual aspects of disease is mostly expressed by authors holding religious office or with a particularly devout agenda; yet, in more subtle ways, it can be seen to have filtered into lay discourse as well. Philippa Maddern's (2018) analysis of the use of the word *merriment* in late medieval English further demonstrates this point. Her study reveals that in the English culture of the period, feeling healthy was closely associated with joy and a rounded sense of well-being which included spiritual health. A similar sentiment is also seen in Italian letters of the fifteenth century (e.g. Nicoud 2000: 411). In such reports of one's state of health, functionality and feelings, as well as hope and faith in future health, are all resolutely interdependent.

PATIENTS' HISTORIES

Friends and family members wrote to each other about their health and illness to receive support and care, to strengthen ties and alliances and to calculate future plans. Alongside these testimonies of sharing pains among lay authors, there were therapeutic encounters which provided their own opportunities for unfolding the narratives of illness. The late medieval 'medical marketplace' was varied and included a range of skills and practices. Patients often turned to several different channels – a barber, saint's shrine, a local healer, itinerant specialist or learned physician – depending on availability and social milieu, though some healers were thought to be experts in particular conditions, such as bone fractures, dentistry (see Figure 6.4), childbirth, episodes of madness, etc. Most of these healing encounters are undocumented due to their oral nature, but some records do exist. The two most substantial are learned physicians' medical consultations and canonization inquest testimonies extant from the thirteenth century onwards. In both cases, inclusion of the sufferer's narrative was of

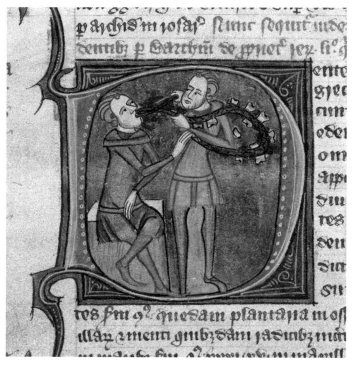

FIGURE 6.4: Dental specialist, James Le Palmer, *Omne bonum* (late-fourteenth century). London, British Library, MS Royal 6 E VI, Vol. 2, fol. 503v (detail). Credit: British Library/Public Domain.

institutional importance and anchored in the development of the academic world. Physicians used written consultations or *consilia* to educate their students in the processes of diagnosis and tailoring prescriptions and regimen. Commitment to the idea of individual complexion required attention to each patient's specific humoural balance and symptoms (Agrimi and Crisciani 1994; Crisciani 2004; Siraisi 1996). Inquisitors collected testimonies of miraculous healing to substantiate sanctity. These procedures emerged as the influence of the legal schools grew, concomitant with a turn towards reliance on witnesses in juridical procedures in general (Goodich 2007: 70–1). Personal experiences, the importance of specific circumstances and situations were thus an integral element of the growing subtlety of medicine and canon law.

Case history as narrative

In a twelfth-century Salernitan treatise on the topic of medical bedside manner, the physician is advised to collect as much information as possible from the patient before sharing his diagnosis with the patient and their family (Sigerist 1960: 131–40; McVaugh 1997; Linden, 1999: 32). Somewhat cynical in tone, the gathering of detail is intended to help the practitioner obtain clues in case his technical procedures of uroscopy or measuring the pulse fail him. While this treatise considers questioning the patient a clever trick, from the thirteenth century on it was deemed an essential part of diagnosis. Surviving case books indicate that this was indeed an elementary part of practice. Tillman de Syberg worked in Strasburg in the second half of the fourteenth century, probably as physician to Cardinal Frederick de Saarwerden, the Archbishop of Cologne, but he also saw both male and female patients with diverse illnesses. An account of his practice is given in a manuscript which lists the cases he handled. Among them was Peter, scribe to the Abbot of Gengenbach, who suffered from headaches and had been constipated for eight days. He also had a pain in the 'mouth of the stomach' (with no swelling), his mouth tasted bitter, he was always thirsty for only cold water, and he had no appetite. Tillman gathered that he was suffering from excess choler (*Ymaginabar coleram esse in causa illius fastisii*) and prescribed him medicine accordingly (Wickersheimer 1939: 80). Through reading the list of symptoms, we hear the echo of the preceding conversation between the physician and his patient. Although probably guided by the physician's questions, it demonstrates an outlook concerned with various aspects of feeling ill, such as inclinations, sensations, specific pains and dysfunctions. Even the diagnosis of humoural imbalance includes some diverse complaints and, in this sense, remains close to the symptomatic language a patient might use.

Describing some particular sensations, physicians often repeated their patients' complaints more precisely. At the turn of the fifteenth century, Guillaume Boucher, a Parisian physician, reported treating a young man who suffered from unbalanced fever, especially around his chest, noting that the patient felt a pressing tightness in his chest (Wickersheimer 1909: 257). Ugo Benzi of Siena (1376–1439) reiterated the contents of a letter sent to him by another physician concerning a young man he had treated for ongoing headaches. Ugo went on to detail the course of the headaches over the previous twenty months, explaining how the pain shifted and changed from nightly pains to palpitations, to seeing spots and additional bouts of fever. In another case he added the patient's description of the pains she suffered which moved from the groin downwards and felt like being touched by fire. While sleeping, he added, she felt as if ants were crawling inside her limbs (Benzi 1518: fols 76v, 67v). Baverio Baviera (d. 1480) tells of a Dominican friar named Marcus of Bologna who was burdened with various nerve problems, including a hearing impediment which created a constant wave-like sound in his ears (Baviera 1489: fol. 37v). Bartolomeo de Montagnana (d. 1452) described the impaired vision of a patient who saw little figures flying around him like flies or gnats, and continually tried to catch them in his hands (Montagnana 1497: fol. 110v). Giovanni Batista de Monte, in the early-sixteenth century, treated a woman for headaches she suffered after childbirth, noting she felt her head to be 'an empty vessel' (Monte 1559: fol. 13v). In all these examples, inclusion of the patient's descriptions of their experience is a necessary part of substantiating the physician's diagnosis. The precise feeling of pain, or the nature of an irregular function, was considered an aspect of the symptom and was therefore also indicative of the contributive cause; thus, the wave-like sound is interpreted as a sign of excessive humidity, the moving pain a sign of a complex humoural disorder and so on (Cohen 2010: 99; Salmón 1996).

Further indication of the importance of patients' experiences is afforded by cases that pertain to emotional disturbance. Ugo Benzi included in his *consilia* the case of a woman from Parma who, for over four years, suffered from a noxious cold complexion in her stomach, which was full of a thick, sticky matter. This caused nausea and loss of appetite and diminished both her vision and her movement; her other cognitive faculties, however, were unimpaired. Fearing she might die, she began to eat frequently without sufficient intervals between meals, but this only weakened her more, increased her incessant fear and led to further illnesses of the brain and heart (Benzi 1518: fol. 42). Fear is seen here to be central to the illness: it is a reaction to it, an aggravating factor and, in itself, a harmful state for cognitive faculties. Cases of melancholic illnesses described by Giovanni Matteo Ferrari da Grado (d. 1472) and by Bartolomeo de Montagnana in their *consilia*, follow a similar integrated approach (Grado 1535: fols 8–9v; Montagnana 1497: fols 78v–79, 92). These emotional disorders highlight a notion that is fundamental to the complexion-based view of health – that the experience of illness is inextricable from the illness itself. This, of course, paints a holistic picture whereby sensations, cognitive faculties, emotions (*accidentia anime* as the medical texts define them), dreams and thoughts are all, according to this medical notion, part of the well-being of the patient. Rather than disease being the defining category of a person's state, this notion focuses on health and its infraction.

Extant letters from the physicians of Bianca Maria Visconti to her son Galeazzo, the Duke of Milan, containing daily observations of her illness, display how this approach would be applied in practice. The doctors – Andriotto del Maino, Benedetto Reguardati, Guido Parato, Cristoforo da Soncino and Ambrogio Griffis – report on the patient's energy, her sleep, her mood, her fever and her appetite, all of which are seen as indicative of her well-being (Nicoud 2000: 381–2, 393). Benedetto Reguardati, together with three other physicians, sent similar letters to Bianca Maria when her son Filippo fell ill. There too, the report includes information about his pains, functionality and mood as indications of the state of his health (Nicoud 2014: 626–8). These letters have their own rules for conversing about health. Directed at lay recipients, they were written by practitioners to ensure that satisfactory health care was provided and to report on the patient's state. They assisted in propagating the medical idea of complexion, and the image of illness that derived from it, yet they provided an

EXPERIENCES

ideal image of professional care. As revealed by the often-optimistic tone with which the physicians describe the patients' *bona voglia* (goodwill), the desire to maintain good ties with the patient's family is highly visible. Furthermore, much like the case histories of the *consilia*, the letters represented a theory of medicine. It is certain that such close scrutiny of the sick was available only to the wealthy and powerful few.

Consilia cases do reveal some exciting stories that spark the reader's imagination with hints of how patients in medieval times conversed about their illness with their physicians. However, the context of routine medieval practice must not be ignored. While the model of individually tailored medicine certainly fuelled medical teaching, the practice of medicine relied no less on the 'off-the-shelf medicine' of the day, on staple recipes for potions and pills, and on disease-focused diagnoses which paid much less attention to the specific cases (see, e.g. the widely distributed (pseudo-)Peter of Spain 1497; Shaw and Welch 2011). Rudimentary recipe collections were far more useful to the common practitioner, as their dissemination shows. The *practica* literature listing ailments from head to toe did include remarks about diverse manifestations for diagnostic purposes, but prescriptions were still primarily directed at treating diseases (Demaitre 2013). In a similar vein, the *consilia* collections, too, provided many chapters of prescriptions for specific problems (Taddeo 1937). The absence of narratives of illness in the majority of the medical literature of the period shows a discrepancy between the highly individually attentive theory and the more rudimentary practice which demanded fit-for-all remedies.

Healing saints

Accounts of disease and illness abound in the inquest procedures for establishing sanctity. The procession of witnesses appearing before inquest committees and testifying to their once-burdensome illness are a valuable source for learning about sufferers. As Finucane (1977: 83–99), Metzler (2006), McCleery (2014), and Powell (2012), among others, have shown, testimonies include detail ranging from circumstances of the afflictions and the feelings involved to the means by which the miracle occurred. Pursuing evidence of complete transformation from sickness to health, these narratives support a clear-cut definition of health as the absence of sickness. This binary position stems from the nature of the records. They are idealized records, written to celebrate the wonders of sanctity; at the same time, they are judicial texts, written according to a designed structure to conform to legal requirements; they are translated texts, heard in vernacular languages and written down in simple Latin. Consequently, it is often debated whether it is suitable to read them as personal narratives at all (Katajala-Peltomaa 2010: 1084). Rather than attempting to settle this debate, my review below considers how canonization inquests structured the narratives, what they included and what they omitted in preparing the necessary dossier. This account highlights that the rhetoric clearly emphasized the indispensable value of the sufferer's narrative. This insistence, exemplified below, is all the more curious if we bear in mind the heavily stylized nature of the source.

Usually, healing was bestowed in return for a votive offering or prayer by the devoted to a specific saint. The shrine of the saint was often the place in which the miracle occurred, but this was not requisite. In less common cases, when the miracle occurred while the blessed person was still alive, a laying-on of hands or even their gaze could transmit their restoring powers. It was, however, clear that not all saints had the ability to eradicate all illnesses. In the majority of narratives, the cure occurred instantly and perfectly, leaving no trace of the prior condition. Yet for some, we learn, previous approaches – whether to other minor saints or to the same saint but made with less generosity – failed. Such was the case of a man from Ascoli (*c.* 1325) who suffered paralysis on one half of his body, while on the other he suffered terrible recurrent tremors. The miserable man made two offerings to Nicholas of Tolentino. His first offering was not complete and his infirmity remained; but, after a second attempt, done with great devotion, his recovery was quick (Occhioni 1984: 358). Detailing the obstacles in the way of healing emphasizes the severity of the malady, which is the predominant feature of these narratives.

Duration was stated to frame the affliction in time and efforts were frequently made to cite the precise dates. Additional detail asserts the nature of the malady and a vicarious account of the veracity of the miracle. Some specify the organ affected or the location of the affliction on the body; others mention the number of days their fever or illness raged. When the illness included seizures, the number of fits and the times they occurred are mentioned. Often witnesses would explain how their malady impinged on their functioning, mainly being unable to walk or to use their hands (Metzler 2006: 126–85).

Testimonies also show various levels of medical knowledge. Witnesses may provide the names of illnesses, explanations of medical terms, medical rationale and accounts of certain medical procedures. In one of Elizabeth of Hungary's (1207–1231) miracles, Gotefrid from Mareburg testified that he suffered from pains in his legs that originated from abundant phlegm. In other testimonies, a functional language that recalls medical contracts is used: e.g. loss of pain, in the case of Gotefrid; and regaining the ability to walk, in the case of one Dieteric of Gelnhausen (Wolf 2011: 173, 175). These signs of the medicalization of the narratives of witnesses was surely supported by the growing reliance, from the thirteenth century, on medical practitioners as expert witnesses in canonization proceedings (Ziegler 1999). Moreover, since the sources present the combined effort of witness, inquisitor and scribe, it is possible that the more professional language was that of the literate men involved and not the sufferers' own voices (Katajala-Peltomaa 2010).

EXPERIENCES 151

Numerous witnesses refer to the gravity of their illness as motivation for turning to the saint. A lady named Thomassia saw her son on the verge of losing his eyesight because of his incessant crying and her votive offering to Nicholas da Tolentino opened her son's eyes (Occhioni 1984: 109). Many others, in addition to stating their illness by name or by symptom (e.g. headaches, stomach pains, shaking) also remark that their offering was made out of fear of further deterioration. In fact, fear of death seems to be an accepted format in such procedures for explaining the supplication to a particular saint (Menestò and Nessi 1984: 318, 365; Occhioni 1984: 168, 170–1, 173, 451, 475, 477; Menestò 2007: 85, 101). Alternatively, it is woven into the narrative of healing, as in the case of the son of Munaldus Aldrude, who enjoyed the healing hand of Nicholas of Tolentino when he was delivered by the prayers of the blessed man from *spasmus*, which involved great pain and deformations of the mouth and hands. It is noted that he escaped imminent death (Menestò 2007: 601–2). Mentioning the inability of physicians to provide assistance was another way of stating the sufferer's grave state. A number of witnesses mention that they consulted physicians and were treated by them to no avail, and as a last resort they sought the saint's help. The chaplain Fredericus of St George testified that he had an illness which had affected his left leg for more than three years but the attending doctor said he could not cure him because his leg had greatly deteriorated. Having heard of the wonders of Nicholas, Fredericus turned to him for help and was indeed restored to health (Occhioni 1984: 411). Mention of this incident was not by chance; its recurrence signals both the gravity of the case and the absence of any natural cure; necessary criteria for demonstrating that the healing was miraculous (Duffin 2007). Angeluctius de Carpena's predicament was so great that he lost faith in physicians and, believing he would soon die, took extreme unction and asked for the litany to be recited. It was only through the miraculous intervention of Chiara de Montefalco that his pains were alleviated (Menestò 1991: 318–19).

One important feature of these inquest stories is the absence of any spiritual justification for illness. In no case is it implied that the person was suffering due to their sins or lack of devotion. Even in cases where the supplicant's illness could be harmful to one's soul as in the case of a woman who harboured malicious thoughts towards the wet-nurse who accidently killed her new-born daughter, they are not regarded as sinners (Cambell, ed. 1978: 458–9; Archambeau 2013). This is very much in contrast to the tradition of *exempla* miracle tales, popular at the time, which celebrated the topos of a notable sinner punished with illness, then healed and saved by penance, devotion to Mary or another saint (Jean Gobi 1991: 434–5; Metzler 2006: 216–17, 221–2). Miracle tales provided an edifying story meant to encourage the devotion of the flock. They served a didactic function of a model path to faith. Indeed, as the above-mentioned writings of Henry of Lancaster and other pious sufferers show, devout authors recollected their own illnesses according to models offered by these tales. The exclusion of such reasoning from the inquest procedures highlights further the juridical and practical role of these collections. Validating sanctity, they focus on the occurrence of the miracle rather than the witness's spiritual life.

In order both to justify turning to the as-yet unofficial saint and to prove the magnitude of the miracle, it was necessary not to blame the recipient of the cure and to assert the terminal or incurable nature of the malady. Healing the simple person against all odds makes for a great story. However, within the canonization proceedings, whether written as judicial records for professional use or as local evidence and commemoration, the detail was not enjoyed (only) for its dramatic purposes. Each witness offers support for the validity of the therapeutic powers of the alleged saint. A detailed narrative is seen as an authoritative testimony that can be corroborated by other witnesses. As Michael Goodich (2005) suggested, it is also a trustworthy format by which the story could then be further spread and the fame of the saint disseminated. Narratives of illness were, therefore, extremely important for building a solid case for canonization; yet, despite the meticulous collection of specific experiences, this source provides a highly categorical idea of illness. After all, the inquest scenario demands testimonies of complete and successful recovery.

CONCLUSION

The search for the experiences of health and illness in medieval times leads us to a wide assortment of sources and yields an extraordinarily complex, even contradictory, picture. In medieval society, health and illness could mean many different things: in certain cases, they would be considered binary categories, in others they were viewed as unattainable extremities of a more fluid continuum. They refer to body, mind or spiritual soul or to any combination of the three. While health was usually equated with joy and well-being and illness evoked great fears and anguish, devotional practice encouraged viewing illness as an opportunity for penance and summoning the spiritual pains of remorse. Health was, at the same time, a private and subjective experience that affected the individual person, and a familial or communal concern measured according to functionality alone.

Sociologists and anthropologists of medicine have long drawn attention to the fact that family and political strategies of conversing about health and handling episodes of illness are an essential part of how communities interact (e.g. Sontag 1978). Extant medieval letters indicate that this was also true during our period. The developing professional and institutional world from the late twelfth century did, however, bring about a new attention to experiences of illness and to the spectrum of health. These became pivotal for the development of medicine and relevant legal (civil or canonical) procedures in the later Middle Ages. The particular manifestation in each individual of disease or ailment, whether physical, mental or spiritual, had to be accounted for in order to develop a theory or strengthen a trusted system. But, in addition to the desire for inclusive systems, another desire, that for clear categories and definitive terms, appears. Medieval treatment of health and illness shifts between the two tensions of individual experience and the accessible model. Another constant shift implicitly shown in this survey of sources is that between explanatory frameworks of understanding health as a state of the body and the soul, which was shared by both the laity and professionals, and was determined in relation to the contexts and the meanings they provided.

NOTES

1. A comprehensive account of the emergence and use of illness narratives appears in Hydén (1997). Key studies with regard to the literary formation of narratives of illness are Scarry (1985), Porter (1985) and Rimmon-Kenan (2002).
2. See, e.g., the critique of the 'authentic' in narratives in Atkinson (1997) and Thomas (2010).
3. The example from Alain of Lille (d. *c.* 1202) is as follows: 'Quod complexio peccatoris sit inspicienda. Complexio etiam peccatoris consideranda est, secundum quod ex signis exterioribus perpendi potest; quia secundum diversas complexiones, unus magis impellitur ad unum peccatum, quam alius. Quia si cholericus magis impellitur ad iram, sed melancholicus magis ad odium.'
4. The Paston family left a large collection of private correspondence over three generations that spans from 1422–1509. The Strozzi family belonged to Florentine nobility and were among the richest families in the city. The surviving letters of Alessandra Macinghi Strozzi (1406–1471) to her sons illustrate the daily strategies of maintaining power and safeguarding family alliances to preserve social influence and economic stature. Fernando Díaz de Toledo was physician and archdeacon of Niebla who corresponded with members of the monastery of Santa María de Guadalupe in the second and third decades of the fifteenth century.

CHAPTER SEVEN

Mind/Brain: Medieval Concepts

WENDY J. TURNER

INTRODUCTION

The mynde is in the Brayne,	The mind is in the Brain,
The vndyerstandyng in the fronte,	The understanding in the front,
The Ire in the gawle,	The ire in the gall [bladder],
Avaryce - in the Kydney.	Avarice: in the kidney.
Love – in the harte,	Love: in the heart,
Brethyng in the lownges.	Breathing in the lungs.
Gladnes in the splene,	Gladness in the spleen,
thought in the harte,	Thought in the heart,
Blode in the body,	Blood in the body,
hope in the sowle,	Hope in the soul,
The mynde in the spyrit,	The mind in the spirit,
The harte in the mynde,	The heart in the mind,
the Feyth in the harte,	The Faith in the heart,
And cryst in the feyth,	And Christ in the faith,
And whylle it noryssh the body –	And while it nourishes the body –
it is cawlyd – Anima – the sowle,	It is called '*Anima*' the soul.
This worde – Anima – hath many significacions,	The word '*Anima*' has many significations,
for when it is in contemplacyon,	For when it is in contemplation,
it is sayde a spyrit, Spritus,	It is said [to be] a spirit, *Spiritus*.
And when it savyrth,	And when it savours,

it is saide Reson or wytte, Animus,	It is said [to be] Reason or wit, *Animus*.
And – when it felith –	And, when it feels,
it is sayde felyng, Sensus,	It is said [to be] feeling, *Sensus*.
and when it understondyth,	And when it understands,
it is callyd mynde, Mens,	It is called mind, *Mens*.
And when it demyth,	And when it deems,
it is callyd Reson – Racio,	It is called Reason, *Racio*.
And when it consentyth,	And when it consents,
it is callyd, wylle, voluntas,	It is called – will, *Voluntas*.
And when it recordyth	And when it records,
it is sayde, mynde, Memoria.	It is said [to be] – mind, *Memoria*.

—London, Lambeth Palace, MS 306, fol. 118r,
from line 28; compare to Furnivall, ed. 1903: 65[1]

Medical understanding of the *mind*, physiological care of the *brain*, religious implications of *thought* and legal opinions on *intent*, all collided within the cultural context of medieval Europe. Many people – writers, poets, physicians, ecclesiastics, judges and academics – tried to understand how humans functioned by considering connections between the brain, mind, heart and soul. In the Middle Ages, the question of where *thoughts* and *memories* resided had not been settled as functions particular to the brain (Clarke and Dewhurst 1996: 3). As the poem that opens this chapter, which begins with the number of bones and teeth before moving to the head, explains, the 'mind' might be 'in the brain' while 'thought' could be 'in the heart' where the good parishioner should hold his or her 'faith' with the heart being 'in the spirit' which is, in turn, 'in the mind'. Circular logic at its finest. Notice that while 'love' and 'breathing' are where readers today would expect them to be, respectively 'in the heart' and 'in the lungs', at the same time '[a]varice [is] in the kidney' (note there is only one), 'ire' or anger is in the bladder and '[g]ladness in the spleen'. In other words, medieval understanding of the relationships between emotions, memories and thought processes was a marked conundrum. Ideas behind the location and function of the soul created much of this confusion and, in combination with the concept of *passions*, only added to the perplexity of how the brain, mind, soul and heart worked together. Certainly, *feelings*, it could be argued, created visceral, almost animalistic, responses. And yet, simultaneously those same feelings interacted with the soul, constructing an awkward synergy between base emotions, bodily desires and those loftier passions of the spirit.

The poem's unknown author, among others, clearly wondered about that same awkward link between emotion, body, mind and soul. *Anima*, which in the poem has many functions and which is the basis for the word 'animate', was for the author and other medieval writers equivalent to the soul, the seat – they said – of life, movement and reason. The soul was the source of, if not the same as, all human emotion and thought well beyond animalistic instinct; it provided the ability to ponder. For the poet, *anima* effected not only as a spirit and as the mind, but also could think, feel, reason, will and remember. The poem explains that 'the mind is in the brain' and also that 'the mind is in the spirit'. The author considers the seat of the soul as much as he attempts to outline connections between the physical brain and heart and the linked associations of the mind, feelings and soul.

This chapter will illuminate the complex medieval connection of the brain and its thinking power to God, to guilt or innocence and to rational social behaviour as well as disentangle medieval connections between thought and emotion and the brain, heart and spirit. The medieval association of the brain with the spiritual being, the emotional person and the animalistic reaction indicates a need for a cultural history of the brain, rather than a simple scientific, medical, or social history of this important organ. Yet, even among these other fields of study, few have focused on the brain.

Many medieval authors of medical texts, academic manuscripts, ecclesiastical poems, religious treatises and other writings considered the mind and brain to be inseparable from the individual. As the poem illustrates, 'the mind is in the brain' but also 'in the spirit' and often, even in this poem, theories of the mind become mingled with issues concerning the heart, will, memory and feelings. Legal authorities in at least English, French, Spanish, German, Dutch and Italian sources held specific views on reasonable behaviour, guilt, responsibility and premeditation among other ideas that relied on the thoughts and subsequent behaviours of individuals (Turner, ed. 2010). Some of these various authorities and authors theorized about how the brain functioned and – to a limited degree among academics, physicians and surgeons – how to fix it if it were damaged. The Church also weighed in on the inextricable concepts of the mind and heart, meaning those things that reflected the soul, which – according to Church doctrine and the poem above – resided somewhat in both the brain and heart. They used the concept of the reasoned mind as that which could be the instigator of sin, the determining factor of the depth and strength of the soul and the identifiable element of the connection of humans to God. Since the Church weighed in as heavily as the medical community on the cultural significance of the brain and legal definitions of guilt and innocence were based on 'premeditation' as much as action, the cultural implications surrounding the function of the brain became tied to medieval concepts of heart, soul, mind and will.

THE UNDERSTANDING IN THE FRONT

In 1996, Edwin Clarke and Kenneth Dewhurst put together an excellent overview of brain images from antiquity through the twentieth century, with an emphasis on medieval and early modern illustrations (Clarke and Dewhurst 1996: 3–53). They, though, like earlier studies of these diagrams (Sudhoff 1913; Leyaker 1927), concentrated on anatomical construction and how various natural philosophers and schools interested in medicine understood how the brain worked. While helpful as an overview and an excellent guide to medieval brain anatomy, it was not their intent to investigate the ripples these understandings had within a wider socio-cultural context.

Beyond anatomical interests, scholars of the Middle Ages have investigated other medical aspects of the brain. They have given ample attention to the ancient and medieval concept of *pneuma*, which for early natural philosophers was air used in the body to transmit motor signals and only later became tangled with the concept of 'breath of life' or *anima*, the soul or spirit (discussed in greater detail below) (van der Eijk 2005: 122–31; Benso 2008). Several recent studies concentrate on surgery and medicine for the brain, highlighting specific procedures or medications rather than providing an overview of techniques or brain anatomy (Niiranen 2014; Krug 2015; Livingston 2015). One of the better works on anatomy and medieval understanding of the inner workings of the mind and brain is by Mary Carruthers (ed. 2002, 2008) on memory. She is one of a group of scholars considering individual functions of the brain – memory, perception, emotion, intelligence, senses – which at times in the Middle Ages might have been assigned to the heart (Geary 1996; Goodey 2011; King 2010; Pender 2010; Rosenwein 1998; Turner 2010; Wheatley 2010). What those studies have found is that by at least 1200, medieval authors interested in the brain began to hypothesize – based on theories from antiquity and on observations of behaviour following head trauma – that the right side of the brain controlled the left side of the body and vice versa. They began to conjecture that the brain controlled common sense, imagination, reason and memory from front to back. They also began to be more confident that the brain controlled the senses – sight, smell, taste, touch and hearing (see Figure 1.1).

Many medieval brain theories maintained that this vital organ held three 'cells' that governed from front to back: senses and activities, fantasy and cogitation and recall and memory. While ancient authors of brain anatomy had started down this path, these ideas continued to be quite muddy into the Middle Ages. The closest any early natural philosopher came to putting cell theory all together was Galen of Pergamon (*c.* 129–200/216 CE) with his dissection of animals. Yet, cell theory would not work without first addressing the issue of dividing the functions of the heart and brain and resolving, to some degree, the questions of soul and feelings.

The Alexandrine schools tackled the question of whether the brain or heart was primary for life, possibly by dissecting cadavers. Herophilus of Chalcedon (*c.* 335–*c.* 280 BCE) and Erasistratus of Ceos (*c.* 304–250 BCE) explained how the nervous system and the circulatory system were both parallel and interconnected in the brain, but it was Ibn al-Nafïs (1213–1288) in 1242 who first correctly identified the circulation of blood from the right ventricle of the heart to the *vena arteriosa* (pulmonary artery) to the lungs and subsequently throughout the body. He also guessed at the existence of the capillary system (West 2008). Herophilus and Erasistratus described the heart as functioning to give the body warmth and 'vital spirit'. Late antique and medieval natural philosophers designated the nervous system, including the brain and its network through the spinal marrow and nerves, as the centre for all neurological functions, sensitivity and motion. This Alexandrine model of physiology for humans, with slight variations on the details, existed until the nineteenth century. Physically, therefore, the blood and the heart accounted for temperature and emotion, while the nervous system and the brain were responsible for movement and thought. For example, anger could both be caused by an excess of heat and could cause the body temperature to rise, leading later to such colloquial phrases as 'his blood boiled' and 'hot under the collar'.

By the central Middle Ages, physicians and other natural philosophers postulated that if the brain administered all movement and thought, including the memory, there must be divisions within the brain for the various functions. Even though this was debated until well after the end of the Middle Ages, most medieval natural philosophers settled on three cells with different functions. For example, Bartholomaeus Anglicus (*c.* 1200–1272), a Franciscan friar working on his encyclopaedia, writes that:

> there is no (physical) distinction between the three cells of which the brain has three concavities as well as ventricles (called) by physicians 'caretakers': (*ventriculi a phisicis noncupantur*) in the anterior cell outside the ventricle the imagination is formed, in the middle reason, (and) in the posterior memory and recollection.

> —Bartholomaeus 1483: 57

Other theories had the imagination on the border between the front 'cell' and the middle 'cell' or outright in the middle part of the brain with *cogitativa* (cogitation) (Clarke and Dewhurst 1996: 8). Bartholomaeus further explains that 'the anterior ventricle of the brain is generated and partially conditioned by the organs of perception' (Bartholomaeus 1483: 36). He summarizes that there is also

> a middle ventricle, namely at the cell (of) logic to perfect understanding, formed before understanding passes to the helm or to the cell (of) memory (where) impressions are made from other cells carried as in the treasury of a memory depository, indeed that is the posterior of the head.

> —Bartholomaeus 1483: 36

In this theory, input from the world entered the anterior of the brain – through the senses – and a combination of common sense and imagination told the individual what he or she was seeing and, if necessary, how to react. According to Bartholomaeus and others working on interpreting the three-cell theory, cogitation, as well as what we might call critical thinking, which included understanding the difference between fantasy and reality, were housed in the middle of the brain. Information gathered and critically analysed was then stored in the posterior brain as memory (Carruthers 2008: 59–69; Millon 2004: 70). Ibn Sīna (also known as Avicenna, 980–1037) in one of his works on the soul: *Kitāb al-Najāt*, suggested a variation of two functions in each of three cells to solve both the issue of imagination and the differences between fantasy and imagination and to add both receptive and retentive categories for each, with the six being: common sense, fantasy, imagination, estimation (or cognition), retention and recollected memory (*sensus communis, fantasia, ymaginativa (al-mutakhayyîlah), cogitativa (qûwah mufakkirah) seu œstimativa (wahm), retentio (dhikr)* and *memorativa (hafizah)*) (see Figure 7.1; Ivry 2012: no. 3). It should be noted that Ibn Sīna used *fantasia* both as a separate category of fantasy and as an umbrella to encompass and connect fantasy to common sense and to imagination (and he transliterated *sensus communis* and *fantasia* from Latin) (Nichols ed. 2008: 41). At times, other theories combined fantasy and imagination making room for *motiva* (motion) (Finger 2001: 19). Among all these medieval thinkers were variations on how the functions were arranged, although all of them agreed that the memory was in the back and all accounted for an exchange between memories and the other operations of the brain (Carruthers 2008: 59; Carruthers ed. 2002; Siraisi 1990: 82–3; Frugard 1994: 1.53).

Later brain theories continued to have the functions in three cells, or what were later called ventricles, with each function connected to multiple tasks. At least one writer, Flemish surgeon Jehan Yperman (1295–1351), split the senses between the front and the middle, indicating that hearing was part of intelligence (Clarke and Dewhurst 1996: 10, fig. 4). Yet, in most medieval theories, the middle brain functioned as the area for cogitation, including estimation and cognition. There are a few medieval brain diagrams and descriptions that divide the brain into four segments instead of three, as in a French manuscript of 1400 depicting a 'disease man' (see Figure 7.2). This image labels the four 'cells' as *sensus communis, cellula imaginativa, cellula aestimativa rationis* and *cellula memorativa* (Clarke and Dewhurst 1996: 11). This idea compartmentalized common sense as the receiver of all sensory input and put all received information in the front of the brain, making it appear as though all information needed to go through the 'ventricle' of common sense to get to the others. In a woodcut of 1503 for his *Margarita Philosophica*, Gregor Reisch (*c.* 1467–1525) labelled the brain from front to back: *sensus communis, fantasia, ymaginativa, vermis, cognitativa, estimativa* and *memorativa* (see Figure 7.3).

MIND/BRAIN

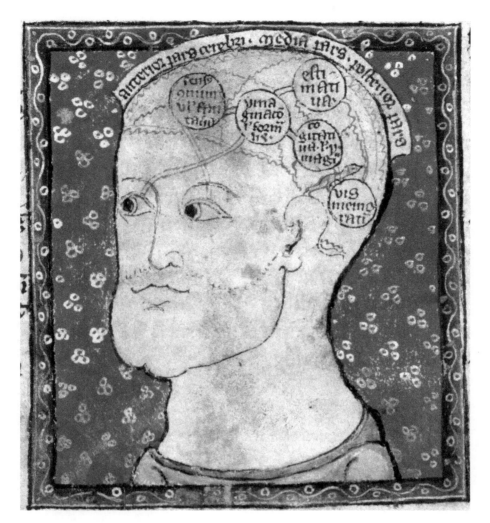

FIGURE 7.1: Ibn Sīna (Avicenna)'s brain theory in his *De generatione embryonica* (dated 1347). Cambridge University Library, MS Gr.g.I.I, fol. 490v. Credit: The Syndics of Cambridge University Library.

The *vermis* (worms) was a narrow area of connection between the front and mid segment of the brain and, while a similar narrow area appears in the image in Figure 7.3 between the middle and back of the brain, there is no label there (Sudhoff 1913, fig. 14; Clark and Dewhurst 1996, 38–9). By contrast, in Augustine's depiction of the brain (Figure 1.1), below *fantasia* and behind the eye a point is labelled *visus* (sight or vision) with other areas similarly labelled (*olfactus, gustus*, etc.). This might help explain the 1503 woodcut in that perhaps the *vermis* was simply a mistake on an illustrator's part – writing *vermis*

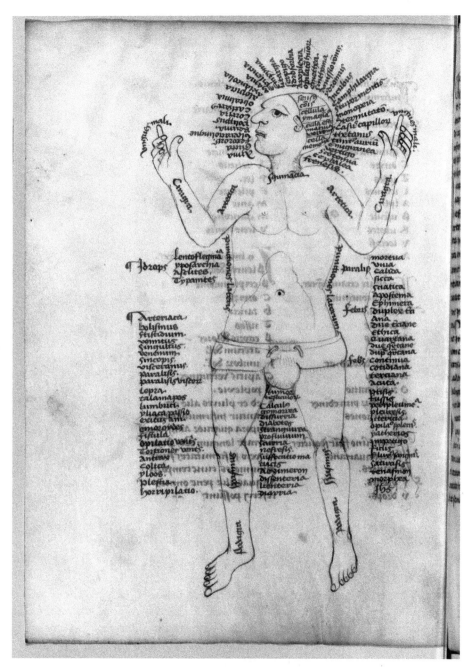

FIGURE 7.2: Disease man, *Petits traités d'hygiène et de médecine* (fifteenth century). Paris, Bibliothèque Nationale, MS Latin 11229, fol. 37v. Credit: Bibliothèque Nationale de France.

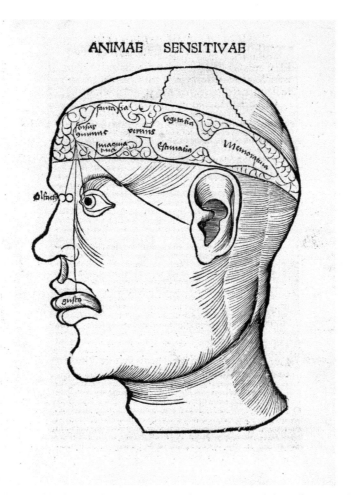

FIGURE 7.3: Cerebral ventricles, Gregor Reisch, *Margarita philosophica* (Freiburg: Johann Schott, 1503), book 10, tractate 2, signature Hii. Credit: Wellcome Collection/ Public Domain.

when he meant *visus* (Clarke and Dewhurst 1996: 32; compare Carruthers 2008: 68), which was copied and recopied after Reisch's original.

Besides the three-cell theory, medieval anatomists and surgeons were aware of what Galen had called the *rete mirabile* (marvellous net) at the base of the brain, which was first described by Herophilus and was based on the brains of animals. Galen postulated that blood – which was a mixture of natural spirits (*pneuma physicon* [Greek] or *spiritus naturalis* [Latin]) and digested food (*chyle*, produced in the liver) – travelled through the body in the veins to the right chamber of the heart and on to the lungs where impurities, *spiritus naturalis* and some blood were exhaled. The body inhaled more *pneuma* (air) or *spiritus* (air) which mixed with and purified the blood and (and this Galen got wrong) returned to the right chamber of the heart, dripping through a hole in the heart to the left chamber, which produced the vital spirit or *pneuma zoticon*. Later, medieval theoreticians, such as Ibn Sīna and al-Nafīs, challenged this idea and put greater emphasis on the heart, not the liver, as the regulator of the pulse and heat in the body; yet, Galen's theories were not fully contradicted until 1543 by Andreas Vesalius (1514–1564) and even then, many continued to put more faith in Galen than Vesalius (Mitchell 2007: 216). In Galen's theory, this *pneuma zoticon* infused the blood concocted 'vital blood' that went from the left chamber through the arteries to (also incorrect) the net of very fine arteries at the base of the brain – the *rete mirabile* – and elsewhere in the brain. There the blood was further improved, creating the highest form of spirits, *pneuma psychikon* (Greek) or *spiritus animalis* (Latin), the psychic or animal spirits, which departed the brain via the nerves; it was these animal spirits produced in the brain that allowed the body to move and to think (Mitchell 2007: 103).

As a corpse lies prone, blood evacuates the arteries, collecting in the heart and veins and leaving the arteries empty; early examiners of corpses must have thought that air or *pneuma* filled the arteries. Many early anatomical drawings are crude, yet they have correctly identified the connection from the bloodstream through the carotid arteries into the cranial cavity. Galen's hypothesis of *pneuma* in the body led to a connection in the writings and philosophies of medieval scholars between the soul or spirit – the 'breath of life' – and the brain, a relationship which fascinated medieval authors with a predilection for science.

BREATHING IN THE LUNGS. THOUGHT IN THE HEART. BLOOD IN THE BODY

Medieval medical recipe books and commonplace books often followed the earlier Egyptian convention of organizing the body from head to toe, localizing functions and symptoms in specific areas. They began with 'headaches' and then went on to what we would describe as mental health concerns, usually located in the head in these texts despite widespread cultural links between rational thought and the heart, as in the opening poem. Then came ear, nose and throat complaints, followed by the trunk of the body (including the lungs and heart), then the limbs, ending with the feet. Physicians treated both injuries and illnesses as interruptions in normal health and wellbeing. If a head injury required surgery, the surgeon was acutely aware that, following the operation, if successful, his patient would need recovery time while the swelling reduced and the head and brain healed. Like a physician, the surgeon, too, had practical reasons for altering an individual's normal regimen or prescribing medicines to aid in the recovery process. Generally, physicians linked all health to having balance within the system of the four humours, a practical reason to suggest rebalancing through diet and exercise, even for their mental health patients. Natural philosophers and physicians suggested regimens for good bodily and spiritual health that included a moderate diet and exercise appropriate for the time of the year and the individual's age and gender.

Prior to the second half of the twentieth century, few scholars had investigated medieval mental health and for those who did so it was almost as an oddity, such as Daniel Hack Tuke who wrote of the 'quaint prescriptions' for the insane in the Middle Ages (Tuke 1882: 6). By the late twentieth century, while some scholars continued to have somewhat romantic ideas about mental health in the Middle Ages (Covey 1998; Foucault 1961; Masters 1977), others started to take the study of medieval mental health and the brain more seriously, writing on such topics as melancholia (Jackson 1986), mental illness (Kroll and Bachrach 1984; Rosen 1964) and insanity (Thiher 1999).

Since 2000, scholarship exploring medieval mental health and the connection to medicine has grown tremendously. Publications explore medieval understandings of mental disorders and care for the mentally disabled in such works as *Origins of Neuroscience: A History of Explorations into Brain Function* (Finger 2001), *Madness in Medieval Law and Custom* (Turner, ed. 2010), *Care and Custody of the Mentally Ill, Incompetent and Disabled in Medieval England* (Turner 2013a); *Mental (Dis)Order in Later Medieval Europe* (Katajala-Peltomaa 2014) and a series of essays in an important volume on wounds and wound treatments (Livingston 2015; Krug 2015; MacInnes 2015) to name a few. Several conferences on the medieval brain specifically, such as that at the University of York (2017), have added to the greater depth and richness of scholarship on our understanding of the medieval conception of thought and brain activity. Other conferences on medieval medicine or medieval disabilities complicate the questions that scholars of mental health are asking of medieval sources, such as *Homo Debilis*, the creative unit organized by Cordula Nolte at the University of Bremen (Nolte 2017) and *Disease, Disability and Medicine* based at the University of Nottingham and run by Christina Lee (Crawford and Lee 2014). These more recent questions include: What did it mean to be disabled (mentally or physically)? While we might categorize neurological, psychological and intellectual conditions into different lists, did medieval society? Are there medieval medications that might be 'rediscovered' to assist modern mental health patients with conditions resistant to current medications? Can the study of medieval mental health help us to unravel the complexities of stress associated with a postmodern existence?

Looking at these most recent studies of mental health from the perspective of medicine it seems that, among medieval brain disorders, the most obvious is a 'broken' head – either through accident or war. Assuming the patient lived, this type of head injury, aside from causing a concussion, could leave a patient with disorientation or, if the trauma to the head was great, with a change in personality (Skinner 2015; MacInnes 2015; Krug 2015; Livingston 2015). If the skull was broken or the head was otherwise injured (a contusion, for example), a repair was necessary. After, the patient might become generally ill, which was why even surgeons proscribed adjustments in regimen for their brain patients, modifying everything from diet to sleep, living spaces, music, exercise or prayer (see the introduction to this volume for more on the underlying theoretical reasons for this).

Surgery on the battlefield was common, but treatment for various types of battle injuries to the brain and head might include herbal treatments and changes in diet as well. Battlefield and other types of injury to the brain from accidents, especially from objects falling on the head or from people falling from a height onto their head, caused brain swellings, seizures, headaches, contusions and broken skulls. Roger Frugard, in his treatise on surgery, *Chirurgia* (*c.* 1180), walked medical students through a head injury that he called *la deverie* (which could be translated as 'devilry', 'possessed', 'thrashing' or 'restless madness') (Gregory 1989: 427, 690). He explained that *la deverie* at times caused or could be *mania* or *melancholia*, both of which we would refer to as mental health conditions; *melancholia* being a condition of 'black bile' overload, which could have an adverse effect on the brain. Frugard set mental health aside, though, to continue his discussion on his patient with *la teste tailleiz* (a damaged head) with *le quir* (a shard, probably a skull fragment) lodged in his brain. Frugard instructed surgeons to

> first bind the patient. Then, by opening the head with a tool that is called trepan, through removal of the material of the malady, is that which is at issue [causing the problem]. It is the healthy wound, as is truly said, [which] is a cure for the previous wound.
>
> —Frugard 1994: 53

Frugard referred to the ancient method of trephining or trepanning a skull as a way to clean up the injury, making the skull edge smoother and removing all broken fragments before closing. The trepan, as a surgical tool, is still in use today. After medieval surgery, the head would be covered with a clean poultice and later closed after any swelling of the brain had receded (assuming the patient lived).

Earlier ancient surgeons articulated their accounts of having cut into or trephined the human head, exposing the brain. Medieval surgeons used this knowledge to save battlefield patients with head trauma or other head injuries, many living years after wounds to the head, skull and/or brain (Arnott, et al 2003; Tracy and DeVries, eds. 2015). For example, medieval surgeons attempted to save the life of King Enrique I of Castile with trepanation after a roof tile fell on his head in 1217; but the thirteen-year-old monarch died soon after. Other

MIND/BRAIN

trephined skulls have been found in medieval Spanish gravesites, where at least one woman appears to have had a successfully trephined skull operation and lived for quite some time (Cohen 2012: 1). For further archaeological evidence for trepanation, see the chapter by Watson and Gilchrist in this volume.

Brain injury, though, was not the only condition treated in the Middle Ages. Other conditions – mental health afflictions – were also considered to be physical and, based on the system of the four humours, treatable. While prayer was often called for as a part of the overall healing process, a more somatic approach was taken by physicians and other care-givers with recommendations of medicines and dietary changes which seemed key to revitalizing mental health in these patients. Susanna Niiranen (2014: 176) writes: 'the main purpose of the recipes is clearly to alleviate pain' and while some early recipes include magical elements, later medieval recipes stuck to allopathic medicines.

Brain malfunctions due to a high fever or some intangible cause were harder to diagnose than a knock on the head. If there was a problem due to illness or an unknown factor, a physician might suggest treatment to rebalance humours through diet, medicines or other therapies including phlebotomy (bleeding the head), baths, extra sleep, dark rooms or changes to living conditions.

Physicians and surgeons, along with a few medically minded monks, priests and natural philosophers, described the areas of the brain responsible for various mental health conditions, which, of course, fell neatly into the three-cell theory described earlier with categories for perception, cogitation and memory. These authors also gave possible reasons for malfunction, including blows to the head, digestive or dietary explanations, environmental descriptions and even spiritual excuses. Neither physicians or surgeons (nor other natural philosophers for that matter) said much about learning disorders or intellectual disabilities, suggesting no cures for an *idiota*, for instance. These issues were only taken up as part of an explanation of how the brain worked if, for instance, an herbal or manual included such an explanation as part of a list of medicines or conditions.

Most medieval physicians recognized that something from within the body, mostly an imbalance of the humours in their system of thinking, could cause a person's brain to function inadequately. Johannes Platearius (1090–1120) explained a relatively widely recognized ailment of *frenesy*, involving agitation and sometimes aggression, writing (taken from an Anglo-Norman translation): 'frenzy is an apostume that is born in the first cell of the head' (Platearius 1994: 171). Platearius wrote about several other conditions of the brain and head, including lethargy, catarrh (runny nose), apoplexy (brain haemorrhage), epilepsy, palsy (which he admits involves more than the brain), mania, melancholy and dolour (sadness). Like other physicians of the later Middle Ages, Platearius described mania as 'a type of frenzy' which affected the imagination while melancholy affected a person's ability to reason (both middle brain). He associated mania with melancholia:

mania is a kind of frenesi, *forsenerie* [another type of humoural madness], and melancholy. Mania, then, is a disease that takes and ill-treats the first cell of the head with the deprivation of the imagination.

Melancholia, he wrote, was 'an infection of the middle cell with deprivation of reason as Constantine said in the book of Melancholia' (Platearius 1994: 180).[2] Platearius proposed several medicines based on the four humours, with ingredients that included *mauves* (mallow), *violat* (violet), *laitues* (lettuce), *mandragore* (mandrake), *rosat* (rose), *sale* (salt) and many others (Platearius 1994: 171–84). All these ingredients are cooling in terms of humoural theory and mallow and mandrake are further soporific; Platearius must have decided that such patients needed sleep and were running too far toward heat. He maintained that no matter the medicine or dietary adjustment – he listed poultices, washes, enemas, oral medicines and others, like salt gently rubbed into the feet – changing a patient's humoural balance rapidly might aggravate a condition.

A change in humoural balance, therefore, was the frequent cause given in medieval texts for shifts in brain health, but the non-naturals such as air quality and food were also named as causes upon occasion and for some maladies more than others. In the case of those born with intellectual impairment, the 'cause' was sometimes blamed on the mother with little to nothing to be done post-birth (Metzler 2016: 5; Kroll and Bachrach 1984: 507–14; Thiher 1999: 44–72). When other causes were to blame, for example, a high fever that might leave a child with limited mental abilities, physicians attempted cures by rebalancing humours toward health – regular cool baths, enemas (clysters) and a changed regimen (Rawcliffe 1997: 64; Nutton 1996: 184–7; Rosen 1964: 278–80; Siraisi 1990: 120–3). Bartholomaeus Anglicus summarized Aristotle's ideas about the malfunction of brain and the physical signs to watch for in the patient: 'the brain that has withered or become too moist will not work, but cools the body or melts the spirit and so illness happens and the loss of intellect and at last dies' (Bartholomaeus 1483: 57).

A near contemporary of Bartholomaeus, Gilbertus Anglicus (mid-thirteenth century), had many suggestions for remedies for brain malfunction based on Galenic and Arabic medical theories. Gilbertus first divided problems with the brain and head into pains of the head, such as headache and problems of the mind. He identified three major categories of mental problems with subcategories, all linked to the three ventricles that medieval physicians envisioned for the brain (Getz 1991: 1–31; Clarke 1975: 86). Gilbertus wrote (taken from a later Middle English translation) that frenzy was in the 'forepart of a man's brain or in the skins of the brain' and that the *comen signes* included 'much waking, and lacking of good wit, wrath, and *woodness* [madness or wild behaviour], and suddenly rising up and suddenly falling down' (Getz 1991: 10). In the middle portion of the brain, Gilbertus identifies mania (Getz 1991: 13). Lethargy was a condition of loss of memory and located in the back of the brain: 'Lethargy is a sickness that makes a man so forgetful, that when he has do a thing, he nay has no mind that he did it' (Getz 1991: 16). Gilbertus considered humours – either too little or too much – to be the cause behind brain malfunctions. He explained that melancholy could be a condition of any of the three areas of the brain, describing it more as a symptom than a condition. In his pharmaceutical treatise, he also covered medicines for three other brain conditions: epilepsy: '*epilencie* is the falling evil'; apoplexy: '*apoplexie* is a sickness that comes of stopping of the principal places that be in a man's brain through some corrupt humor'; and *scotomeye*: '*scotomye* is such a sickness of the brain that it makes a man to seem that he sees flies or black things in the eyes' (Getz 1991: 7). Much like Bartholomaeus, Gilbertus detailed recipes for cures, medicines and therapeutic exercises.

THE MIND IN THE SPIRIT . . . IT IS CALLED ANIMA, THE SOUL

A cluster of recent scholars emphasize the artistic, literary and social perceptions of mental health (Huot 2003; Metzler 2016; Nutton 1996; Rosen 1964), sometimes aligning sin with psychological and neurological disorders (Clarke 1975; Kroll and Bachrach 1984; Thiher 1999), which many medieval authors wrote of as a metaphor for improper 'human' behaviour (as opposed to animal-like behaviour) and which might reflect social attitudes. This type of metaphysical explanation for mental affliction – that the brain was somehow 'guilty' of a sin of the mind and therefore punished – is, for the most part, a literary phenomenon (Harper 2003; Doob 1974; Neaman 1975). It shows up in legal records, letters or wills with extreme rarity. For example, in approximately 1,000 administrative records, court cases, wills and letters in England from 1200–1550 dealing with mental health issues, references to 'devils' appeared only twice (Turner 2013a).

Most literary examples of mental health in the later Middle Ages associate sins of the mind – lust, pride, coveting, disrespect, abuse, etc. – with mental disorder, describing loss of mental ability as a punishment from God (Flanagan 2005; Caciola 2000; Sprunger 2002). Writers employed a trope of the madman, without any actual reference to mentally impaired persons with specific symptoms, to depict a characterization of unpredictability attributed to the sinful person – a portrait of chaos in lives of normally sane persons. The cultural construction for sins of the mind was that unrighteous thinking – brain sins – led to God's punishment of that organ (and in a few tales God stopped protecting a person and devils tormented the sinner), meaning a loss of the ability to perceive the difference between fantasy and reality, or to reason, or to remember.

Other writers, although far less often, describe the intellectually impaired and a few other mental health conditions as innocents protected from (and therefore not understanding) the evils of the world (Huot 2003). Medieval authors, especially but not exclusively those writing ecclesiastical literature, used the image of the innocent, mentally impaired individual to make their audiences think further about their own faults by comparing wise gestures of the mentally incapacitated, no matter the intention, with unwise displays by the supposedly sensible. These characters were innocent of all wrongdoing and many people wrote of them as being protected, having been placed in a mental cocoon away from traumatic harm.

Writers and poets alike compared mental impairment to drunkenness. For example, John Lydgate (1370?–1451?) in his secular poem 'Tyde with a Lyne' writes:

> A mournyng myrth, sobrenes savage [sober when drunk],
>   Prudent foly, stidefast [steadfast] wildenesse;
> Providence conveyed ay with rage;
>   A dronken sadnesse, and a sad drunkenesse;
>   A woode [mad] wisdom, and wise woodenesse [madness];
> Is this fortune, or is it infortune?
> Though I go loose, I tyed am with a lyne.
>
> —Lydgate 1934: 832

Geoffrey Chaucer (1343–1400) wrote something similar in the *Romaunt of the Rose*: 'Wise *woodnesse* and *vode* reason; a sweet peril, into frown; A heavy burden, light to bear' (Chaucer 1899: 212). In other words, if a person were mad, he would not know or care about his state for he could not comprehend otherwise even though it might seem a terrible thing to the bystander. Other medieval authors echoed Lydgate's comparisons between drunkenness and madness, emphasizing the connection between the physical, mental and emotional stemming from the brain. John Gower (1330–1408), for instance, writes: 'Men sein ther is non evidence, / Wherof to knowe a difference / Betwen the drunken and the wode [madman], / For thei be nevere nouther goode; / For wher that wyn doth wit aweie, / Wisdom hath lost the rigte weie . . .' (Gower 1900: 182). Here Gower pointed out the close connection between wit and the mind's ability to think and how the intoxicated individual acts and certainly thinks much like the 'wode' without the ability to reason or to think clearly, much less cogitate.

WHEN IT SAVOURS, IT IS SAID [TO BE] REASON OR WIT, 'ANIMUS'

Within medieval legal and medical records and most commentaries on law, including ecclesiastical law, many mental health conditions can be identified and, for the most part, medieval authors described health conditions of the mind in terms of physiological illness of the brain rather than of spiritual causes. Medieval mental afflictions other than head trauma could be congenital, a result of illness or triggered by unexplainable forces. These ailments included the medical conditions of *mania*, symptomatic of *demencia, amencia, frenesis* and *furiosus*, as well as those individuals suffering from an inability to discern and, therefore, not knowing the difference between good and bad (*sciens nec bonum nec malum*) (Turner 2013b: 135–8). Some individuals were identified as having some type of intermittent disorder with phases like the moon, being a *lunaticus*. Others were simply described as mentally unhealthy (*insanus*) or mentally suffering (*passione*). The general term *non compos mentis* (not of sound mind) was used as a stand-alone term when a patient's or criminal's mental health was uncertain yet also clearly compromised, or with other descriptors to refine exactly what was wrong. The Jewish biblical commentator and philosopher Abraham Ibn Ezra (1089–1167) wrote that being naked in body was closely linked to loss of mental health and might provide evidence of insane behaviour (Shoham-Steiner 2014: 94). Within Jewish medieval sources 'it was up to family members, religious leaders and physicians of sorts to diagnose the mentally ill' (Shoham-Steiner 2014: 89). Generally within the mostly non-literate society of the Middle Ages, a good memory was important; as the opening poem explains, '[a]nd when it records, [i]t is said [to be] mind, *Memoria*.' Being *non sanus memoria* (without a healthy memory), therefore, was a serious condition, which might affect an individual's cultural interactions and standing (Turner 2013b: 143–5).

Medieval legal and administrative records also include references to learning disabilities: those persons who were *fatuus* (fatuous, socially inappropriate), *ignorans* (ignorant) or *idiota* (idiots, intellectually disabled) (Turner 2013b: 138–43). For example, in 1353, John Heton is described as 'an idiot . . . he is not of sound mind in all matters relevant to human thoughts, [unable to] discern [. . . and without] a good memory, he neglects himself (TNA C 135/125, mem 25; Stamp et al 1921: 132–3). Landholders in medieval England labelled *idiota*, such as John Heton, were legally and socially considered as children. They would have been granted a guardian to manage their properties and legal affairs, as discussed further below (Turner 2013a: 161–210). Other mentally impaired individuals without real property would have been in the care of their family (Pfau 2010b: 96). This same general treatment of the mentally incapacitated can be seen in the medieval legal and medical records of cultural contexts outside of 'Christendom'. For example, in Ottoman Arab legal records, those individuals who had a 'departure of reason' (*zawal al-'aql*) had the status 'of a minor child' (Scalenghe 2014: 117). Treatment for all these conditions, while imperfect, was generally to the benefit of the mentally impaired or intellectually disabled individual across Europe and beyond.

WHEN IT CONSENTS, IT IS CALLED WILL, 'VOLUNTAS'

Within the medieval fields of law and disabilities, a few scholars have analysed medieval understandings of the brain with an eye to perceiving differences in interpretation and classification between epilepsy, intellectual disabilities and psychological and neurological disorders, including *phrenitis/frenesis*, lethargy, *melancholia* and *mania* (the last two could manifest as positive or negative). The present author's early work on mental health in medieval England paved the way for broader discussions about how mental health conditions fit within the wider conversation of disability studies (Turner 2010; Turner 2013a; Turner 2013b). New investigations connect mental health to law or medicine but rarely both (Bruhrer 2014; Butler 2015; Pfau 2010a; Pfau 2010b). Generally, all of these scholars have concentrated on what the brain produced – the emotion, the mental health condition, the sin and so on – rather than on how or why the brain or other body part (heart, liver, etc.) produced that condition or what, if anything, the medieval community thought might be happening.

Medieval legal commentators were likely unaware of the details of study in those circles fascinated by the brain. Yet, within the law, persons who could not think clearly, could not therefore *intend* to do something and, as such, were not subject to punishment under the law. Consequently, writers of commentary on law took up their own study and categorization of mental health and intellectually disabling conditions (Butler 2015: 198–200; Turner 2013a: 63–90). In the *Decretum Gratiani* (Gratian's Decretum, *c*.1140s), Gratian explains that certain people could not plead on behalf of themselves: 'insane persons, fools, mutes, the deaf, prodigals [spendthrifts] and children' [*furioso, furiosa, fatuo, fatua, muto, surdo, prodigo, et adolescente*] (Gratian 1861: decreti II, causa XVI, quest. 1–3). The mad also could not enter marriage, but if an individual became mad after already having been married, he or she was not to be removed from the marriage. However, if the sane spouse wanted a divorce, loss of mental health in a partner was one ground on which divorce might be granted in many places (Butler 2015: 160; Scalenghe 2014: 118; Pfau 2008). In terms of the sacraments, most ecclesiastics agreed that the individual should be given the host, since it might act as a medicine, and if she could indicate 'yes' to baptism, even through hand signs, she should be baptized (Goodey 2011: 201–4).

In civil law, those without the full use of their brain were, at times, treated differently in medieval society. French customary law assigned the wardship of mentally impaired individuals to relatives, rather than making them wards of the king as was the case in England. Philippe de Beaumanoir (1250–1296) elucidated on the French context:

[I]f the oldest is completely insane, the right of firstborn should pass to the oldest after him, for it would be a bad thing to leave anything in the possession of such a man; but he should be properly [*honestement*] supported out of what would have been his if he had been a person who could hold land. But we mean this to apply to those who are so insane that they would not know how to behave if they were married or not for if a person had enough intelligence to be married, without more, so that he could have heirs, he and his property should be under guardianship until the heir came of age.

—Beaumanoir 1992: 591

French society considered disinheritance and/or guardianship with 'honest' care appropriate for those without the ability to think clearly (Pfau 2010b: 97–8). Beginning in the mid-thirteenth century, English law upheld the right of all mentally incapacitated persons – no matter their condition – to inherit real property. Landholding mad-persons and intellectually disabled persons were granted royal guardians to assist in the care of these individuals, including oversight of their legal and property-related issues (Turner 2013a: 161–210).

Late fourteenth-century English property owners in boroughs and chartered cities started indicating their state of mind when writing wills; furthermore, they also indicated that, in spite of the law, mentally incompetent heirs should be circumvented in favour of heirs with 'sound minds'. For example, while in 1387 Robert Corn began his will quite simply: 'In the name of god, Amen . . . I Robert Corn, Ceteseyn [citizen] of London, be-quethe my sowle to god, to lygge in the chirch of our lady of abbechirch. Also y be-quethe my goodes [etc.]' (Furnivall ed. 1964: 1), in 1437, John Nottingham deemed it necessary to include a statement in his will that he was 'of sound mind and good memory' [*sane mente ac bona memoria*] (Tymms, ed. 1850: 5). John Baret, in another example, wrote not only that he was of sound mind and memory, but also willed that all 'idiots and fools' should be skipped over and that if one in the future was to be the heir, the executors should 'refuse him and take another that is next' (Tymms, ed. 1850: 15–44). Generally, those who had trouble thinking clearly or remembering would have been left alone as long as they could function day to day with little assistance. If, however, their condition left them a burden to their families or neighbours, there was a possibility they would be given a guardian, but they could not engage in any legal contracts, including marriage, without the ability to think, to will, or to reason.

Criminals without a clear mind at the time of their crimes were also granted special treatment under the law. Persons committing crimes with mental health conditions in England as well as elsewhere in Europe could have been granted a pardon for felonies or trespasses. In France, mentally ill criminals generally had to seek a pardon from the king. Relatives or neighbours often wrote remission letters (*lettres de remission*) with the assistance of a royal clerk on behalf of the mentally ill or impaired individual asking for a remission of punishment (Pfau 2010a: 97–122). According to Ephraim Shoham-Steiner, the Jewish medieval community concentrated on being *impudens* (shameless), rather than examining intent; the *mashugga* (madman) or *insipiens* (exposed individual) was seen as animal-like (Shoham-Steiner 2014: 89–94). Until the later thirteenth century, the English king continued to travel the country giving advice on cases that did not easily fit into the norms of judgment; some involved the mentally incapacitated. For example, in 1212 the king was consulted on the case of an insane man (*stulto*) who was in prison because 'he knows himself to be mad' and 'he confesses himself a thief, while in reality he is not guilty' (Kaye, ed. 1966: 66–7). In cases of murder, normally a convicted killer would lose his or her life, but if mentally unable rationally to make the decision to commit homicide, the accused would be found guilty but not punished. He or she was often jailed until calm and recovered, but otherwise was not corporally punished. There was no 'insanity plea', but there was the common law practice to pardon those without the capacity of intent to harm (Butler 2015: 75–83; Turner 2010: 93; Turner 2018).

CONCLUSION: IT IS CALLED REASON, 'RACIO'

The medieval history of the brain and mind is complicated. Those persons working to understand the brain first had to contend with the conceptualization of *thinking* as being fused to the ideas of *feelings*, which traditionally had been attributed to the heart, while the soul, which some said resided in both the heart and mind, seemed to be infused in the whole person. Mary Carruthers points out that while the memory as a function might have been located in the brain, 'the metaphoric use of *heart* for memory persisted' (Carruthers 2008: 59) and much the same, it could be argued, was true for the soul.

Most medieval natural philosophers, physicians and others illustrating or describing the brain after about 1200 conceptualized it as having three cells with corresponding functions that included the senses and imagination, cognitive ability and thought and recall and memory. These writers – be they professors, medical authors of textbooks, physicians with commonplace books, ecclesiastical authors or others pondering through their pens the seat of the soul – all had an interest in how the brain made connections between the various elements of sense, action, instinct, thought and memory. Some suggested non-natural interference – bad air, the wrong food, excretions or retentions, too much or too little exercise, over- or under-sleeping and, of course, stresses that weighed on the mind – as possible causes for malfunction (Pender 2010). Others searched for reasons within the body (natural reasons) and the balance of the humours.

As early anatomists began to unravel bits of the whole – the left and right hemispheres and whether there truly was a *rete mirabile* in humans – other interested parties from physicians to ecclesiastics hypothesized about how the brain worked, including a variety of functions, three or more 'cells' or 'ventricles' and the seats of the senses in their writings. At the same time, authors writing about the law also categorized mental health conditions, including intellectual disabilities. Overall, the cultural understanding of the brain and the mind was one of an organ which controlled thought and actions. A drunken person looked and acted much the same as one who was mentally impaired. The brain was connected to the soul and, with this intimate attachment, the brain was integral to the self, to the personality of the individual and to the spiritual standing of the person. Without the heart, the body would die and, while the body might live if the head and, therefore, the brain were damaged, without the head, the body would die. Medieval anatomists and other writers, such as the poet who wrote the opening lines to this chapter, conjectured that while there was 'blood in the body' and 'hope in the soul', the mind was 'in the spirit' and 'in the brain'.

NOTES

1. The poem is in a different hand to the rest of the manuscript in which it is inserted; a fifteenth- and sixteenth-century miscellany. The modern translation is by Wendy J. Turner.
2. This is a reference to Constantine the African. For more on this author, see the chapter in the present volume by F. Eliza Glaze and also Kwakkel and Newton (2019).

CHAPTER EIGHT

Authority: Trusting the Text in the Early Middle Ages

F. ELIZA GLAZE

INTRODUCTION

Authority (*auctoritas*) is, historically, a multivalent concept; in the medieval world, it referred equally to trusted authors of written works, as well as to living persons with highly specialized knowledge. Another type of authority rested in governing bodies who wielded the power to regulate societal practices, such as medical licensing or public health, as was seen in the chapters on environment and animals earlier in this volume. In what we would today call the rational medical tradition (i.e. medicine based upon philosophically grounded textual authorities of the ancient and medieval world) the authority of a remedy was validated by the esteem in which the therapeutic agent or author was held, regardless of whether that healer-author was a long-dead medical writer or a living practitioner whose therapies were based upon experience and expertise. Reputation conferred authority and vice versa. Practitioners of great experience, including unlettered empirics whose skills derived from the oral transmission of knowledge and from repeated practice, also earned a steady following within their communities, although often little is known about them. Moreover, in addition to authoritative book medicine and acquired expertise, appeals for assistance from saintly or divine power were believed to lead to cures sanctioned by religious authorities (Flint 1989). Trust in all such types of authorities was often simultaneous at every level of society among those suffering from illness and injury.

Under the influence of Christianity's strict monotheism, the history of medicine could so easily have developed quite differently, allowing only Christian authorities to have been preserved in medieval Europe. This did not happen. Instead, classical pagan foundations were carried forward and confidence in Hippocratic and Galenic medicine survived the transition from an open polytheistic pagan faith tradition to one that was more exclusionary and restrictively monotheistic. A similar process took place in the Islamicate world as described in Chapter Three of this volume on disease. This chapter will focus on this transition during the early Christian Middle Ages, arguing for both continuity and innovation in textual authority.

FROM LATE ANTIQUITY INTO THE EARLY MIDDLE AGES

It is worth emphasizing from the start that there are almost no signs of heated competition between medical knowledge derived from or attributed to ancient sources and the Christian religion that was embraced and imposed throughout the West during the same period, although many types of pagan or superstitious healing practices were prohibited as the conversion of populations was undertaken during these same centuries. In the earliest Christian centuries, some Church fathers had railed against popular faith in physicians and other types of healers and some Christian authorities described illness as the outward consequence of sin and spiritual corruption, but recent research suggests that even the most ardent early Christians accepted disease as a natural phenomenon that was part of the divine order and therefore allowed for natural as well as spiritual remedies in order to relieve suffering (Temkin 1991; Ferngren 2009; Lindberg 2002). Some early Christian leaders who studied and/or practised medicine, such as Bishops Nemesius of Emesa and Theodotus of Laodicea (both *fl.* fourth century CE), gave further authority to physical medicine. The early Christian martyrs, Zenobius of Sidon, Pantaleon, and Cosmas and Damian (all killed under the Emperor Diocletian, 284–305 CE), were also seen as learned physicians, as was the Apostle Luke (Nutton 2004: 302–3).

In the tradition of rational medicine that had been established in the ancient Mediterranean (i.e. medical thought and therapy based upon explanations of health and disease rooted in the philosophical principles and textual traditions of famous author-practitioners) the authority of a treatment or regimen derived from the esteem in which that ancient author-practitioner was held. This sense of the authoritative knowledge of texts later exerted an enormous influence, especially in a world where textuality soon became associated with religious legitimacy and governing bodies' authentic powers. Thus, medical texts

AUTHORITY 179

bearing the names of lofty authorities like Hippocrates (*fl.* 420–380 BCE), Herophilus (d. *c.* 280 BCE), Democritus (*fl.* 420 BCE), Dioscorides (*fl.* 70 CE), Galen (129–200/216 CE), Soranus (*fl.* second century CE), Oribasius (*c.* 325–400 CE) and Alexander of Tralles (*c.* 525–*c.* 605 CE) resonated down the centuries, conveying a sense of confidence and trustworthiness to those medieval people who received and revered these traditions of textuality (Nutton 2004: 292–309).

That said, it is worth noting that other texts, which look to our eyes rather less rational, were also inherited from antiquity. Small works, like the anonymous, magical *Letter of the Vulture*, were copied in Christian monastic scriptoria right alongside works by Dioscorides and others. Texts that refer to 'cynomancy' – prognosticating the outcome of a patient's illness or demise by a black dog's (or the tick of a black dog's) response to certain rituals – derived ultimately from Pliny the Elder's (d. 79 CE) *Natural History*. These were not early medieval illiterate or 'folk' practices working their way into learned medical tradition, but were firmly part of that tradition with a range of apotropaic and scientific functions (Horden 2009; MacKinney 1942a, 1942b; Van Arsdall 2005, 2007).

Most emphasis, however, was placed on canons of the aforementioned great authors' texts, especially those from the 'Rational Sect' represented most strongly by Galen and Hippocrates. These canons had been taught by philosophically minded educators in cities like Alexandria and Ravenna, but although sections of pedagogical texts and lectures upon them survived into the early Middle Ages – some of which were translated into Latin – these experienced only a limited circulation. The poverty of this tradition was due primarily to the fact that the forum for which such canons had been created (i.e. organized centres for medical education) had already disappeared in the West before the middle of the eighth century (Beccaria 1959, 1961, 1971; Izkander 1976; Palmieri 2005, 2008; Agnellus of Ravenna; Glaze 2007). Even very popular pedagogical texts attributed to Galen, like a Latin translation of the *Introduction, or the Physician*, barely survived at all within medieval Europe (Petit 2013).

Take the example of the physician Soranus of Ephesus, a contemporary of Galen's also active in Rome but of the 'Methodist Sect' – a medical-philosophical tradition widely popular in the Roman Empire – but whose authentic texts were almost entirely unknown in medieval Europe. Instead, later Roman authors Caelius Aurelianus and Muscio (both *fl.* fifth century CE), summarized Soranus' writings, inspiring an indirect tradition that wielded a more enduring influence in the Latin West well into the early-modern period. The illustrations of Muscio's *Gynaecology*, a text based on Soranus', were even reproduced in later centuries without any text, underscoring the extent to which images conveyed authority in their own right (Hanson and Green, 1994; Green 2017). Summaries, images and excerpts of ancient authorities often sufficed to convey a concise core of ideas to early medieval readers.

Another example of what could happen to an influential body of work can be seen in the case of Oribasius, who served as physician to Emperor Julian the Apostate (d. 363 CE). Oribasius assembled a massive text which he called the *Collectiones medicae* (Medical Collections) in either seventy or seventy-two books. Recognizing the unwieldy nature of his own production, Oribasius created his own abbreviations in two forms: the *Synopsis* in nine books for Eustathius and a text often called *Euporista* (Easy Remedies) for his friend Eunapius. Both of these survive in Greek and in two different Latin renditions. Of the massive *Collectiones* we have only fragments (Fischer 2013: 37–9; Grant, ed. 1997: 1–22; Beccaria 1956: 475). As this example shows, neatly organized medical anthologies geared towards the practical enumeration of signs/symptoms, therapeutic rationale and appropriate treatments became much more useful than a great scholar's *magnum opus*.

During the sixth century, a new context opened up for medical textual authority: the monastery. Around the year 570, the Roman Senator Cassiodorus, having retired from service to the Ostrogothic rulers of Italy, created a reading guide for the monks of the new monastic foundation that he established on his familial estates in southern Italy, a place known as the Vivarium. In the *Institutes of Divine and Human Learning* Cassiodorus advised his monks that, if knowledge of Greek letters was unknown to them, they could readily find on the shelves of their establishment the most useful works of medical authorities in Latin renditions. These included 'the herb book of Dioscorides, depicted [illustrated] with remarkable accuracy'; versions of the Latin translations of Hippocrates and Galen, noting specifically Hippocrates' *On Herbs and Cures* and Galen's *Method of Healing, to Glaucon* – a treatise on fevers – and the text of 'Caelius Aurelius', *On Medicine* (Glaze 2000: 59–65). One leading scholar on ancient medicine has called Cassiodorus' list 'a meagre harvest from Classical Antiquity' (Nutton 2004: 300). Indeed it is; but it is also highly instructive.

There are several noteworthy aspects to this first explicit inventory of medical authorities whose writings were carefully preserved in a Christian monastic setting. The list implies that much more medical literature was still, at that time, accessible elsewhere for those proficient in Greek, but the titles and descriptions of the Latin texts given here are unusual, making them difficult to identify. Dioscorides' main work on pharmaceutical agents had been translated into Latin by this time, but there was also another illustrated text circulating under his name, now known as Pseudo-Dioscorides' *Book of Medicine from Feminine Herbs*, of which many early copies survive (Riddle 1980; Collins 2000: 25–147). Similarly, a range of Hippocratic texts had also been Latinized, most notably the very popular *Aphorisms* and *Prognostics*, but none of them was entitled *On Herbs and Cures*. However, a popular ensemble of Latin texts known today as the *Herbarium* complex – including a wide range of herbal and

AUTHORITY

animal-based medicines attributed to Antonius Musa (*fl.* first century BCE), one Apuleius Platonicus and a Sextus Placitus – had been assembled probably in the fourth or fifth century. 'Caelius Aurelius' in Cassiodorus' list might well signify Caelius Aurelianus, although his massive text *On Acute and Chronic Diseases* was not often copied and only survives today in one early fragment (Hanson and Green 1994). Much more popular was a text attributed to one Aurelius known as *On Acute Diseases*. The text identified as Galen's *Method of Healing, to Glaucon*, might represent that text in two books, or it might signify a very popular 'third book', not by Galen, that often travelled with the *Method of Healing, to Glaucon* as the *Liber tertius* (Collins 2000: 148–238; Nutton 2004: 300; Fischer 2003).

It was already an established tradition by the sixth century, that pseudonymous texts attributed to famous medical authorities of the ancient past populated the shelves of readers interested in literate medicine and that the most learned variety of authority depended upon access to and familiarity with these texts and the ideas within them. Although the expansive theories that distinguished members of different medical 'sects' had long since been largely attenuated, these names and their affiliations still had the power to convey confidence and provide a sense of the continuity between medieval readers and ancient learned traditions. This manuscript tradition (i.e. the preservation, reproduction and circulation of medical texts within monastic networks) may also have become a pattern by the time Cassiodorus established the Vivarium. Donating medical books to the monastic foundation in which one found spiritual and physical shelter became a time-honoured tradition which spread across Europe hand-in-hand with the expansion of Christianity (Glaze 2000: Table 1). The Italian peninsula and Rome itself initially played a central role in this transmission of texts (McCormick 2001: 696–728). Continued respect for the value of written medical knowledge in Christian communities represents an important aspect of this transitional period, at a time when the ancient world's centres of book production, its large urban centres and their markets still served as a conduit for products that would be transmitted to and consumed in far more rural realms to the north and west. Christianity, as a culture of the book, placed great value on all varieties of written knowledge.

After the early seventh century, there is little evidence of formal schools dedicated to the study of medicine either in the eastern Roman Empire (Byzantium) or in the Latin West. Yet during the ninth to eleventh centuries, ancient ideals of the educated, authoritative physician were perpetuated by the copying and recopying of various versions of late-antique deontological texts, describing how the practitioner should comport himself (in the texts, the *medicus* is always a 'he') and what kind of educational foundation he should have in order to support ethical medical practice. These brief guides directed that the would-be physician should begin his studies early and should master the fundamental components of the Seven Liberal Arts; one version advocated the study of grammar, astronomy, arithmetic, geometry and music, but stated that rhetoric is not useful to the physician as it encourages an undesirable loquacity (MacKinney 1952a: 1–31; Laux 1930: 417–34, 419–20; Fischer 2000b).

To take just one example: the *Isagoge Sorani* (Introductory text of Soranus) was a text stripped of any obvious Methodist philosophical orientation. It described how the ideal student or practitioner should adhere to one version or another of the Hippocratic Oath. He must be a practitioner who follows the rules of professional etiquette. His bedside manner and moral rectitude had to be preserved and maintained throughout his career. The *Isagoge* devoted a chapter to distinguishing between the true physician and false doctors whose practice might be driven by base instincts and imperfect knowledge; the true physician needed to be able to recognize and relate a single patient's condition or symptoms to larger, universal categories and their function. He ought to have a thorough understanding of humoural theory, anatomy and physiology; the function of the senses; the operation of conception and reproduction; the behaviour of diseases; the utility of phlebotomy, diet and regimen to correct humoural imbalances; the function of medicinal agents and how to compound them; and the likely outcomes of diseases and their treatments for the patient (Fischer 2000b). This would have been a tall order for any medieval literate physician to fulfil; but a grounding in textual authority was an established expectation and remained so throughout the period.

Nearly all these deontological texts agreed that the advanced discipline of philosophy should be studied at the same time as medicine (Laux 1930: 419–20; Fischer 2000b; Rose 1963: 244–5). In his *Etymologies*, Isidore, Bishop of Seville (d. 636 CE), drew on these guides in his placing of medicine alongside philosophy as one of the more advanced fields of study requiring a strong foundation in the Liberal Arts (Isidore 2010: 109–15). Isidore surveyed in twenty books the origins of everything from grammar to medicine, the cosmos and all its various parts and all types of human endeavour. His work soon became a canonical staple of education across Latinate Europe, a tradition that lasted well into the early modern period. Books 4 and 11 of the *Etymologies* dealt specifically with medicine, medical history and the human body (anatomy and physiology), while other books included passages on the medicinal value of plants, trees and minerals (Sharpe, ed. 1964; Isidore 1911; Isidore 2010).

In book 4, Isidore defined medicine (see the introduction to this volume) and then went on to identify the inventors of medicine: Apollo and his son Asclepius (whom he saw as men), Hippocrates (a member of the Asclepiad clan) and the three main ancient sects of medicine – the Methodists, Empiricists and Rationalists. He then detailed the four Hippocratic humours of the body, a list

AUTHORITY   183

of acute and chronic illnesses, superficial illnesses and remedies and medications. These last few included the ancient triad of pharmacy, diet/regimen and surgery. Isidore proceeded to categorize the types of books useful to physicians as aphorisms, prognostics, *dynamidia* (a type of text describing the powers or strengths of plants and other medicinal ingredients) and herbals where ingredients would be suitably described for collection (Isidore 2010: 109–115; MacKinney 1952b). Entire books and chapters of Isidore's *Etymologies* were often extracted, supplemented and circulated with medical texts and would certainly have been familiar to most clerically educated individuals (Beccaria 1956: 466–7; Codoñer 2008). Isidore's recognized authority surely underpinned and endorsed the general understanding that medical literature and medical philosophy based upon ancient models was to be considered the pre-eminent ideal among literate members of society. Texts derived from ancient pagan sources were deemed entirely appropriate guides to the preservation of human health and the alleviation of suffering within the Christian world.

MEDICINE IN CAROLINGIAN CENTRES OF LEARNING

By the time of the onset of the Carolingian age in Christian Europe, late in the eighth century, medical literature and medical practice were just as respected as the study of other ancient *artes*, including grammar, rhetoric and dialectic. Approximately forty monastic library catalogues that survive from the period prior to the year 1100 include medical books, most of which are listed with the grammar texts of classical authors available for study in the monastic schoolroom (Glaze 2000: Table 1 and chapters 2–3). Among the writings of great book collectors at the Carolingian court, we find positive assertions about the dignity of learned medicine and physicians (*medici*). In a poem sent to Charlemagne (r. 768–814), for instance, Alcuin, Abbot of St. Martin at Tours (d. 804), describes the worthy authorities whom Charlemagne has promoted and deployed across his empire, such as administrative officers and priests. In describing the authorities of the royal court, he ranks physicians as secondary in dignity and merit only to the clergy.

> Then the physicians process in, the Hippocratic sect [i.e. the rational sect],
> This one opens veins [surgery], this one mixes herbs in a mortar [pharmacy],
> That one prepares porridge [diet], that one proffers the medicinal drinking-cup
> [therapeutics].
> And nevertheless, O physicians, deliver all for free,
> That Christ's blessing may fall upon your hands:
> These acts are all pleasing to me; such the praiseworthy order.
>
> —Alcuin 1881: 245; compare to Wallis, ed. 2010:
> 80; Leja 2018: 8

184   A CULTURAL HISTORY OF MEDICINE IN THE MIDDLE AGES

With these lines, Alcuin establishes that the physicians of the Carolingian court were masters of all the areas of rational medicine, including surgery, pharmacy, diet and therapeutics. And that by practising charitably, their art imitated Christ's own *caritas,* marking them second only to the priesthood in this imagined courtly *ordo.* Alcuin explicitly invokes the doctors to engage in Christian charity without charging high fees, thus denying greed and earning Christ's blessing.

Another example of this easy peace between rational medicine and Christian values in ecclesiastical contexts is provided by the so-called *Lorscher Arzneibuch* (Lorsch Book of Remedies), a handbook also discussed in Stearn's chapter on Disease in this volume, which was produced at the Abbey of Lorsch in the Rhineland, one of Carolingian Europe's foremost monastic houses. This interesting manuscript – now Bamberg, Staatsbibliothek, MS cod. med. 1 (L.III.8) – dates to *c.* 800. It is a slender volume identified explicitly as a 'posy' – a florilegium or anthology – taken from various medical books (Beccaria 1956: 195–7; MacKinney 1952a; Stoll, ed. 1992; Fischer 2010; Leja 2018: 9–16). The manuscript begins by observing that God in his plenitude created the heavens and the earth, the universe and humanity and then continues with a brief excursus on the nature of performing good works (Keil and Schnitzer, eds. 1991: 1–27; Fischer 2010). There then follows a three-fold division of philosophy, based on Isidore, dividing it into *aethica* (ethics), *loica* (logic) and *phisica* (knowledge of the natural world). *Phisica* is further divided into seven disciplines: arithmetic, geometry, music, astronomy, astrology, mechanics and medicine (Bylebyl 1990). Medicine itself is defined as 'the knowledge of curing . . . and of the bodily temperaments, and the recovery of health, which is not unknown in divine books' (Stoll, ed. 1992: 58). The text goes on to quote from the biblical book of *Ecclesiasticus* (38: 1) to the effect that one should 'honour the doctor, for he too is created by the highest God'. The anonymous author then provides more than fifty examples of this agreement between the outlook of medicine and religion, including references from the early Church Father Jerome (d. 420 CE) and from the biblical books of Isaiah, Jeremiah, Paul, Job, Acts, Tobias, Romans and Timothy (Stoll, ed. 1992: 58; MacKinney 1952a).

This defence of medicine in the *Lorscher Arzneibuch* closes with the author excerpting verbatim Cassiodorus' guidance to his monks on the reading of Latin texts attributed to Dioscorides, Hippocrates, Galen and Aurelius. 'Read these, therefore' the *Lorscher Arzneibuch* commands, 'and just as they say, make medicines'. It is scarcely possible to imagine a more resounding endorsement than this for the study and use of inherited medical literature in a Christian environment. Even in the absence of formal medical schools, medical knowledge and literature gathered together with an eye to therapeutics was deemed to hold a legitimate and authoritative place within European society.

At another important centre for learning in this period, the great Abbey of Monte Cassino in southern Italy, an early medieval reader would have found the following variety of texts in the Abbey's library: *The Wisdom of the Art of Medicine* (similar to the *Isagoge Sorani* described earlier); Hippocrates' *Prognostics*; a short treatise on how a physician ought to behave while visiting the sick; another on the cure of fevers; Vindicianus Afer's *Gynaecia* (a treatise on embryology composed in the fourth century CE); Hippocrates' *On Phlebotomy*; extracts from Isidore of Seville's fourth book of the *Etymologies* on medicine; Aristotle's *Problems*; Hippocrates' *Letter to King Antiochus*, followed by a series of other such letters; Galen's *On Pulses and Urines* (i.e. standard Rationalist diagnostic tools); Galen and Pseudo-Galen's *Method of Healing, to Glaucon*, Books 1 to 3; a fourth book attributed to Galen, but really taken from Theodorus Priscianus (*fl.* 400 CE); Aurelius' *On Acute Diseases*; Esculapius on chronic diseases; a commentary on the *Aphorisms* of Hippocrates; 180 pages of Alexander [of Tralles]; an alphabetically arranged book of herbal cures attributed to Galen that begins: 'in the name of the Holy Trinity, here begins the *Alfabeta*'; an illustrated *Herbarium* attributed to Apuleius Platonicus (including cures allegedly used by the Emperor Augustus); Pseudo-Dioscorides' *Book of Medicine from Feminine Herbs*; an illustrated book of medicines from animals; the *Book of Medicines from the Badger* (these last four collectively the core of the *Herbarium* complex mentioned earlier); a second, different version of the *Alphabet of Galen*; and miscellaneous recipes copied into blank and marginal spaces (Beccaria 1956: Monte Cassino cod. 97, 297–303; Everett 2012: 125–7; Voigts 1978; Langslow 2006: 45–6). Whether these texts preserved the original words of their great authors was of little concern to an early medieval audience; the authorities' names were enough to inspire trust and to ensure that such texts would be copied, added to and circulated down through the centuries. Very similar anthologies were transmitted all across Europe and preserved by various monastic foundations.

The aforementioned collection of medical texts at Monte Cassino included letters said to have been written by great medical authorities to family members or patrons. There are indeed authentic ancient examples of these. They comprised a predominantly practical genre that connected medieval readers to the ancient authorities in imagined traditions of shared understandings (Langslow 2007). Letters giving medical advice remained popular throughout the Middle Ages, as can be seen from Naama Cohen-Hanegbi's chapter in this volume. In addition to the psychological appeal of this rhetorically created sense of intimacy, the epistolary genre created a space where great authorities might convey important life-saving information to novices across great distances, thus serving both didactic and therapeutic roles.

The letters themselves might comprise the pedagogical and therapeutic communications on their own; or they might introduce lengthier practical manuals. In every case, the appeal of medical letters to later readers interested in connecting to the past and learning from respected authors was entirely effective (Langslow 2007; Morello and Morrison 2007). In all such cases, the utility of a text was more important than its authenticity (Nutton 2011: 7–18). Augusto Beccaria's great catalogue of 145 surviving Latin medical manuscripts copied prior to *c.* 1100 discloses a whole panoply of letters offering medical and dietetic advice, purporting to be by famous authorities (Beccaria 1956). Examples include the *Epistula peri hereseon* (Letter on the Sects) – gathered together with material from a late-antique scholastic commentary on Galen's *De sectis* (Peri hereseon; On Sects); Cassius Felix's (*fl.*mid-fifth century CE) prefatory letter to his 'dearest son' that headed his treatise *On Medicine* (Glaze 2007); and the epistolary prologue to the popular alphabetically arranged text called *Alfabetum Galieni* (The Alphabet of Galen), which is addressed to 'dearest Paternianus' (Everett, ed. 2012: 141).

MEDICAL AUTHORITY AND THE NEED FOR SELF-HELP

One of the reasons why medical authorities in the early Middle Ages focused upon the circulation of predominantly shorter practical materials was the need for self-reliance in a largely ruralized world which, following the decline of Roman imperial authority, suffered from shrinking urban centres and collapsing governmental infrastructures. These factors made therapeutic handbooks, letters, herbal and pharmaceutical manuals and abbreviated question-and-answer dialogues the most concise and essentially valuable forms of medical textuality. This need for efficacy, which privileged proven remedies over abstruse theories, was true of both the Latin half of the former Roman Empire and, by the eighth century, also of much of the Greek-speaking Byzantine East (Nutton 2013: 7–18; Andorlini 2007, Fischer 2012; Zipser 2009, Zipser, ed. 2013; Bouras-Vallianatos 2018, 194–7). In the absence of a diverse population of trained medical practitioners – and educational centres able to produce significant numbers of them – and in areas where markets selling ingredients from distant realms in volume and at reasonable prices became rarer and rarer, it became ever more imperative that literate persons be able to educate themselves to a modest degree, to identify alternative healing agents and to care for themselves and their communities (Fischer 2012; McCormick 2001, 696–728).

The simplifying process of therapeutics can be seen with medical authors like Marcellus of Bordeaux (*fl.* early-fifth century CE) who constructed manuals that were accessible to a population of self-medicating family members and dependents in late ancient Gaul, employing proven, simple remedies. Gone were the theriacs (see Chapter 4 above on Animals for more on these complex drugs) and antidotes with dozens of expensive, exotic ingredients that had been favoured by Rome's imperial elites (Totelin 2004; Stannard 1972). Such self-help manuals remained popular throughout the Christianization of Europe and enjoyed an ever-wider circulation as more and more book-owning monastic and ecclesiastical foundations were established.

What is surprising within this context, is that no equivalent textual tradition emerged for surgery. Aside from very brief phlebotomy guides for bloodletting, a list of surgical instruments' names, so badly corrupted as to be unintelligible and one short excerpt surviving in a single manuscript, surgery is hardly represented at all in the Latin tradition (Meaney 2000: 229; Green 2015). The only surgical tradition that seems to circulate is a series of cautery illustrations (see Figure 8.1), possibly of late antique Alexandrian or early Byzantine origin (Glaze 2007; Maion 2007; Beccaria 1956: 281–4; Collins 2000: 180–3; Jones 1998: 76–79). It may be that textual knowledge was insufficient for some aspects of practice and consequently had to be supplemented by the communication of tacit knowledge between practitioners through forms of apprenticeship (Van Arsdall 2007a; 2007b: 415–34; 2011: 201–16; Banham and Voth 2015:

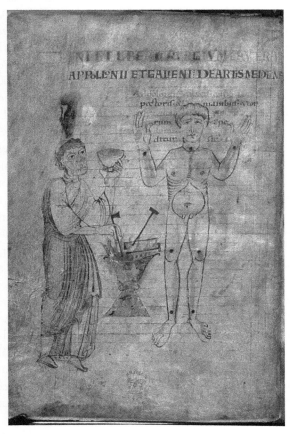

FIGURE 8.1: Cautery illustration (*c.*1100). London, British Library MS Sloane 2839, fol. 1v. Credit: British Library/Public Domain.

169–74). Archaeology shows that the bones of some early medieval men and women were carefully set and that trepanation was employed to alleviate intracranial pressure (Skinner 2015; Roberts 2014: 445–7). There is a wealth of non-medical sources – law codes, saints' lives, chronicles, poetry – for injuries, broken bones and other disabling conditions (Pilsworth 2014). Yet it was only from the late-eleventh century that an entire book (in the earliest version of the *Pantegni Practica* – see below) discussing surgery at length became authoritative in the Latin tradition (Corner 1927; Jones 1998: 76–82; Green 2015). The first explicit reference to any illustrated surgical text in monastic and cathedral libraries dates from the mid-twelfth century catalogue of the Abbey of St Amand in northern France (Glaze 2000: 282). It was not until *c.* 1240–1320 that a series of authors working primarily in northern Italy managed to bring surgery close to par with other types of theoretically grounded medical knowledge (McVaugh 2006).

The aforementioned process of simplification affected the size as well as the content of medical manuscripts designed for practical ends. Although there were occasionally longer compilations – such as the *Liber passionalis* (The Book of Diseases) and the *Tereoperica* (Therapeutics), both put together before the turn of the millennium – these were extremely rare and involved a major investment in valuable parchment (Fischer 2013; Fischer 2007, 105–25; Fischer 2000a; Langslow 2006; Glaze 2007). One eighth-century medical manuscript produced in northern Italy and later owned by the Abbey of Lorsch is more typically 'pocket-sized', with only 66 leaves, measuring just 18 × 12 cm, with a writing space in single columns of just 14.5 × 9.5 cm. It preserves a copy of the *Alphabet of Galen*, a Psalter and a few medical recipes (McCormick 2001: 713; Everett 2012: 121–3).[1] The dimensions of this and several other surviving medical books attest to their intended portability as manuals, rather than as works of reference for desk-top or lectern consultation. Another unique survivor copied in northern Italy during the first half of the ninth century was originally carried without any binding at all and was later, upon arrival at the Abbey of St Gall in Switzerland, folded over rather as one would a modern soft-cover magazine (Bischoff 1966).[2] A number of medical books were recorded in monastic and cathedral library catalogues in such an unbound state. This one is typically practical in nature: it opens with a question-and-answer treatise on phlebotomy, miscellaneous recipes, a therapeutic treatise in head-to-foot order, an alphabetized list of synonyms of medicinal agents in two linguistic traditions and a version of the *Herbarium* complex for which the illustrations of herbs and animals were never filled in. Even without the illustrations completed, this would have been a very useful manuscript, especially to an experienced practitioner, perhaps a monk or secular cleric.

Several similarly practical folding almanacs have survived from the late Middle Ages in a rather fragile state. They contained chiefly diagnostic and

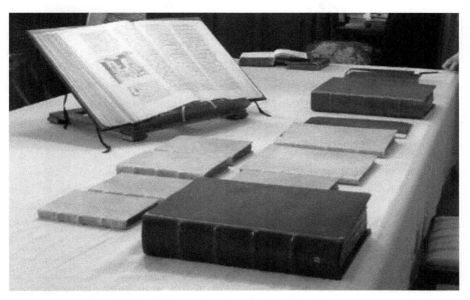

FIGURE 8.2: Photograph of the medieval medical books of Monte Cassino. Credit: F. Eliza Glaze.

prognostic guides, diagrams and calendars and would have hung from a belt about the waist, sometimes protected in a cloth cover or bag (Jones 1998: 53–7). In the early-medieval northern European world, with monastic houses few and far between and even fewer urban centres, clerics and missionaries versed in medical knowledge may well have been highly itinerant; the loss rate for anything they carried with them would therefore have been very high. Compare instead codex 97 from the Abbey of Monte Cassino, which measures 41.4 x 30 cm and extends to more than 550 pages in length. Codices of that size and weight would never have been very portable; in fact, the two oldest medical books at Monte Cassino are far and away the largest of the dozen pre-modern medical manuscripts that survive there. Anyone wanting or needing to travel with useful references from larger volumes needed to produce something much smaller.[3]

Such portable ephemera would have been much less likely to survive unless bound together deliberately and stored away on some foundation's shelves. This appears to be something akin to what Walahfrid Strabo, Abbot of Reichenau, produced when, prior to his death in 849, he gathered together a series of notebooks, mostly in his own handwriting but written over the course of many years. Interspersed through this personal collection of favourite works on grammar, computation, theology and history are thirty-two pages of medical literature, including excerpts on diet, a dietary calendar, a phlebotomy text—

detailing the dangerous *dies caniculares* (dog days) when bloodletting should be avoided—recipes against illnesses associated with cold weather and passages from Roman agricultural manuals. There are even some rare Old High German glosses offering vernacular terms for Latin ones (Bischoff 1967).

In general, texts listing a variety of equivalent, local or inexpensive ingredients to replace hard-to-find and expensive ones (a genre known generally as *quid pro quo*) abounded in a world which needed self-help manuals. There is good evidence that costly ingredients available only from exotic locales – including pepper, cumin, cinnamon, ginger, cloves, camphor, incense and mastic – continued a limited currency as desirable commodities in the great abbeys of Carolingian Europe, where they were received as gifts, purchased as precious medicines and dispersed along with a dying person's other valuables to friends and family (McCormick 2001: 708–19; Stannard 1972, 1974; Riddle 1965). Thus, medicinal glossaries or lists of synonyms for the many types of pharmaceutical agents, where one linguistic tradition was equated with others, became a truly essential genre in medical literature (Burnett 2013; García González 2007; Glaze 2012). Late-antique medical authorities like Oribasius or Theodorus Priscianus, had already written treatises of *euporista* or 'easily procurable remedies'. Theodorus stated hyperbolically that, using his text of accessible remedies, the sick 'need not head off straightaway to Pontus [the Black Sea] or scour the deep interior of Arabia to obtain storax or castoreum or other riches from distant parts of the globe' (Everett 2012: 27; Brodersen 2017; Baader 1984). This tradition continued well into the Middle Ages. The portable north Italian manuscript already discussed above, later at St Gall, included a list of synonyms of medicinal agents and its herbal section derived from Pseudo-Apuleius includes an additional twenty-six unique chapters of plants whose names are almost entirely unrecognizable; their earliest editor suggested that they may have signified local alpine plants (Landgraf 1928; Voigts 1979; Collins 2000: 183–4; García González 2008).

TEXTUAL AUTHORITIES ADAPTED TO LOCAL LANGUAGES AND USAGES, C. 1000

In one region of Europe, England, the status of medical texts as esteemed repositories of valued knowledge can be seen in the very unusual translation of Latin medicinal texts into a European vernacular, Old English. Although most of these Old English texts survive in manuscripts dating from the turn of the millennium or after, it is likely that the translations were produced earlier. The best-attested texts in terms of the numbers of copies surviving in Old English are the ensemble of works popular also at Monte Cassino, the *Herbarium* complex. In addition to the herbal attributed to Apuleius Platonicus, Pseudo-Dioscorides' *Book of Medicine from Feminine Herbs* and the short text on the

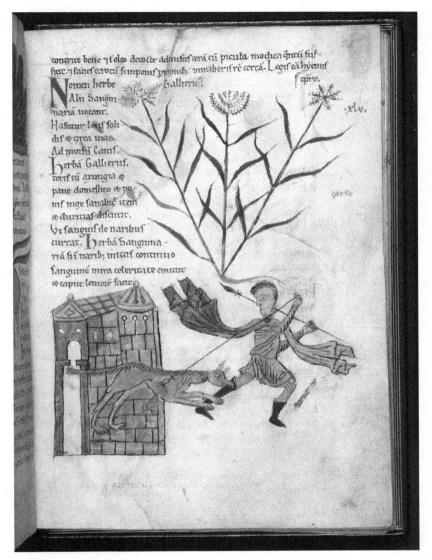

FIGURE 8.3: Crowsfoot and dog bite, Pseudo-Apuleius Platonicus, *De medicaminibus herbarum* (late-twelfth century). London, British Library, MS Harley 5294, fol. 25. Credit: British Library/Public Domain.

medicinal uses of the badger, this group of works included a brief treatise on the medicinal uses of betony, another on the mulberry, one on medicine from quadrupeds and another attributed to Sextus Placitus on medicines derived from animals. Most of the surviving Old English copies descend from the illustrated Latin textual tradition or were at least prepared to receive illustrations

(Collins 2000: 148–238; Jones 1998: 58–67). These included not only illustrations of the medicinal agents themselves, but also scenes showing humans being bitten by rabid dogs or serpents for which the simple ingredient in question provided treatment; in slightly later traditions, additional images showing human figures attacking the dogs or serpents in question with sword or spear conveyed a sense of human effort combating the source of the injury in question (see Figures 4.3 and 8.3).

Scholars who have studied the Old English vernacular tradition intensively are quick to point out that the unknown translators did not simply produce a direct translation, but rather selected and adapted their renditions, revealing 'acute intelligence, thorough knowledge of the matter treated and a good . . . [mastery] of Latin' (D'Aronco 2007: 38). In many cases, the Mediterranean plant materials were supplied with their English names; it is likely that many of these medicinal plants were capable of being cultivated in England at the time and, for the more exotic items, English travellers or their intermediaries would have been capable of acquiring them through trade across the Alps (Voigts 1979, 1976; McCormick 2001: 678–88). In one copy, a colour-coded table of chapters noting each ingredient and the ailments it treated, made navigating the book particularly useful to the practitioner; to augment it further, additional recipes were copied into blank spaces in the manuscripts (Jones 1998: 61).

That the Old English *Herbarium* was actually utilized by practitioners is further evident from the use of these Old English translations as sources in a series of practical recipe collections also written in Old English and known as *Leechbooks* (Physicians' Books) and *Lacnunga* (Remedies). One of the *Leechbooks* carries a unique statement about the owner or author of the book, identifying him by name as Bald and his scribe as Cild. *Bald's Leechbook* is distinctive not only for this author identification, but also because it represented a unique arrangement of material based upon some of the best Latin medical literature circulating in the early medieval period. In the *Lacnunga* text, the recipes are arranged by the bodily location of the ailment or its primary symptoms and are bound with a copy of the Old English *Herbarium*, making it a particularly useful manual for medical practice (D'Aronco 2007; Meaney 2000).

Scholars have now established that, far from representing a collection of mere 'folk' medicine, these translations into Old English reveal that well before the Norman Conquest in the eleventh century, English practitioners were quick to adopt the best and most popular versions of practical medical literature available on the continent and to adapt it to their usage (Van Arsdall 2005, 2007; Cameron 1983a, 1983b, 1993). Very little is known about these practitioners, but it has been posited that the use of the vernacular implies the owners and users of these manuscripts were not churchmen, but rather laymen lacking a facility in Latin (Banham 2006: 237–9). Scholars working on other regions of Europe have also attempted to argue that certain features of surviving manuscripts suggest they, too, were lay-practitioners' personal manuals, but that such practitioners would surely have known Latin (Meaney 2000; Pilsworth 2014: 81–100). However, as one scholar points out, based upon textual evidence, 'how exactly these various healers acquired their skills is irrecoverable. All we can say with confidence is that little of it involved schools' (Horden 2009: 18). We have just one surviving example of text-based medical instruction from the *Histories* of Richer of Rheims of *c*. 1000. Richer explains that as a young man he went to the cathedral of Chartres to study the logic of Hippocrates under the tutelage of a master Heribrand, who was said to be so skilled in medicine that the arts of 'pharmacology, botany, and surgery' were well understood by him (Richer 2011: 305–11).

In contrast, we know from documentary sources that there were numerous self-designating *medici* who signed documents as witnesses or were themselves involved in property transactions, especially in northern and southern Italy (Pilsworth 2009; 2014: 177–215; Skinner 1997). The majority of such signatories identify themselves as *clericus et medicus* (cleric and physician), implying both a degree of literacy and a sense of professional identity as physicians. A significant number do not provide any religious title, designating themself merely as *medicus*, especially in southern Italy, where there are also several Jewish *medici* documented (Skinner 1997: 79–107). The involvement of all these *medici* in documentary culture indicates they were held in fairly high esteem within their communities. They are all men. Women are almost invisible in the medical marketplace of the early Middle Ages, in contrast to the roles they played in antiquity (Nutton 1992; Flemming 2000: 33–46; Totelin 2011; Pilsworth 2014: 151–62).

Research of this kind on the medical practitioners of other parts of early medieval Europe is still much needed. What it shows so far is the importance of geographical location and population diversity. Southern Italy, for example, had populations of resident Greeks, including Greek monks and clerics, Byzantine administrative officials, Lombard natives, Jewish communities, itinerant merchants from several parts of North Africa and Sicily, and slaves. The result is much closer to what is seen in contemporary documents from Cairo in Egypt than in monastic archives elsewhere (Skinner 1997; Pilsworth 2014). England, in contrast, was much less urbanized with fewer centres of learning, although it would be a mistake to see it as lacking diversity. However, following the Norman conquests of England, southern Italy and Sicily in the second half of the eleventh century, England was influenced very quickly by southern Italian learning; for example, both the cautery illustrations in Figure 8.1 and the new texts and translations described below from Salerno and Monte Cassino became almost immediately popular in Anglo-Norman England and northern France (Burnett, ed. 1987; Glaze 2000: chapters 4–5, Table 1; Banham 2006; Wallis 2011).

TRANSFORMATIONS IN TEXTUAL MEDICAL AUTHORITY IN SALERNO (ELEVENTH–TWELFTH CENTURY)

Aside from the remarkable assimilation of ancient and late-ancient trust in medical authority based upon pre-Christian texts that we have seen effected prior to the eighth century, the most remarkable transformation of medical textuality, along with a political and public sense of authoritative knowledge and practice, took place in southern Italy between *c.* 1025 and 1200, within the broad ambit of the city of Salerno. Already by *c.* 1055–1075, Salerno played a new role in what we might call the 'authoritative textual turn'. This process set the city of Salerno at the international nexus of medical innovation and textually rooted practice for well over a century, until it was eclipsed by other centres in *c.* 1225 (Demaitre 2003; Black 2012). During that century a community of medical authors and practitioners working in or associated with Salerno appear to have grasped the importance of producing new medical books and new practical manuals attributed to themselves as a method for garnering both fame and economic success. Activities undertaken there set the entire West upon a new intellectual trajectory in regard to the knowledge of publicly embraced, medical practices legitimized by the knowledge of books.

Several factors in eleventh-century southern Italy played significant roles in framing a cultural environment in which such a transformation could take place most fruitfully. Chief among these were the multi-cultural, multi-confessional and multi-linguistic populations interacting in the region; the historic role of Italian centres in the transmission and preservation of written medical knowledge; the rise of southern Italy as the dominant trading sector in the Mediterranean, at the expense of Egypt and Ifriqiya (modern Tunisia) (Smith 2015); a long-standing tradition and reputation for medical therapeutic excellence in the city of Salerno itself; and the close relationship between political and ecclesiastical leadership that emerged in the region between *c.* 1055 and 1087, particularly between Salerno and the Abbey of Monte Cassino (Newton 1999: 11–13; Kwakkel and Newton 2019).

One of the first stages of this process took place in Salerno prior to the mid-eleventh century when a medical practitioner named Gariopontus of Salerno put together a synthetic head-to-foot therapeutic medical manual based upon the popular early medieval ensemble of texts derived primarily from the works of Galen, Pseudo-Galen, Aurelius, Esculapius, Theodorus Priscianus and Alexander of Tralles. Gariopontus' existence as a citizen-donor and cleric are recorded in the 'book of memory' of the confraternity attached to the Salernitan Cathedral of St Matthew, as well as in the records of the Abbey of La Trinità in neighbouring Cava de' Tirreni. Although there is no sound evidence of a medical school or any formal medical pedagogy in Salerno or its vicinity prior to *c.* 1100, Gariopontus is nonetheless referred to in eleventh-century

AUTHORITY

manuscripts as 'the master'. Each chapter of his manual contained for each condition a range of treatments, as well as diets and baths; the text began with the diseases of the head and went straight through to the foot, ending with two lengthy books on fevers that preserved and repackaged core elements of Galenic fever theory. In the earliest manuscripts of the *Passionarius* there were also additional marginal and interlinear glosses further explaining technical terminology and the identities of pharmaceutical ingredients. The chapters of each book were from the outset carefully detailed in tables at the head of each of the seven books, thereby rendering the whole easily accessible and navigable (Glaze 2008, 2012).

Efforts like Gariopontus' were fairly unusual for his day and for this region (compare the *Tereoperica*, *Liber passionalis* and *Lorscher Arzneibuch* mentioned above: all much earlier products from north of the Alps). Yet Gariopontus was by no means the only famed practitioner of medicine in Salerno and its hinterland. Passing references in chronicles, poetry and romances invoked the practical abilities of Salernitan practitioners and would continue to do so for decades. Salerno was renowned before the mid-eleventh century as a healthy city with excellent medical practitioners. It was, moreover, the seat of an archbishopric, an active port and the capital of the southern Lombard princes. After the Norman conquest of the city in 1077, it became the seat of the Norman dukes of Calabria, Apulia and Sicily (Metcalfe 2009, 2003).

Two noteworthy figures associated with Salerno in the second half of the eleventh century helped to effect the elevation of that city into a territory even more closely allied to both political and religious authority, namely Desiderius of Benevento, later Abbot of Monte Cassino (r. 1058–1086) and in his final year of life Pope Victor III (d. 1087), and Alfanus of Salerno, first a monk of Monte Cassino and, from 1058, the Archbishop of Salerno (d. 1085). Desiderius had first come to Salerno seeking treatment for illness due to its fame as a centre of medical practice. By 1058, Alfanus was known for his medical ability as well as his theological acumen and his literary skills, which may have helped win him the gratitude of the pope who appointed him archbishop of his native city in that year (Newton 1999: 13). Monte Cassino and the members of the community affiliated with the Abbey show every sign of having been already preoccupied with the accumulation of recipes for several centuries; the *antidotaria* (remedy collections) of early medieval Monte Cassino and its affiliates stretch to hundreds of pages – for example Monte Cassino manuscript 69 (ninth century), preserves more than 500 pages of remedies and Monte Cassino manuscript 225 and Vatican Barb. Lat. 160 (both eleventh century) add hundreds more pages of new recipes featuring exotic pharmacopoeia from the east (Beccaria 1956: 293–297, 303–5, 324–31; Glaze 2018). Ingredients like lapis lazuli, whole ground pearls, the incense of Constantinople, musk, sugar, tamarind and costly items imported from the Arabian Peninsula and Indian

Ocean begin to appear for the first time in the medical recipes of the Latin West (Glaze 2018).

Thus, a taste for exotic ingredients transmitted by various routes from the Islamicate world was already well established in the region, by the time the great Arabic-to-Latin translator of medical texts, Constantine the African (of Ifriqiya) arrived in Salerno prior to 1076 as a refugee from war-torn North Africa. He arrived at the very moment the city was enduring an ultimately successful Norman siege which caused significant damage and subsequent political change. It is no surprise that medical practitioners like Johannes the 'Abbot of the Court', brother of the last Lombard prince and brother-in-law to the Norman conqueror Robert Guiscard (d. 1085), and Archbishop Alfanus, both of whom had already employed the new exotica in their own practical remedies, stepped forward to serve as the newly-arrived Constantine's colleagues and patrons (Kwakkel and Newton 2019).

Constantine the African (d. *c.* 1098/99) is frequently considered by historians as something of 'a bolt from the blue', a one-man watershed who turned the medicine of Christendom in a new direction almost single-handedly, bringing it more in line with the traditions of medicine in the Islamicate world. He is, unquestionably, the single most recognized medical authority of the eleventh century. However, it is important to understand the aforementioned political and cultural context in which Constantine found southern Italy in general at the time of his arrival and the city of Salerno in particular. This reveals a more finely nuanced set of circumstances and conditions that provided the broader background to his intellectual and therapeutic contributions (Glaze 2019).

Constantine is known for rendering more than twenty-four complex Arabic medical works into Latin, a language in which Constantine would have been only partially competent. The most important translations were the *Kitāb Kāmil aṣ-ṣināʿa aṭ-ṭibbīya* (The Complete Book of the Medical Art) by the Persian physician 'Alī b. al-'Abbās al-Majūsī (d. *c.* 990) – which became known as the *Pantegni*; the *Kitab Zād al-musāfir wa-qūt al-ḥāḍir* (Provision for the Traveller and Sustenance for the Settled) by Ibn al-Jazzār (d. 979), from al-Qayrawān in North Africa, Latinized as the *Viaticum*; and highly influential works on urines and diet by Ishāq al-Isrā'īlī (d. 955), a Jewish author-practitioner also from al-Qayrawān (Burnett and Jacquart, eds. 1994). Constantine began this challenging work in busy Salerno, but completed it at the nearby Abbey of Monte Cassino, a place much more conducive to study, where he became a monk. There he found the most brilliant scriptorium in Europe, busily producing the most innovative rhetorical, classical, theological, mathematical and musical texts of the period and also the aforementioned *antidotaria* featuring the new pharmacopoeia (Newton 2011). Only at Monte Cassino could Constantine have found the considerable human and material resources that he needed: assistant-scribes fluent in Latin and with rhetorical abilities, as well as abundant

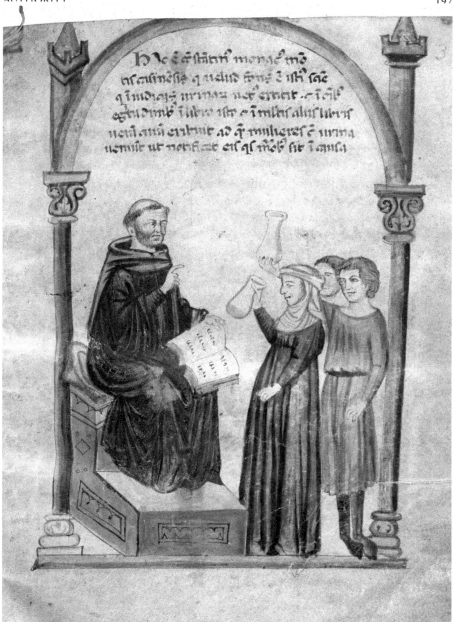

FIGURE 8.4: Constantine the African judging urines, *Various medical treatises* (fourteenth century), Oxford, Bodleian Library, MS Rawlinson C. 328, fol. 3. Credit: Bodleian Library.

time, quietude and parchment. The few portrayals we have of Constantine from illustrated manuscripts usually show him in the robes of a Benedictine monk, either book in hand, judging urines (i.e. constructing diagnoses and prognoses) or sitting at a table surrounded by books (see Figure 8.4).

Constantine's translation programme may have been influential in the appearance of an entirely new corpus of texts primarily dedicated to expert medical practice based upon the authoritative tradition of Hippocratic-Galenic principles – the so-called *Articella* (Little Art of Medicine). This corpus included the *Isagoge* of Johannitius (an introductory text by Ḥunayn ibn Isḥāq (d. 873), a Christian physician of Baghdad, to the *Tegni* of Galen), the Hippocratic *Aphorisms* with Galen's commentary, the Hippocratic *Prognostics, On Urines* by Theophilus and *On Pulses* by Philaretus (both the latter were obscure Greek authors of the seventh century). Traditional understandings of the formation of the *Articella* and its origins have sometimes suggested a Monte Cassino connection, while more recent work also perceives the influence of Archbishop Alfanus (Nutton 1995: 142; Wallis 2011). However, the recent palaeographical redating of the earliest manuscript of the *Articella*, placing its production in the final quarter of the eleventh century and localizing it to Monte Cassino, ties the introduction of this core canon of texts more closely to Constantine and his group of colleague-assistants than has hitherto been realized. It is also noteworthy that this earliest copy from the late-eleventh century includes both Galen's *Tegni* with contemporary marginal glosses and the Hippocratic *Regimen in Acute Diseases*; older scholarship formerly considered these texts to have been added to the *Articella* only after *c.* 1150 (Kwakkel and Newton 2019).

This new canon of texts became the chief focus of medical study at Salerno in the twelfth century and soon, thereafter, at the schools of Montpellier, Paris and elsewhere. By the close of the Middle Ages, more than fifty universities across Europe offered very similar curricula in medicine (Demaitre 2013: 4–33; O'Boyle 1998). In areas rich in Jewish populations there were also translations into Hebrew, thereby allowing Jews to continue as expert medical authorities despite not being permitted to attend universities (Shatzmiller 1995; Fidora et al 2013). The *Articella* remained an essential part of the literate practitioner's specialized training well into the sixteenth century, even after many new textual authorities had been translated from Greek and Arabic into Latin and made widely available, many via the Iberian Peninsula, which was similar to southern Italy in its multiculturalism and political complexity. Constantine was followed by other prolific translators such as Stephen of Pisa/Antioch (*fl.* first half of twelfth century), Gerard of Cremona (d. *c.* 1187), Burgundio of Pisa (d. 1193) and Niccolò da Reggio (*fl.* first half of fourteenth century).

From the twelfth century onwards, the primary method of teaching the *Articella* and other texts was to have the masters of schools – and universities after the late-twelfth century – provide Salernitan-style commentary lectures upon them. In so doing, the new masters established themselves as living and textual authorities in their own rights. As a result, the Salernitans' reputation across Europe achieved legendary status and copies of their commentary texts, the texts upon which they commented and the new translations of Constantine and his circle spread across Europe with surprising speed (Glaze 2000). Many of the same twelfth-century masters in Salerno also appreciated the power of textuality to convey therapeutic authority. They composed practical manuals (*Practicae*), much as Gariopontus had done earlier, but integrating the newest theoretical and therapeutic materials. They named their manuals after themselves – one *Practica* by Platearius (d. *c.* 1161), another by Archimattheus (*fl.* mid-twelfth century) and still others by Copho and Bartholomaeus (*fl.* early and mid-twelfth century respectively). Nearly all of these masters appreciated anew the opportunity to present to a public audience and wider marketplace their therapeutic expertise and to ground that expertise in the knowledge of canonical texts and ancient authorities which they themselves taught in a classroom setting (Wallis 2005; Recio Muñoz 2016).

One of the earliest new texts to appear in twelfth-century Salerno – a text that was neither a translation nor a compilation of other works – was the *Antidotarium Nicolai* (*The Antidotary of Nicholas of Salerno*). This text, beginning with an author's first-person statement and ending with a section on standard weights and measures, contained more than 100 named remedies. Another new Salernitan text was the *Circa instans* attributed to Platearius. Where the *Antidotarium Nicolai* prescribed compound remedies made up of several ingredients listed carefully in precise weights and measures, the *Circa instans* described the powers or 'strengths' of each simple ingredient – whether plant, animal, or mineral in origin – and the precise degree of coldness, hotness, dryness or wetness. Using this text would allow the mixing of multiple ingredients, carefully calculated to combat a patient's precise illness. The *Antidotarium Nicolai* and the *Circa instans* were widely used for centuries – indeed, they became required reading in the pharmacies of many regions into the fifteenth century and were translated into nearly every vernacular (Roberg 2002, 2007, 2011; Ventura 2012).

Perhaps the most famous of the new author-practitioners was a woman known as Trota (or Trocta) of Salerno. Her practical expertise harnessed the traditional wisdom of the *mulieres Salernitanae* (the women of Salerno), skilled in treating the conditions of women both before and after childbirth, as well as cosmetics and what we might call dermatological complaints. Trota's fame as a *magistra*, or female authority, became even greater when the text called *De curis mulierum* (On the Cures of Women) which preserves her therapies, was joined by two others on women's medicine to form what later became known as the *Trotula* (Green, ed. 2001). Subsequent confusion between the title of the book and the woman herself resulted in the woman and the text fusing into one so that she became known as Trotula. Trota is a virtually unique case of a woman

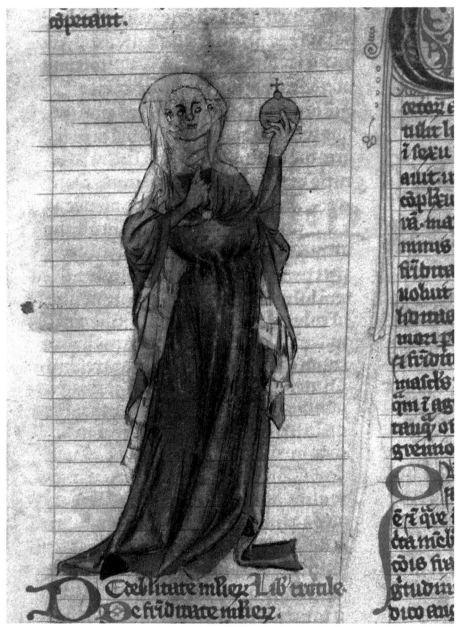

FIGURE 8.5: Trota, *Miscellanea Medica XVIII* (early-fourteenth century). London, Wellcome Library, MS 544, p. 65. Credit: Wellcome Library/Public Domain.

AUTHORITY

practitioner's expertise earning her lasting and widespread fame. It is ironic that, in spite of Trota's role as medieval Europe's first author of medicine for women written by a woman, with the growth of the universities and the exclusion of women from enrolment in them, obstetrics and gynaecology became an increasingly masculine specialization (Green 2008).

CONCLUSION

This chapter has shown that, by the end of the twelfth century, there was widespread popular trust in the authority of written medical knowledge and especially the great medical *auctores*, both of antiquity and from more recent times, from several religious traditions. Medical reputations continued to be constructed throughout the early Middle Ages based on a combination of experience and the skilful compilation of texts adapted to new times and places. Early medieval textual authority thrived because it was based on ancient medical texts yet was able to innovate continually and draw in new ideas, practices and materials. With the formation of the *Articella* and the production of related commentaries and new compositions, a group of set texts were unquestionably created that placed knowledge of the human body, in health and in disease and the therapeutic care of everyone squarely within a Hippocratic-Galenic theoretical orientation. Emphasis was placed on training practitioners in the essential elements of medical theory in order to aid, support and intellectually ground therapeutic practice. With a firm foundation in Galenic theory, which situated the human within a complex universal order, the Salernitans and their successors elsewhere emphasized that the accurate diagnosis, prognosis and treatment of illness rested upon and was validated by a thorough-going knowledge of medical books (Demaitre 2003). The best medical practice, from *c*. 1100 forward, was to be rooted in theoretical, bookish and philosophical knowledge. Yet it is undeniable that this embracing of pagan, Muslim and Jewish medical authorities only happened because it was not considered at odds with Christian religion. Without this acceptance and the continued Christian focus on the merits of learning within monasteries and a few urban contexts, long after the decline or disappearance of ancient Roman educational centres, rational and scientific medicine might never have developed and predominated throughout the West.

NOTES

1. Vatican Library, MS Pal. lat. 187, s. 8, N, available at: http://bibliotheca-laureshamensis-digital.de/bav/bav_pal_lat_187/0015 (accessed 29 June 2020).
2. St Gallen, Switzerland, Stiftsbibliothek MS Cod Sang 217, available at: www.e-codices.unifr.ch/en/list/one/csg/0217) (accessed 29 June 2020).

202   A CULTURAL HISTORY OF MEDICINE IN THE MIDDLE AGES

3. Figure 8.2 is a photograph of codices 69 and 97, dating from the ninth to tenth centuries; the two largest volumes with brown covers lying closed upon the table, the nearest being codex 69. The large volume open upon the lectern is codex 132, an eleventh-century illustrated copy of Hrabanus Maurus' (d. 856) encyclopaedia *De rerum naturis* (On the Natures of Things). It measures 49 x 35cm, only slightly larger than codices 69 and 97.

BIBLIOGRAPHY

Abreu, Laurinda and Sally Sheard, eds (2013), *Hospital Life: Theory and Practice from the Medieval to the Modern*, Oxford: Peter Lang.

Abu-Lughod, Lila (1991), 'Writing Against Culture', in Richard Fox (ed.), *Recapturing Anthropology: Working in the Present*, 137–62, Santa Fe: School of American Research Press.

Abu Zayd, Nasr Hamid (2002), 'Illness and Health', in Jane McAuliffe (ed.), *The Encyclopedia of the Qur'ān*, vol. 2, 501–2, Leiden: Brill.

Addyman, Peter (1989), 'The Archaeology of Public Health at York, England', *World Archaeology*, 21: 244–64.

Agnellus of Ravenna (1981), *Lectures on Galen's 'De sectis'*, ed. David Davies, Leendert Westerink, et al., Buffalo: State University of New York Department of Classics.

Agresta, Abigail (2020), 'From Purification to Protection: Plague Response in Late Medieval Valencia', *Speculum*, 95: 371–95.

Agrimi, Jole and Chiara Crisciani (1994), *Les consilia médicaux*, trans. Caroline Viola, Turnhout: Brepols.

Ahmed, Shahab (2016), *What is Islam? The Importance of Being Islamic*, Princeton: Princeton University Press.

Aitchison, Briony (2009), 'Holy Cow! The Miraculous Cures of Animals in Late Medieval England', *European Review of History: Revue européenne d'histoire*, 16: 875–92.

Alain of Lille (1965), *Liber poenitentialis*, ed. Jean Longère, Louvain: Éditions Nauwelaerts.

Albala, Ken (1998), 'Fish in Renaissance Dietary Theory', in Harlan Walker (ed.), *Fish: Food from the Waters: Proceedings of the Oxford Symposium on Food and Cookery 1997*, 9–19, Totnes: Prospect Books.

Albala, Ken (2002), *Eating Right in the Renaissance*, Berkeley: University of California Press.

Albala, Ken (2012), 'Food for Healing: Convalescent Cooking in the Early-Modern Era', *Studies in History and Philosophy of Biological and Biomedical Sciences*, 43: 323–8.

Albertus Magnus (1999), *On Animals*, trans. Kenneth Kitchell and Irven Resnick, Baltimore: Johns Hopkins University Press.

Alcuin (1881), *Carmina*, no. 26, ed. Ernst Dümmler, *Monumenta Germaniae Historica. Poetae latini aevi carolini*, vol. 1, 245–46, Berlin: Weidman.

Aldobrandino of Siena (1911), *Le régime du corps de Maître Aldebrandin de Sienne*, ed. Louis Landouzy and Roger Pepin, Paris: Librairie Ancienne Honoré Champion Éditeur.

Alexander, Michelle, Christopher Gerrard, Alejandra Gutiérrez, and Andrew Millard (2015), 'Diet, Society and Economy in Late Medieval Spain: Stable Isotope Evidence from Muslims and Christians from Gandía, Valencia', *American Journal of Physical Anthropology*, 156: 263–73.

Alfani, Guido and Tommy Murphy (2017), 'Plague and Lethal Epidemics in the Pre-Industrial World', *Journal of Economic History*, 77: 314–43.

Álvarez Fernández, Maria (2009), 'Abastecimiento y consumo de pescado en Oviedo a finales de la Edad Média', in (no editor), *La pesca en la Edad Media*, 71–86, Madrid: Xunta de Galicia, Sociedad Española de Estudios Medievales, Universidad de Murcia, CSIC.

Amasuno, Marcelino (2004), 'El saber médico tras el prólogo del Libro de buen amor: "loco amor" y "amor héroes"', in Francisco Toro Ceballos and Bienvenido Morros (eds), *Juan Ruiz, Arcipreste de Hita, u el "Libro de buen amor": Actas del Congreso Internacional del Centro para la Edición de los Clásicos Españoles*, 247–70, Alcalá la Real: Ayuntamiento/Centro para la Edición de los Clásicos Españoles.

Andorlini, Isabella (2007), 'Teaching Medicine in Late Antiquity: Methods, Texts and Contexts', in Patrizia Lendinara, Loredana Lazzari, and Maria D'Aronco (eds), *Form and Content of Instruction in Anglo-Saxon England in the Light of Contemporary Manuscript Evidence*, 401–14, Turnhout: Brepols.

Andrén, Anders (1986), 'I städernas under värld', in Anders Andrén, Marit Anglert, Mats Anglert, et al (eds), *Medeltiden och arkeologin: Festskrift till Erik Cinthio*, 259–70, Lund: Lund University.

Anthimus (2007), *On the Observation of Foods*, ed. Mark Grant, Totnes: Prospect Books.

Aquinas, Thomas (1921), *The 'Summa Theologica' of St Thomas Aquinas, Second Part of the Second Part, Questions 141–70*, vol. 13, trans. by the Fathers of the English Dominican province, London: Burns Oates & Washbourne.

Arano, Luisa Cogliati (1996), *The Medieval Health Handbook: Tacuinum Sanitatis*, New York: George Braziller.

Archambeau, Nicole (2013), 'Tempted to Kill: Miraculous Consolation for a Mother after the Death of her Infant Daughter', in Elena Carrera (ed.), *Emotions and Health, 1200–1700*, 47–66, Leiden: Brill.

Armstrong, Edward (1900), 'The Sienese Statutes of 1262', *English Historical Review* 15: 1–19.

Arnau de Vilanova (1996), *Regimen sanitatis ad Regem Aragonum*, ed. Luis García Ballester, et al., Barcelona: Fundació Noguera/Universitat de Barcelona.

Arnau de Vilanova (1999), *De esu carnium*, ed. Dianne Bazell, Barcelona: Fundació Noguera/Universitat de Barcelona.

Arner, Timothy (2019), 'The Disappearing Scar of Henry V: Triage, Trauma, and the Treatment of Henry's Wounding at the Battle of Shrewsbury', *Journal of Medieval and Early Modern Studies*, 49: 347–76.

BIBLIOGRAPHY 205

Arnold, Ken, Roy Porter, and Lise Wilkinson (1994), *Animal Doctor: Birds and Beasts in Medical History: An Exhibition at the Wellcome Institute for the History of Medicine*, London: Wellcome Trust.

Arrizabalaga, Jon (2002), 'Problematizing Retrospective Diagnosis in the History of Disease', *Asclepio*, 54: 51–70.

Asfora, Wanessa (2011), 'Aspects of the Incorporation of a Cookery Book in the Early Middle Ages', unpublished paper presented at the International Medieval Congress, University of Leeds, 11–14 July 2011, originally available from the author's academia.edu page (accessed 6 July 2018).

Asfora Nadler, Wanessa (2016), 'Apicius in the Early Medieval Manuscripts: Medieval or Roman Cookery book?' in (no editor), *L'Alimentazione nell'Alto Medioevo: pratiche, simboli, ideologie*, Atti delle Settimane 63: 493–513, Spoleto: Fondazione Centro Italiano di Studi sull'Alto Medioevo.

al-ʿAsqalānī, Ibn Ḥajar (1990), *Badhl al-Māʿūn fī faḍl al-ṭāʿūn*, ed. Aḥmad ʿAṣṣām ʿAbd al-Qādir al-Kātib, Riyad: Dar al-ʿĀṣīma.

Aston, Mick, ed. (1988), *Medieval Fish, Fisheries and Fishponds in England*, 2 vols, Oxford: BAR Publishing.

Atat, Ayman Yasin (2020), 'Bathtubs as a Healing Approach in Fifteenth-Century Ottoman Medicine', in Sara Ritchey and Sharon Strocchia (eds), *Gender, Health and Healing, 1250–1550*, 245–63, Amsterdam: University of Amsterdam.

Atkinson, Paul (1997), 'Narrative Turn or Blind Alley?' *Qualitative Health Research*, 7: 325–44.

Attewell, Guy (2007), *Refiguring Unani Tibb: Plural Healing in Late Colonial India*, New Delhi: Orient Longman.

Augustine of Hippo (1996), *De doctrina Christiana*, trans. Roger Green, Oxford: Clarendon Press.

Ausécache, Mireille (2006), 'Des aliments et des médicaments', *Cahiers de recherches médiévales*, 13: 249–58.

Avicenna (1556), *Liber canonis medicinae*, Basel: Ioannes Heruagios.

Aymer, Alphonse (1926), 'Le sachet accoucheur et ses mystères', *Annales du Midi*, 38: 273–347.

Azman, Josip, Amir Muzur, Vedran Frkovic, H. Pavletic, Adriana Prunk, and Ante Skrobonja (2006), 'Public Health Problems in the Medieval Statutes of Vinodol, Vrbnik and Senj (West Croatia)', *Journal of Public Health*, 28: 166–7.

Baader, Gerhard (1984), 'Early Medieval Latin Adaptations of Byzantine Medicine in Western Europe', *Dumbarton Oaks Papers*, 38: 251–9.

Bailey, Anne (2017), 'Miracles and Madness: Dispelling Demons in Twelfth-Century Hagiography', in Siam Bhayro and Catherine Rider (eds), *Demons and Illness from Antiquity to the Early-Modern Period*, 233–55, Leiden: Brill.

Bailey, Charles (1856), *Transcripts from the Municipal Archives of Winchester*, Winchester: Hugh Barclay.

Banham, Debby (2006), 'A Millennium in Medicine? New Medical Texts and Ideas in England in the Eleventh Century', in Simon Keynes and Alfred Smyth (eds), *Anglo-Saxons: Studies Presented to Cyril Roy Hart*, 230–42, Dublin: Four Courts Press.

Banham, Debby and Christine Voth (2015), 'The Diagnosis and Treatment of Wounds in the Old English Medical Collections: Anglo-Saxon Surgery?' in Larissa Tracy and Kelly DeVries (eds), *Wounds and Wound Repair in Medieval Culture*, 153–74, Leiden: Brill.

Barker, Hannah (2019), *That Most Precious Merchandise: The Mediterranean Trade in Black Sea Slaves, 1260–1500*, Philadelphia: University of Pennsylvania Press.

Barrett, James, Alison Locker, and Callum Roberts (2004), '"Dark Age Economics" Revisited: the English Fish Bone Evidence AD 600–1600', *Antiquity*, 78: 618–36.

Barrett, James, and nineteen others (2011), 'Interpreting the Expansion of Sea Fishing in Medieval Europe Using Stable Isotope Analysis of Archaeological Cod Bones', *Journal of Archaeological Science*, 38: 1516–24.

Barrett, James and David Orton, eds (2016), *Cod and Herring: The Archaeology and History of Medieval Sea Fishing*, Oxford: Oxbow.

Bartholomaeus Anglicus (1483, spine reads 1482), *De proprietatibus rerum*, ed. Petrus Ungarus, London: Anton Koberger.

Bartolomeo de Montagnana (1497), *Consilia CCCV in quibus agitur de universis fere aegritudinibus, humano corpori evenientibus, & mira facilitate, curandi eas adhibetur modus*, Venice: Bonetus Locatellus.

Baumgarten, Elisheva (2019), 'Ask the Midwives: A Hebrew Manual on Midwifery from Medieval Germany', *Social History of Medicine*, 32: 712–33.

Baverio Baviera (1489), *Consilia medica*, Bologna: Franciscus dictus Plato de Benedictis.

Bayless, Martha (2012), *Sin and Filth in Medieval Culture: The Devil in the Latrine*, London: Routledge.

Beaumanoir, Philippe de (1992), *The Coutumes de Beauvaisis of Philippe de Beaumanoir*, ed. and trans. F.R.P. [Ron] Akehurst, Philadelphia: University of Pennsylvania Press.

Beccaria, Augusto (1956), *I codici di medicina del periodo presalernitano (secoli IX, X e XI)*. Rome: Edizioni di storia e letteratura.

Becher, Tony and Paul Trowler (2001), *Academic Tribes and Territories: Intellectual Enquiry and the Culture of Disciplines*, 2nd edn, Buckingham: Society for Research into Higher Education/Open University Press.

Benedek, Thomas (2007), 'Historical Background of Discoid and Systemic Lupus Erythematosus', in Daniel Wallace and Bevra Hahn (eds), *Dubois' Lupus Erythematosus*, 2–15, Philadelphia: Lippincott Williams & Wilkins.

Benito i Monclús, Pere, ed. (2013), *Crisis alimentarias en la Edad Media: modelos, explicaciones y representaciones*, Lleida: Editorial Milenio.

Benso, Silvia (2008), 'The Breathing of the Air: Presocratic Echoes in Levinas', in Brian Schroeder and Silvia Benso (eds), *Levinas and the Ancients*, 9–23, Bloomington, IN: Indiana University Press.

Bergqvist, Johanna (2014), 'Gendered Attitudes Towards Physical Tending Amongst the Piously Religious of Late Medieval Sweden', in Effie Gemi-Ioranou, et al (eds), *Medicine, Healing and Performance*, 86–105, Oxford: Oxbow.

Berlin, Adele, Marc Zvi Brettler, and Michael Fishbane (2014), *The Jewish Study Bible*, New York: Oxford University Press.

Bernard de Gordon (1486), *Lilium medicine*, Ferrara: Andreas Belfortis, Gallus.

Bhayro, Siam and Catherine Rider, eds (2017), *Demons and Illness from Antiquity to the Early-Modern Period*, Leiden: Brill.

Biblia Vulgata (1965), *Biblia Vulgata iuxta Vulgata Clementinam*, ed. Alberto Colunga and Laurentio Turrado, 4th edn, Madrid: La Editorial Católica.

Birrell, Jean (2015), 'Peasants Eating and Drinking', *Agricultural History Review*, 63: 1–18.

Bischoff, Bernard (1966), 'Über gefaltete Handschriften, vornehmlich hagiographischen Inhalts', in Idem (ed.), *Mittelalterliche Studien: Ausgewählte Aufsätze zur Schriftkunde und Literaturgeschichte*, vol. 1, 93–100, Stuttgart: Anton Hiersemann.

BIBLIOGRAPHY

Bischoff, Bernard (1967), 'Eine Sammelhandschrift Walahfrid Strabos (cod. Sangall. 878)', in Idem, (ed.), *Mittelalterliche Studien: Ausgewählte Aufsätze zur Schriftkunde und Literaturgeschichte*, vol. 2: 34–51, Stuttgart: Anton Hiersemann.

Black, Winston (2012), '"I will add what the Arab once taught": Constantine the African in Northern European Medical Verse', in Anne Van Arsdall and Timothy Graham (eds), *Herbs and Healers from the Ancient Mediterranean through the Medieval West: Essays in Honor of John Riddle*, 153–86, Farnham: Ashgate.

Blake, Hugo (2015), 'Italian Wares', in Roberta Gilchrist and Cheryl Green (eds), *Glastonbury Abbey: Archaeological Investigations 1904–79*, 270–2, London: Society of Antiquaries of London.

Blumenthal, Debra (2014), 'Domestic Medicine: Slaves, Servants and Female Medical Expertise in Late Medieval Valencia', *Renaissance Studies*, 28: 515–32.

Boddington, Andy (1996), *Raunds Furnells: The Anglo-Saxon Church and Churchyard*, London: English Heritage.

Bonfield, Christopher (2017), 'The First Instrument of Medicine: Diet and Regimens of Health in Late Medieval England', in Linda Clark and Elizabeth Danbury (eds), *'A Verray Parfit Praktisour': Essays presented to Carole Rawcliffe*, 99–120, Martlesham: The Boydell Press.

Bonfield, Christopher, Jonathan Reinarz, and Teresa Huguet-Termes, eds (2013), *Hospitals and Communities, 1100–1960*, Oxford: Peter Lang.

Bonneuil, Christophe and Jean-Baptiste Fressoz (2017), *The Shock of the Anthropocene: The Earth, History and Us*, trans. David Fernbach, London: Verso.

Booth, Christopher (2017), 'Holy Alchemists, Metallurgists, and Pharmacists: The Material Evidence for British Monastic Chemistry', *The Journal of Medieval Monastic Studies*, 6: 195–215.

Bos, Kirsten, and fourteen others (2011), 'A Draft Genome of *Yersinia Pestis* from Victims of the Black Death', *Nature*, 478: 506–10.

Bouras-Vallianatos, Petros (2018), 'Reading Galen in Byzantium: The Fate of *Therapeutics to Glaucon*', in Petros Bouras-Vallianatos and Sofia Xenophontos (eds), *Greek Medical Literature and its Readers: From Hippocrates to Islam and Byzantium*, 180–230, Abingdon: Routledge.

Boyd, Kenneth (2000), 'Disease, Illness, Sickness, Health, Healing and Wholeness: Exploring Some Elusive Concepts', *Medical Humanities*, 26: 9–17.

Boyde, Patrick (1993), *Perception and Passion in Dante's Comedy*, Cambridge: Cambridge University Press.

Brabant, Rosa Kuhne (2002), 'Al-Razi on When and How to Eat Fruit', in David Waines (ed.), *Patterns of Everyday Life*, 317–27, Aldershot: Ashgate.

Brasher, Sally (2017), *Hospitals and Charity: Religious Culture and Civic Life in Medieval Northern Italy*, Manchester: Manchester University Press.

Brenner, Elma (2013), 'Leprosy and Public Health in Late Medieval Rouen', in Linda Clark and Carole Rawcliffe (eds), *The Fifteenth Century XII: Society in an Age of Plague*, 123–38, Woodbridge: The Boydell Press.

Brenner, Elma (2015), *Leprosy and Charity in Medieval Rouen*, London: Royal Historical Society.

Brentjes, Sonja, Taner Edis, and Lutz Richter-Bernburg, eds (2016), *1001 Distortions: How (Not) to Narrate History of Science, Medicine, and Technology in Non-Western Cultures*, Würzburg: Ergon.

British Archaeology news item (2016), 'Britain in Archaeology', *British Archaeology*, 149, July–August: 10–11.

Brodersen, Kai (2017), review of *Popular Medicine in Graeco-Roman Antiquity: Explorations*, ed. William Harris. Leiden, Brill, 2017, *Bryn Mawr Classical Review* (25.09.2017). Available online: http://bmcr.brynmawr.edu/2017/2017-09-25.html (accessed 29 June 2020).

Brody, Saul (1974), *The Disease of the Soul: Leprosy in Medieval Literature*, Ithaca: Cornell University Press.

Brown, Jonathan (2007), *The Canonization of al-Bukhārī and Muslim: The Formation and Function of the Sunnī Hadīth Canon*, Leiden: Brill.

Brown, Peter ([1971] 1989), *The World of Late Antiquity*, London: Norton.

Brumann, Christoph (1999), 'Writing for Culture: Why a Successful Concept Should Not Be Discarded', *Current Anthropology*, 40: 1–27.

Bürgel, Johann Christoph ([1968] 2016), *Ärztliches Leben und Denken im arabischen Mittelalter*, Leiden: Brill.

Buhrer, Eliza (2014), 'Law and Mental Competency in Late Medieval England', *Reading Medieval Studies*, 40: 82–100.

Buquet, Thierry (2016), 'De la pestilence à la fragrance: l'origine de l'ambre gris selon les auteurs arabes', *Bulletin d'études orientales*, 64: 113–33.

Burnett, Charles, ed. (1987), *Adelard of Bath: An English Scientist and Arabist of the Early Twelfth Century*, London: Warburg Institute.

Burnett, Charles (2001), 'The Coherence of the Arabic-Latin Translation Program in Toledo in the Twelfth Century', *Science in Context*, 14: 249–88.

Burnett, Charles (2013), 'Simon of Genoa's Use of the *Breviarium* of Stephen, the Disciple of Philosophy', in Barbara Zipser (ed.), *Simon of Genoa's Medical Lexicon*, 67–78, London: Versita.

Burnett, Charles and Danielle Jacquart, eds (1994), *Constantine the African and Ali ibn al-Abbas al-Maǧūsī: The Pantegni and Related Texts*, Leiden: Brill.

Burridge, Claire (2020), 'Incense in Medicine: Early Medieval Perspectives', *Early Medieval Europe*, 28: 219–55.

Butler, Sara (2015), *Forensic Medicine and Death Investigation in Medieval England*, New York: Routledge.

Bylebyl, Jerome (1990), 'The Medical Meaning of *Physica*', *Osiris*, 2nd series, 6: 16–41.

Bynum, Caroline Walker (1995), *The Resurrection of the Body in Western Christianity, 200–1336*, New York: Columbia University Press.

Caciola, Nancy (2000), 'Mystics, Demoniacs, and the Physiology of Spirit Possession in Medieval Europe', *Comparative Studies in Society and History*, 42: 268–306.

Caesarius of Heisterbach (1851), *Dialogus miraculorum: Textum ad quatuor codicum manuscriptorum editionisque principis fidem*, ed. Joseph Strange, Cologne: J.M. Heberle.

Cambell, Jacques, ed. (1978), *Enquête pour le procès de canonization de Dauphine de Puimichel comtesse d'Ariano*, Torino: Bottega d'Erasmo.

Cameron, Malcolm (1983a), 'The Sources of Medical Knowledge in Anglo-Saxon England', *Anglo-Saxon England*, 11 (1983): 135–55.

Cameron, Malcolm (1983b), 'Bald's *Leechbook*: its Sources and their Use in its Compilation', *Anglo-Saxon England*, 12: 153–82.

Cameron, Malcolm (1993), *Anglo-Saxon Medicine*, Cambridge: Cambridge University Press.

Campbell, Bruce (2016), *The Great Transition: Climate, Disease and Society in the Late Medieval World*, Cambridge: Cambridge University Press.

BIBLIOGRAPHY

Campbell, James (2002), 'Domesday Herrings', in Christopher Harper-Bill, Carole Rawcliffe and Richard Wilson (eds), *East Anglia's History: Studies in Honour of Norman Scarfe*, 5–17, Woodbridge: The Boydell Press/Centre of East Anglian Studies, University of East Anglia.

Cardwell, Peter (1995), 'The Hospital of St Giles by Brompton Bridge, North Yorkshire', *The Archaeological Journal*, 152: 109–245.

Carpenter, Christine and Charles Lethbridge Kingsford, eds (1996), *The Stonor Letters and Papers, 1290–1483*, Cambridge: Cambridge University Press.

Carr, David (2008), 'Controlling the Butchers in Late Medieval English Towns', *The Historian*, 70: 450–61.

Carraway Vitiello, Joanna (2014), 'Forensic Evidence, Lay Witnesses and Medical Expertise in the Criminal Courts of Late Medieval Italy', in Wendy J. Turner and Sara Butler (eds), *Medicine and the Law in the Middle Ages*, 133–56, Leiden: Brill.

Carr-Riegel, Leslie (2016), 'Waste Management in Medieval Krakow: 1257–1500', MA diss., Central European University, Budapest, Hungary.

Carruthers, Mary, ed. (2002), *Medieval Craft of Memory: An Anthology of Texts and Pictures*, Philadelphia: University of Pennsylvania Press.

Carruthers, Mary (2008), *The Book of Memory: A Study of Memory in Medieval Culture*, Cambridge and New York: Cambridge University Press.

Castle, Jo, Brendan Derham, Jeremy Montagu, Robin Wood, and Jon Hather (2005), 'The Contents of the Barber-Surgeon's Cabin', in Julie Gardiner with Michael Allen (eds), *Before the Mast: Life and Death Aboard the Mary Rose*, 189–225, Portsmouth: The Mary Rose Trust Ltd.

Cátedra García, Pedro, ed. (1994), *Sermón, Sociedad y Literatura en la Edad Media: San Vicente Ferrer en Castilla (1411–12)*, Valladolid: Junta de Castilla y León.

Cavadini, John (1993), *The Last Christology of the West: Adoptionism in Spain and Gaul, 785–820*, Philadelphia: University of Pennsylvania Press.

Cavallo, Sandra (2017), 'Conserving Health: The Non-Naturals in Early-Modern Culture and Society', in Sandra Cavallo and Tessa Storey (eds), *Conserving Health in Early-Modern Culture: Bodies and Environment in Italy and England*, 1–19, Manchester: Manchester University Press.

Cavallo, Sandra and Tessa Storey (2013), *Healthy Living in Late Renaissance Italy*, Oxford: Oxford University Press.

Celestine III (1853), *Epistolae et Privilegia*, Patrologia Latina 206, ed. Jacques-Paul Migne, Paris: Imprimerie Catholique.

Cessford, Craig (2015), 'The St. John's Hospital Cemetery and Environs, Cambridge: Contextualizing the Medieval Urban Dead', *The Archaeological Journal*, 172: 52–120.

Chakrabarty, Dipesh (2007), *Provincializing Europe: Postcolonial Thought and Historical Difference*, 2nd edn, Princeton: Princeton University Press.

Champollion-Figeac, Jacques-Joseph, ed. (1839), *Lettres de Rois, Reines et autres Personnages des Cours de France et d'Angleterre*, Paris: Imprimerie Royale.

Charleston, Robert (1975), 'Introduction', in Colin Platt and Richard Coleman-Smith, *Excavations in Medieval Southampton 1953–1969*, Volume 2, 204–15, Leicester: Leicester University Press.

Chaucer, Geoffrey (1899), 'Romaunt of the Rose: Minor Poems', in Walter Skeat (ed.), *The Complete Works of Geoffrey Chaucer*, vol. 1, Oxford: Clarendon Press.

Chaucer, Geoffrey (1933), *Romaunt of the Rose*, in Fred Robinson (ed.), *The Complete Works of Chaucer*, 664–739, Boston: Houghton Mifflin.

Chew, Helena and William Kellaway (1973), *London Assize of Nuisance 1301–1431: A Calendar*, London: London Record Society.

Childs, Wendy and Maryanne Kowaleski (2000), 'Fishing and Fisheries in the Middle Ages' and 'The Internal and International Fish Trades of Medieval England and Wales', in David Starkey, Chris Reid and Neil Ashcroft (eds), *England's Sea Fisheries: The Commercial Sea Fisheries of England and Wales Since 1300*, 19–35, London: Chatham Publishing.

Chipman, Leigh, Peter Pormann and Miriam Shefer-Mossensohn (2017), 'Introduction', Special Issue on Medicine, Part 1, *Intellectual History of the Islamicate World*, 5: 201–209.

Chipman, Leigh (2018), 'Islamic Medicine: Refractions of the Classical Past', in Roberta Casagrande-Kim, Samuel Thrope and Raquel Ukeles (eds), *Romance and Reason: Islamic Transformations of the Classical Past*, 64–83, Princeton: Princeton University Press.

Chiquart (2010), *Du fait de cuisine: On Cookery of Master Chiquart (1420)*, ed. Terence Scully, Tempe AZ: ACMRS.

Chouin, Gérard, ed. (2018), 'Sillages de la peste noire en Afrique subsaharienne: une exploration critique du silence/Black Death and its Aftermaths in Sub-Saharan Africa: A Critical Exploration of Silence', *Afriques*, 9. Available online: https://doi.org/10.4000/afriques.2084 (accessed 29 June 2020).

Choyke, Alice and Gerhard Jaritz, eds (2017), *Animaltown: Beasts in Medieval Urban Space*, Oxford: BAR Publishing.

Ciecieznski, Natalie (2013), 'The Stench of Disease: Public Health and the Environment in Late-medieval English Towns and Cities', *Health, Culture and Society*, 4: 91–104.

Cifuentes, Lluis and Carmel Ferragud (1999), 'El Libre de la menescalia de Manuel Díes: de espejo de caballeros a manual de albéitares', *Asclepio*, 60: 93–127.

Citrome, Jeremy (2006), *The Surgeon in Medieval English Literature*, New York: Palgrave Macmillan.

Clark, John Willis, ed. (1897), *The Observances in Use at the Augustinian Priory of St Giles and St Andrew at Barnwell, Cambridgeshire*, Cambridge: Macmillan and Bowes.

Clarke, Basil (1975), *Mental Disorder in Earlier Britain: Exploratory Studies*, Cardiff: University of Wales Press.

Clavel, Benoît (2001), 'L'Animal dans l'alimentation medieval et moderne en France du Nord (XIIIᵉ-XVIᵉ siècles)', special whole issue, *Revue Archéologique de Picardie*, 19.

Clover, Helen and Margaret Gibson, eds (1979), *The Letters of Lanfranc, Archbishop of Canterbury*, Oxford: Clarendon Press.

Cockayne, Emily (2007), *Hubbub: Filth, Noise and Stench in England, 1600–1770*, New Haven: Yale University Press.

Codoñer, Carmen (2008), 'Textes médicaux insérés dans les *Etymologiae* isidoriennes', *Cahiers de recherches médiévales*, 16: 17–37.

Cohen, Esther (2010), *The Modulated Scream: Pain in Late Medieval Culture*, Chicago: University of Chicago Press.

Cohen, Jennie (2012), 'Perforated Skulls from Middle Ages Found in Spain', *History in the Headlines*, 9 May, A+E Networks. Available online: www.history.com/news/perforated-skulls-from-middle-ages-found-in-spain (accessed 29 June 2020).

Cohen-Hanegbi, Naama and Uri Melammed (2013), 'Appendix: Jean of Avignon's Introduction to his Translation of *Lilium medicine*, an Annotated Critical Edition

BIBLIOGRAPHY

and Translation', in Gad Freudenthal and Resianne Fontaine (eds), *Latin into Hebrew, vol. 1: Studies*, 146–59, Leiden: Brill.

Cohen-Hanegbi, Naama (2016), 'Jean of Avignon: Conversing in Two Worlds', *Medieval Encounters*, 22: 165–92.

Cohen-Hanegbi, Naama (2017), *Caring for the Living Soul: Emotions, Medicine and Penance in the Late Medieval Mediterranean*, Leiden: Brill.

Cohn, Samuel (2013), 'The Historian and the Laboratory: The Black Death Disease', in Linda Clark and Carole Rawcliffe (eds), *Society in an Age of Plague*, 195–212, Woodbridge: The Boydell Press.

Collins, Minta (2000), *Medieval Herbals: The Illustrated Traditions*, London: British Library.

Connell, Brian, Amy Gray Jones, Rebecca Redfern, and Don Walker (2012), *A Bioarchaeological Study of Medieval Burials on the Site of St Mary Spital: Excavations at Spitalfield Market, London E1, 1991–2007*, London: Museum of London Archaeology.

Connelly, Erin and Stefanie Künzel, eds (2018), *Disease, Disability and Medicine in Medieval Europe*, Oxford: Archaeopress.

Cook, Michael (1986), 'Early Islamic Dietary Law', *Jerusalem Studies in Arabic and Islam*, 7: 217–77.

Cooke, Rachel (2016): 'Too Many Cookbooks Not Enough Broth', *The Guardian*, food and drink feature, Sunday 17 April. Available online: www.theguardian.com/commentisfree/2016/apr/17/too-many-cookbooks-not-enough-broth-gwyneth-paltrow (accessed 29 June 2020).

Condrau, Flurin (2007), 'The Patient's View Meets the Clinical Gaze', *Social History of Medicine*, 20: 525–40.

Coomans, Janna (2018), 'In Pursuit of a Healthy City: Sanitation and the Common Good in the Late Medieval Low Countries', PhD thesis, University of Amsterdam, Amsterdam, Netherlands.

Coomans, Janna (2019), 'The King of Dirt: Public Health and Sanitation in Late-Medieval Ghent', *Urban History*, 46: 82–105.

Coomans, Janna and Guy Geltner (2013), 'On the Street and in the Bathhouse: Medieval Galenism in Action?' *Anuario de Estudios Medievales*, 43: 53–82.

Cormack, Margaret, ed. (2012), 'Approaches to Childbirth in the Middle Ages', special issue, *Journal of the History of Sexuality*, 21: 201–324.

Corner, George (1927), *Anatomical Texts of the Earlier Middle Ages: A Study in the Transmission of Culture*. Washington DC: Carnegie.

Corporation of Nottingham (1882), *Records of the Borough of Nottingham*, vol. 1, London: Bernard Quaritch.

Cosman, Madeline (1973), 'Medieval Medical Malpractice: The *Dicta* and the Dockets', *Bulletin of the New York Academy of Medicine*, 49: 22–47.

Cosnet, Bertrand (2015), 'La transmission de l'iconographie des vertus dans les manuscrits italiens du XIVe siècle: La réinvention de la *Somme le roi*', in Joris Heyder and Christine Seidel (eds), *Re-Inventing Traditions: On the Transmission of Artistic Patterns in Late Medieval Manuscript Illumination*, 33–47, Berlin: Peter Lang.

Coste, Joël, Danielle Jacquart, and Jackie Pigeaud, eds (2012), *La rhétorique médicale à travers les siècles*, Geneva: Droz.

Crawford, Sally and Christina Lee, eds (2014), *Social Dimensions of Medieval Disease and Disability*, Oxford: Archaeopress.

Crisciani, Chiara (2004), 'Consilia, responsi, consulti: I pareri del medico tra insegnamento e professione', in Carla Casagrande, Chiara Crisciani, and Silvana Vecchio (eds), *Consilium: Teorie e pratiche*, 259–79, Florence: SISMEL/Edizioni del Galluzzo.

Cunningham, Andrew (2002), 'Identifying Disease in the Past: Cutting the Gordian Knot', *Asclepio*, 54: 13–34.

Curth, Louise Hill (2013), *A Plaine and Easie Waie to Remedy a Horse: Equine Medicine in Early Modern England*, Leiden: Brill.

Curtis, Valerie and Adam Birna (2001), 'Dirt, Disgust, and Disease: Is Hygiene in Our Genes?' *Perspectives in Biology and Medicine*, 44: 17–31.

Daileader, Philip (2016), *Saint Vincent Ferrer, His World and Life*, New York: Palgrave Macmillan.

Dam, Raymond van (1985), *Leadership and Community in Late Antique Gaul*, Berkeley: University of California Press.

D'Aronco, Maria (2007), 'The Transmission of Medical Knowledge in Anglo-Saxon England: The Voices of the Manuscripts', in Patrizia Lendinara, Loredana Lazzari and Maria D'Aronco (eds), *Form and Content of Instruction in Anglo-Saxon England in the Light of Contemporary Manuscript Evidence*, 35–58, Turnhout: Brepols.

Davis, Norman, ed. (1971), *Paston Letters and Papers of the Fifteenth Century*, part 1, Oxford: Oxford University Press.

De Groote, Koen (2005), 'The Use of Ceramics in Late Medieval and Early Modern Monasteries: Data from Three Sites in East Flanders (Belgium)', *Medieval Ceramics*, 29: 31–43.

Demaitre, Luke (1998), 'Medieval Notions of Cancer: Malignancy and Metaphor', *Bulletin of the History of Medicine*, 72: 609–37.

Demaitre, Luke (2003), 'The Art and Science of Prognostication in Early University Medicine', *Bulletin of the History of Medicine*, 77: 765–88.

Demaitre, Luke (2007), *Leprosy in Premodern Medicine: A Malady of the Whole Body*, Baltimore: Johns Hopkins University Press.

Demaitre, Luke (2013), *Medieval Medicine: The Art of Healing, from Head to Toe*, Santa Barbara: Praeger.

Demaitre, Luke (2015), 'Review of *Walking Corpses: Leprosy in Byzantium and the Medieval West*', *Bulletin of the History of Medicine*, 89: 339–40.

Deputy Keeper of the Records (1911), *Calendar of Close Rolls Preserved in the Public Record Office: Edward III*, vol. 13, 1369–1374, London: HMSO.

Deputy Keeper of the Records (1914), *Calendar of Patent Rolls Preserved in the Public Record Office: Edward III*, vol. 15, 1370–1374, London: HMSO.

Derham, Brendan (2002), 'The *Mary Rose* Medical Chest', in Robert Arnott (ed.), *The Archaeology of Medicine: Papers Given at a Session of the Annual Conference of the Theoretical Archaeology Group Held at the University of Birmingham on 20 December 1998*, 105–11, Oxford: BAR Publishing.

DeWitte, Sharon and Maryanne Kowaleski (2017), 'Black Death Bodies', *Fragments*, 6. Available online: http://hdl.handle.net/2027/spo.9772151.0006.001 (accessed 29 June 2020).

DeWitte, Sharon and Philip Slavin (2013), 'Between Famine and Death: England on the Eve of the Black Death: Evidence from Paleoepidemiology and Manorial Accounts', *Journal of Interdisciplinary History*, 44: 37–60.

Dickson, Camilla (1996), 'Food, Medicinal and Other Plants from the 15th Century drains of Paisley Abbey, Scotland', *Vegetation History and Archaeobotany*, 5: 25–31.

BIBLIOGRAPHY

DiMeo, Michelle and Sara Pennell, eds (2013), *Reading and Writing Recipe Books, 1550–1800*, Manchester: Manchester University Press.

Dixon, Piers, Ian Rogers, and Jerry O'Sullivan (2000), *Archaeological Excavations at Jedburgh Friary, 1983–1992*, Edinburgh: Scottish Trust for Archaeological Research.

Dobson, Mary (1997), *Contours of Death and Disease in Early Modern England*, Cambridge: Cambridge University Press.

Dols, Michael (1977), *The Black Death in the Middle East*, Princeton: Princeton University Press.

Doob, Penelope (1974), *Nebuchadnezzar's Children: Conventions of Madness in Middle English Literature*, New Haven: Yale University Press.

Douglas, Mary (1969), *Purity and Danger: An Analysis of the Concepts of Pollution and Taboo*, 2nd impression with corrections, London: Routledge & Kegan Paul.

Drobnick, Jim, ed. (2006), *The Smell Culture Reader*, Oxford and New York: Berg.

Duarte, King of Portugal (2011), *Leal Conselheiro*, ed. João Dionísio, Ibero-American Electronic Texts Series, Madison: University of Wisconsin-Madison. Available online: http://digicoll.library.wisc.edu/cgi-bin/IbrAmerTxt/IbrAmerTxt-idx?type=header&id=IbrAmerTxt.LealConsel (accessed 29 June 2020).

Dufeu, Val (2018), *Fish Trade in Medieval North Atlantic Societies: An Interdiscplinary Approach to Human Ecodynamics*, Amsterdam: Amsterdam University Press.

Duffin, Jacalyn (2007), 'The Doctor Was Surprised; Or How, to Diagnose a Miracle', *Bulletin of the History of Medicine*, 81: 699–729.

Dunning, Gerald (1969), 'The Apothecary's Mortar from Maison Dieu, Arundel', *Sussex Archaeological Collections*, 107: 77–8.

Durham, Brian (1992), 'The Infirmary and Hall of the Medieval Hospital of St John the Baptist at Oxford', *Oxoniensia*, 56: 17–75.

Dyer, Christopher (2006), 'Gardens and Garden Produce in the Later Middle Ages', in Christopher Woolgar, Dale Serjeantson and Tony Waldron (eds), *Food in Medieval England: Diet and Nutrition*, 27–40, Oxford: Oxford University Press.

Eamon, William and Gundolf Keil (1987), '"Plebs amat empirica:" Nicholas of Poland and his Critique of the Mediaeval Medical Establishment', *Sudhoffs Archiv*, 71: 180–96.

Ebner, Margaret (1993), *Major Works*, ed. Leonard Hindsley, New York: Paulist Press.

Egan, Geoff (1998), *The Medieval Household: Daily Living*, c. *1150–c. 1450*, London: HMSO.

Egan, Geoff (2007), 'Material Culture of Care for the Sick: Some Excavated Evidence from English Medieval Hospitals and Other Sites', in Barbara Bowers (ed.), *The Medieval Hospital and Medical Practice*, 65–76, Aldershot: Ashgate.

Egan, Geoff (2019), 'The Accessioned Finds', in Chiz Harward, Nick Holder, Christopher Phillpotts, and Christopher Thomas, *The Medieval Priory and Hospital of St Mary Spital and Bishopsgate Suburb: Excavations at Spitalfields Market, London E1, 1991–2007*, 256–83, London: MOLA Monograph.

Egan, Geoff and Frances Pritchard (2002), *Dress Accessories*, c. *1150–c. 1450*, Woodbridge: The Boydell Press.

Eijk, Philip van der (2005), 'The Heart, the Brain, the Blood and the *Pneuma*: Hippocrates, Diocles and Aristotle on the Location of Cognitive Processes', in Idem, *Medicine and Philosophy in Classical Antiquity: Doctors and Philosophers on Nature, Soul, Health and Disease*, 119–38, Cambridge: Cambridge University Press.

Eliav-Feldon, Miriam, Benjamin Isaac, and Joseph Ziegler, eds (2009), *The Origins of Racism in the Medieval West*, Cambridge: Cambridge University Press.

Ereshefsky, Marc (2009), 'Defining "Health" and "Disease"', *Studies in History and Philosophy of Biological and Biomedical Sciences*, 40: 221–27.

Ermacora, Davide (2015), 'Pre-Modern Bosom Serpents and Hippocrates, *Epidemiae* 5: 86: A Comparative and Contextual Folklore Approach', *Journal of Ethnology and Folkloristics*, 9: 75–119.

Eyler, Joshua, ed. (2010), *Disability in the Middle Age: Reconsiderations and Reverberations*, Farnham: Ashgate.

Fagan, Brian (2006), *Fish on Friday: Feasting, Fasting and the Discovery of the New World*, New York: Basic Books.

Fancy, Nahyan (2013), *Science and Religion in Mamluk Egypt: Ibn al-Nafis, Pulmonary Transit and Bodily Resurrection*, New York: Routledge.

Ferngren, Gary (2009), *Medicine and Health Care in Early Christianity*, Baltimore: Johns Hopkins University Press.

Ferragud, Carmel (2013), 'The Role of Doctors in the Slave Trade During the Fourteenth and Fifteenth Centuries within the Kingdom of Valencia', *Bulletin of the History of Medicine*, 87: 143–69.

Ferragud, Carmel (2014), 'Expert Examination of Wounds in the Criminal Court of Justice in Cocentaina (Kingdom of Valencia) During the Late Middle Ages', in Wendy J. Turner and Sara Butler (eds), *Medicine and the Law in the Middle Ages*, 109–32, Leiden: Brill.

Ferrer, Saint Vincent (1932–1938), *Sermons*, eds Josep Sanchis Sivera and Gret Schib, Editorial Barcino: Barcelona, 6 vols.

Ferrer, Saint Vincent (1973), *Sermons de Quaresma*, ed. M. Sanchs Guarner, 2 vols, Albatross Editions, Valencia.

Fidora, Alexander et al (2013), 'Introducing a Neglected Chapter in European Cultural History', in Resianne Fontain and Gad Freudenthal (eds), *Latin-into-Hebrew*, vol. 1: *Studies*, 9–18, Leiden: Brill.

Finger, Stanley (2001), *Origins of Neuroscience: A History of Explorations into Brain Function*, Oxford: Oxford University Press.

Finucane, Ronald (1977), *Miracles and Pilgrims: Popular Beliefs in Medieval England*, London: Dent.

Finucane, Ronald (1997), *The Rescue of the Innocents: Endangered Children in Medieval Miracles*, New York: St Martin's Press.

Fischer, Klaus-Dietrich (2000a), 'Dr. Monk's Medical Digest', *Social History of Medicine*, 13: 239–51.

Fischer, Klaus-Dietrich (2000b), 'The *Isagoge* of Pseudo-Soranus', *Medizinhistorisches Journal*, 35: 3–30.

Fischer, Klaus-Dietrich (2003), 'Der pseudogalenische *Liber tertius*', and 'Galeni qui fertur ad Glauconem Liber tertius ad fidem codicis Vindocinensis 109', in Ivan Garofalo and Amneris Roselli (eds), *Galenismo e Medicina tardoantica: fonti greche, latine e arabe*, 101–32 and 283–346, Naples: Annali dell'Istituto Universitario.

Fischer, Klaus-Dietrich (2007), 'Die Quellen des *Liber passionalis*', in Arsenio Ferraces Rodríquez (ed.), *Tradición griega y textos médicos latinos en el período presalernitano*, 105–25, A Coruña: Universidade da Coruña, Servicio de publicaciones.

Fischer, Klaus-Dietrich (2010), 'Das *Lorscher Arzneibuch* im Widerstreit der Meinung', *Medizinhistorisches Journal*, 45: 165–88.

Fischer, Klaus-Dietrich (2012), 'Wenn kein Arzt erreichbar ist: medizinische Literatur für Laien in der Spätantike', *Medicina nei Secoli: Arte e Scienza*, 24: 379–401.

BIBLIOGRAPHY

Fischer, Klaus-Dietrich (2013), 'Two Latin Pre-Salernitan Medical Manuals, the *Liber passionalis* and the *Tereoperica (Ps. Petroncellus)*', in Barbara Zipser (ed.), *Medical Books in the Byzantine World*, 35–56, Bologna: Eikasmós Online II.

Fissell, Mary (2004), 'Making Meaning from the Margins: The New Cultural History of Medicine', in Frank Huisman and John Harley Warner (eds), *Locating Medical History: The Stories and their Meanings*, 364–89, Baltimore: Johns Hopkins University Press.

Flanagan, Sabina (2005), 'Heresy, Madness, and Possession in the High Middle Ages', in Ian Hunter, John Laursen and Cary Nederman (eds), *Heresy in Transition: Transforming Ideas of Heresy in Medieval and Early Modern Europe*, 29–41, Aldershot: Ashgate.

Flandrin, Jean-Louis (2013): 'Seasoning, Cooking and Dietetics in the Late Middle Ages', in Jean-Louis Flandrin and Massimo Montanari (eds), *Food: A Culinary History*, trans. Albert Sonnenfeld, 313–27, New York: Columbia University Press.

Flemming, Rebecca (2000), *Medicine and the Making of Roman Women: Gender, Nature and Authority from Celsus to Galen*, Oxford: Oxford University Press.

Flint, Valerie (1989), 'The Early Medieval *medicus*, the Saint – and the Enchanter', *Social History of Medicine*, 2: 127–45.

Forcada, Miquel (2011), *Ética e ideología de la Ciencia: el medico-filósofo en al-Andalus*, Almería: Fundación Ibn Tufayl.

Foscati, Alessandra (2019), '"Nonnatus dictus quod caeso defunctae matris utero prodiit:" Postmortem Caesarean Section in the Late Middle Ages and Early Modern Period', *Social History of Medicine*, 32: 465–80.

Foucault, Michel (1961), *Histoire de la Folie*, Paris: Librairie Plon.

Fowden, Garth (1993), *Empire to Commonwealth: Consequences of Monotheism in Late Antiquity*, Princeton: Princeton University Press.

Fowden, Garth (2014), *Before and After Muḥammad: The First Millennium Refocused*, Princeton: Princeton University Press.

Foxhall, Katherine (2014), 'Making Modern Migraine Medieval: Men of Science, Hildegard of Bingen and the Life of a Retrospective Diagnosis', *Medical History*, 58: 354–74.

Franklin-Lyons, Adam (2009), 'Famine: Preparation and Response in Catalonia after the Black Death', PhD diss., Yale University, New Haven, USA.

Frantzen, Allen (2014), *Food, Eating and Identity in Early Medieval England*, Woodbridge: The Boydell Press.

Freedman, Paul (2008), *Out of the East: Spices and the Medieval Imagination*, New Haven: Yale University Press.

Freidenreich, David (2011), *Foreigners and their Food: Constructing Otherness in Jewish, Christian and Islamic Law*, Berkeley: University of California Press.

French, Katherine (2016), 'The Material Culture of Childbirth in Late Medieval London and its Suburbs', *Journal of Women's History*, 28: 126–48.

Frioux, Stéphane (2012), 'At a Green Crossroads: Recent Theses in Urban Environmental History in Europe and North America', *Urban History*, 39: 529–39.

Frohne, Bianca (2015), 'Performing Dis/ability? Constructions of "Infirmity" in Late Medieval and Early Modern Life Writing', in Christian Krötzl, Katariina Mustakallio and Jenni Kuuliala (eds), *Infirmity in Antiquity and the Middle Ages: Social and Cultural Approaches to Health, Weakness and Care*, 51–70, Farnham: Ashgate.

Frugard, Roger (1994), *Chirurgia*, in Tony Hunt (ed.), *Anglo-Norman Medicine*, vol. 1, 1–145, Cambridge: D.S. Brewer.

Fulbert of Chartres (1976), *The Letters and Poems of Fulbert of Chartres*, ed. and trans. Frederick Behrend, Oxford: Clarendon Press.

Furnivall, Frederick, ed. (1903), 'Of the Seats of the Passions', in Idem (ed.), *Political, Religious, and Love Poems*, London: Kegan Paul.

Furnivall, Frederick, ed. (1964), *Fifty Earliest English Wills in the Court of Probate, London: A. D. 1387–1439*, London, New York and Toronto: Oxford University Press. Available online: http://quod.lib.umich.edu/c/cme/EEWills (accessed 30 June 2020).

Galloway, James (2017), 'Fishing in Medieval England', in Michel Balard (ed.), *The Sea in History: The Medieval World*, 629–41, Woodbridge: The Boydell Press.

García Ballester, Luis (2002), 'On the Origins of the Six Non-Natural Things in Galen', in Idem, *Galen and Galenism: Theory and Medical Practice from Antiquity to the European Renaissance*, article IV, Aldershot: Ashgate Variorum Reprints.

García González, Alejandro, ed. (2007), *Alphita*, Florence: SISMEL/Edizioni del Galluzzo.

García González, Alejandro (2008), '*Hermeneumata medicobotanica vetustiora*: apuntes para una edición completa de los glosarios médico-botánicos altomedievales (siglos VIII–XI)', *Studi medievali*, 49: 119–39.

García Marsilla, Juan Vicente (2013), 'Alimentación y salud en la Valencia medieval: teorías y prácticas', *Anuario de Estudios Medievales*, 43: 115–58.

García Marsilla, Juan Vicente (2018), 'Food in the Accounts of a Travelling Lady: Maria de Luna, Queen of Aragon, in 1403', *Journal of Medieval History*, 44: 569–94.

Garden, Kenneth (2014), *The First Islamic Reviver: Abū Ḥāmid al-Ghazālī*, Oxford: Oxford University Press.

Gasper, Giles (2004), '"A Doctor in the House"? The Context for Anselm of Canterbury's Interest in Medicine with Reference to a Probable Case of Malaria', *Journal of Medieval History*, 30: 245–61.

Gasper, Giles and Faith Wallis (2016), '*Salsamenta Pictavensium*: Gastronomy and Medicine in Twelfth-Century England', *English Historical Review*, 131 (2016): 1353–85.

Geary, Patrick (1996), *Phantoms of Remembrance: Memory and Oblivion at the End of the First Millennium*, Princeton: Princeton University Press.

Gell, Alfred (1998), *Art and Agency: An Anthropological Theory*, Oxford: Clarendon Press.

Geltner, Guy (2011), 'Public Health and the Pre-Modern City: A Research Agenda', *History Compass*, 10: 231–45.

Geltner, Guy (2013), 'Healthscaping a Medieval City: Lucca's *Curia viarum* and the Future of Public Health History', *Urban History*, 40: 395–415.

Geltner, Guy (2014), 'Finding Matter Out of Place: Bologna's Fango ("Dirt") Notary in the History of Premodern Public Health', in Rosa Smurra, Hubert Houben and Manuela Ghizzoni (eds), *Lo sguardo lungimirante delle capitali: saggi in onore di Francesca Bocchi / The Far-sighted Gaze of Capital Cities: Essays in Honour of Francesca Bocchi*, 307–21, Rome: Viella.

Geltner, Guy (2018), 'Public Health', in Sarah Rubin Blanshei (ed.), *A Companion to Medieval Bologna*, 103–28, Leiden: Brill.

Geltner, Guy (2019a), 'In the Camp and on the March: Military Manuals as Sources for Studying Premodern Public Health', *Medical History*, 63: 44–60.

Geltner, Guy (2019b), *Roads to Health: Infrastructure and Urban Wellbeing in Later Medieval Italy*, Philadelphia, University of Pennsylvania Press.

BIBLIOGRAPHY

Gentilcore, David (2016), *Food and Health in Early Modern Europe: Diet, Medicine and Society, 1450–1800*, London: Bloomsbury.

Gerrard, Chris and David Petley (2013), 'A Risk Society? Environmental Hazards, Risk and Resilience in the Later Middle Ages in Europe', *Natural Hazards*, 69: 1051–79.

Getz, Faye, ed. (1991), *Healing and Society in Medieval England: A Medieval Translation of the Pharmaceutical Writings of Gilbertus Anglicus*, Wisconsin: University of Wisconsin Press.

al-Ghazali (2001), *Faith in Divine Unity and Trust in Divine Providence*, trans. David Burrell, Louisville: Fons Vitae.

Gilbertus Anglicus (1510), *Compendium medicine Gilberte Anglici*, Lyons: Jacobus Sacconus.

Gil Sotres, Pedro (1998), 'The Regimens of Health', in Mirko Grmek, (ed.), *Western Medical Thought from Antiquity to the Middle Ages*, coord. Bernardino Fantini, trans. Antony Shugaar, 291–318, Cambridge MA: Harvard University Press.

Giladi, Avner (2015), *Muslim Midwives: The Craft of Birthing in the Pre-Modern Middle East*, New York: Cambridge University Press.

Gilchrist, Roberta (1992), 'Christian Bodies and Souls: The Archaeology of Life and Death in Later Medieval Hospitals', in Steven Bassett (ed.), *Death in Towns: Urban Responses to the Dying and the Dead, 100–1600*, 101–18, London and New York: Leicester University Press.

Gilchrist, Roberta (1995), *Contemplation and Action: The Other Monasticism*, London and New York: Leicester University Press.

Gilchrist, Roberta (2005), *Norwich Cathedral Close: The Evolution of the English Cathedral Landscape*, Woodbridge: The Boydell Press.

Gilchrist, Roberta (2008), 'Magic for the Dead? The Archaeology of Magic in Later Medieval Burials', *Medieval Archaeology*, 52: 119–59.

Gilchrist, Roberta (2012), *Medieval Life: Archaeology and the Life Course*, Woodbridge: The Boydell Press.

Gilchrist, Roberta (2020), *Sacred Heritage: Monastic Archaeology, Identities, Beliefs*, Cambridge: Cambridge University Press.

Gilchrist, Roberta and Barney Sloane (2005), *Requiem: The Medieval Monastic Cemetery in Britain*, London: Museum of London Archaeology Service.

Gilmour, Brian and David Stocker (1986), *St Mark's Church and Cemetery*, London: Council for British Archaeology.

Giovanni Battista da Monte (1559), *Consilia Medica Omnia*, Nuremberg: in officina Ioannem Montanum, & Vlricum Neuberum.

Giovanni Matteo Ferrari da Grado (1535), *Consilia*, Lyon: In aedibus Jacobi Giunti.

Glaze, F. Eliza (2000), 'The Perforated Wall: The Ownership and Circulation of Medical Books in Medieval Europe, *c.* 800–1200', PhD diss., Duke University, Durham, USA.

Glaze, F. Eliza (2005), 'Galen Refashioned: Gariopontus of Salerno's *Passionarius* in the Later Middle Ages and Renaissance', in Elizabeth Lane Furdell (ed.), *Textual Healing, Essays in Medieval and Early Modern Medicine*, 53–77, Leiden: Brill.

Glaze, F. Eliza (2007), 'Master-Student Medical Dialogues: The Evidence of London, BL Sloane 2839', in Patrizia Lendinara, Loredana Lazzari and Maria D'Aronco (eds), *Form and Content of Instruction in Anglo-Saxon England in the Light of Contemporary Manuscript Evidence*, 467–94, Turnhout: Brepols.

Glaze, F. Eliza (2008), 'Gariopontus and the Salernitans: Textual Traditions in the Eleventh and Twelfth Centuries', in Danielle Jacquart and Agostino Paravicini

Bagliani (eds), *La 'Collectio Salernitana' di Salvatore De Renzi*, 149–90, Florence: SISMEL/Edizioni del Galluzzo.

Glaze, F. Eliza (2012), 'Medical Wisdom and Glossing Practices in and around Salerno, *c.* 1040–1200', in Anne Van Arsdall and Timothy Graham (eds), *Herbs and Healers from the Ancient Mediterranean through the Medieval West: Essays in Honor of John M. Riddle*, 63–107, Farnham: Ashgate.

Glaze, F. Eliza (2018), 'Salerno's Lombard Prince: Johannes "Abbas de Curte", as Medical Practitioner', *Early Science and Medicine*, 23: 177–216.

Glaze, F. Eliza (2019), 'Introduction. Constantine the African and the *Pantegni* in Context', in Erik Kwakkel and Francis Newton, *Medicine at Monte Cassino: Constantine the African and the Oldest Manuscript of his 'Pantegni'*, 1–29, Turnhout: Brepols.

Glaze, F. Eliza and Brian Nance, eds (2011), *Between Text and Patient: The Medical Enterprise in Medieval and Early Modern Europe*, Florence: SISMEL/Edizioni del Galluzzo.

Gläser, Manfred, ed. (2004), *Lübecker Kolloquium zur Stadtarchäologie im Hanseraum IV: Die Infrastruktur*, Lübeck: Schmidt-Römhild.

Gomes, Sandra Rute Fonseca (2011), 'Territórios medievais do pescado do Reino de Portugal', MA diss., University of Coimbra, Coimbra, Portugal.

Goodey, Christopher (2011), *A History of Intelligence and 'Intellectual Disability': The Shaping of Psychology in Early Modern Europe*, Farnham: Ashgate.

Goodich, Michael (2005), 'Microhistory and the *Inquisitiones* into the Life and Miracles of Philip of Bourges and Thomas of Hereford', in Werner Verbeke, Ludo Milis and Jean Goossens (eds), *Medieval Narrative Sources: A Gateway into the Medieval Mind*, 91–106, Leuven: Leuven University Press.

Goodich, Michael (2007), *Miracles and Wonders: The Development of the Concept of Miracle, 1150–1350*, Aldershot: Ashgate.

Gordon, Stephen (2014), 'Disease, Sin and the Walking Dead in Medieval England, *c.* 1100–1350: A Note on the Documentary and Archaeological Evidence', in Effie Gemi-Ioranou, et al (eds), *Medicine, Healing and Performance*, 56–70, Oxford: Oxbow.

Gordon, Stephen (2015), 'Medical Condition, Demon or Undead Corpse? Sleep Paralysis and the Nightmare in Medieval Europe', *Social History of Medicine*, 28: 425–44.

Govantes-Edwards, David, Chloë Duckworth, and Ricardo Córdoba (2016), 'Recipes and Experimentation? The Transmission of Glassmaking Techniques in Medieval Iberia', *Journal of Medieval Iberian Studies*, 8: 176–95.

Gower, John (1901), 'Confessio Amantis', Book 6, in George Macaulay (ed.), *The English Works of John Gower*, vol. 2, London: Kegan Paul, Trench, Trubner & Co.

Gowland, Rebecca and Bennjamin Penny-Mason (2018), 'Overview: Archaeology and the Medieval Life Course', in Christopher Gerrard and Alejandra Gutiérrez (eds), *The Oxford Handbook of Later Medieval Archaeology in Britain*, 759–73, Oxford: Oxford University Press.

Grainger, Ian, Duncan Hawkins, Lynn Cowal, and Richard Mikulski (2008), *The Black Death Cemetery, East Smithfield, London*, London: Museum of London.

Grant, Edward, ed. (1974), *A Source Book in the History of Science*, Cambridge, MA: Harvard University Press.

Grant, Mark, ed. (1997), *Dieting for an Emperor: A Translation of Books 1 and 4 of Oribasius' Medical Compilations with an Introduction and Commentary*, Leiden: Brill.

Grant, Mark, ed. (2000), *Galen on Food and Diet*, London: Routledge.

BIBLIOGRAPHY

Gratian (1861), *Decretum*, Patrologia Latina 187, ed. Jacques-Paul Migne, Paris: Imprimerie Catholique.

Graves, C. Pamela (2008), 'From an Archaeology of Iconoclasm to an Anthropology of the Body: Images, Punishment and Personhood in England, *c*. 1500–1660', *Current Anthropology*, 49: 35–60.

Greco, Gina and Christine Rose, eds (2009), *The Good Wife's Guide:* Le Ménagier de Paris, *A Medieval Household Book*, Ithaca: Cornell University Press.

Green, Monica (1989), 'Women's Medical Practice and Health Care in Medieval Europe', *Signs: Working Together in the Middle Ages: Perspectives on Women's Communities*, 14: 434–73.

Green, Monica (2005), 'Bodies, Gender, Health, Disease: Recent Work on Medieval Women's Medicine', *Studies in Medieval and Renaissance History*, 3rd series, 2: 1–49.

Green, Monica (2008), *Making Women's Medicine Masculine: The Rise of Male Authority in Pre-Modern Gynaecology*, Oxford: Oxford University Press.

Green, Monica (2009), 'Integrative Medicine: Incorporating Medicine and Health into the Canon of Medieval European History', *History Compass*, 7: 1218–45.

Green, Monica (2010), 'The Diversity of Human Kind', in Linda Kalof (ed.), *A Cultural History of the Human Body in the Middle Ages*, 173–90, Oxford: Berg.

Green, Monica (2011), 'History of Medicine or History of Health?' *Past and Future*, 9: 7–9. Available online: www.academia.edu/5219204/Monica_H._Green_History_ of_Medicine_or_History_of_Health_Past_and_Future_issue_9_Spring_ Summer_2011_7-9 (accessed 29 June 2020).

Green, Monica (2012), 'The Value of Historical Perspective', in Ted Schrecker (ed.), *The Ashgate Research Companion to the Globalization of Health*, 17–37, Aldershot: Ashgate.

Green, Monica (2015), 'Crafting a (Written) Science of Surgery: The First European Surgical Texts', REMEDIA: The History of Medicine in Dialogue with its Present. Available online: https://remedianetwork.net/2015/10/13/crafting-a-written-science-of-surgery-the-first-european-surgical-texts/ (accessed 29 June 2020).

Green, Monica (2017), ''Cliff-Notes' on the Circulation of the Gynecological Texts of Soranus and Muscio in the Middle Ages', available online: www.academia. edu/7858536/Monica_H._Green_Cliff_Notes_on_the_Circulation_of_the_ Gynecological_Texts_of_Soranus_and_Muscio_in_the_Middle_Ages_2017 (accessed 29 June 2020).

Green, Monica (2018), 'Medical Books', in Erik Kwakkel and Rodney Thomson (eds), *The European Book in the Twelfth Century*, 277–92, Cambridge: Cambridge University Press.

Green, Monica, ed. (2001), *The Trotula: A Medieval Compendium of Women's Medicine*, Philadelphia: University of Pennsylvania Press.

Green, Monica, ed. (2014), *Pandemic Disease in the Medieval World: Rethinking the Black Death*, Kalamazoo: Arc Medieval Press.

Gregory, Stewart, ed. (1990), *The Twelfth-Century Psalter Commentary in French for Laurette D'Alsace (An Edition of Psalms I–XXXV)*, vol. 1, London: Modern Humanities Research Association.

Gutas, Dimitri (1998), *Greek Thought, Arabic Culture: The Graeco-Arabic Translation Movement in Baghdad and Early 'Abbāsid Society (2nd–4th/8th–10th centuries)*, New York: Routledge.

Haider, Najam (2014), *Shīʿī Islam: An Introduction*, Cambridge: Cambridge University Press.

Hanawalt, Barbara (1986), *The Ties that Bound: Peasant Families in Medieval England*, New York: Oxford University Press.

Handley, Sasha (2016), *Sleep in Early-Modern England*, New Haven: Yale University Press.

Hanson, Ann Ellis and Monica Green (1994), 'Soranus of Ephesus: *Methodicorum Princeps*', *Aufstieg und Niedergang der Römischen Welt*, Teil 2, Band 37.2: 968–1075.

Harper, Stephen (2003), *Insanity, Individuals, and Society in Late-Medieval English Literature: The Subject of Madness*, Lewiston: Edwin Mellen.

Harris, Marvin (1976), 'History and Significance of the Emic/Etic Distinction', *Annual Review of Anthropology*, 5: 329–50.

Harris, Mary Dormer (1907–1913), *The Coventry Leet Book: Or Mayor's Register, Containing the records of the City Court Leet or View of Frankpledge, A.D. 1420–1555, with Divers other matters*, 4 parts, London: Kegan Paul, Trench, Trübner & Co.

Harris, Nichola E. (2016), 'Loadstones are a Girl's Best Friend: Lapidary Cures, Midwives and Manuals of Popular Healing in Medieval and Early-Modern England', in Barbara Bowers and Linda Keyser (eds), *The Sacred and the Secular in Medieval Healing: Sites, Objects, and Texts*, 182–218, New York: Routledge.

Harris-Stoertz, Fiona (2014), 'Midwives in the Middle Ages? Birth Attendants, 600–1300', in Sara Butler and Wendy J. Turner (eds), *Medicine and the Law in the Middle Ages*, 58–87, Leiden: Brill.

Hartnell, Jack (2017a), 'Surgical Saws and Cutting Edge Agency', in Grażyna Jurkowlaniec, Ika Matyjaszkiewicz and Zuzann Sarnecka (eds), *The Agency of Things in Medieval and Early Modern Art: Materials, Power and Manipulation*, 156–71, Abingdon: Routledge.

Hartnell, Jack (2017b), 'Tools of the Puncture: Skin, Knife, Bone, Hand', in Larissa Tracy (ed.), *Flaying in the Pre-Modern World: Practice and Representation*, 20–50, Woodbridge: The Boydell Press.

Hartnell, Jack (2018), *Medieval Bodies: Life, Death and Art in the Middle Ages*, London: Wellcome Collection.

Harvey, Barbara (1993), *Living and Dying in England 1100–1540: The Monastic Experience*, Oxford: Clarendon Press.

Harward, Chiz, Nick Holder, Christopher Phillpotts, and Christopher Thomas (2019), *The Medieval Priory and Hospital of St Mary Spital and Bishopsgate Suburb: Excavations at Spitalfields Market, London E1, 1991–2007*, London: MOLA Monograph.

Hasse, Dag Nikolaus (2016), *Success and Suppression: Arabic Sciences and Philosophy in the Renaissance*, Cambridge MA: Harvard University Press.

Havlíček, Filip, Adéla Pokorná and Jakub Zálešák (2017), 'Waste Management and Attitudes Towards Cleanliness in Medieval Central Europe', *Journal of Landscape Ecology*, 10: 266–87.

Heng, Geraldine (2018), *The Invention of Race in the European Middle Ages*, Cambridge: Cambridge University Press.

Henri de Mondeville (1893), *Chirurgie de maître Henri de Mondeville*, ed. Edouard Nicaise, Paris: Felix Alcan.

Henry of Grosmont (2014), *The Book of Holy Medicines*, ed. Catherine Batt, Tempe: ACMRS.

Hieatt, Constance and Sharon Butler, eds (1985), *Curye on Inglysch: English Culinary Manuscripts of the Fourteenth Century (Including the Forme of Cury)*, London: Early English Text Society/Oxford University Press.

BIBLIOGRAPHY

Hildburgh, Walter (1908), 'Notes on Some Amulets of the Three Magi Kings', *Folklore*, 19: 83–7.

Hillson, Simon (1996), *Dental Anthropology*, Cambridge: Cambridge University Press.

Hoeniger, Cathleen (2006), 'The Illuminated *Tacuinum sanitatis* Manuscripts from Northern Italy *c.* 1380–1400: Sources, Patrons, and the Creation of a New Pictorial Genre', in Jean Givens, Karen Reeds and Alain Touwaide (eds), *Visualizing Medieval Medicine and Natural History, 1200–1550*, 51–81, Aldershot: Ashgate.

Hoffman, Richard (1996), 'Economic Development and Aquatic Water Systems in Medieval Europe', *American Historical Review*, 101: 631–69.

Holmbäck, Åke and Elias Wessen, eds (1966), *Magnus Erikssons Stadslag i Nusvensk Tolkning*, Lund: Carl Bloms Boktryckeri.

Holmes, Catherine and Naomi Standen, eds (2018), 'The Global Middle Ages', *Past & Present*, 238, supplement 13.

Holton-Krayenbuhl, Anne (1997), 'The Infirmary Complex at Ely', *Archaeological Journal*, 154: 118–72.

Hooper, Jill (2006), 'Waste and its Disposal in Southwark', *The London Archaeologist*, 11: 95–100.

Hopwood, Nick, Rebecca Flemming, and Lauren Kassell, eds (2018), *Reproduction: Antiquity to the Present Day*, Cambridge: Cambridge University Press.

Horden, Peregrine (2007), 'A Non-natural Environment: Medicine Without Doctors and the Medieval European Hospital', in Barbara Bowers (ed.), *The Medieval Hospital and Medical Practice*, 133–46, Aldershot: Ashgate.

Horden, Peregrine (2008), 'Sickness and Healing', in Thomas Noble and Julia Smith (eds), *The Cambridge History of Christianity. Volume 3: Early Medieval Christianities, c. 600–c. 1100*, 416–32, Cambridge: Cambridge University Press.

Horden, Peregrine (2011), 'What's Wrong with Early Medieval Medicine?' *Social History of Medicine*, 24: 5–25.

Horden, Peregrine and Elisabeth Hsu, eds (2013), *The Body in Balance: Humoral Medicines in Practice*, New York: Berghahn.

Howell, Martha (2000), 'The Spaces of Late Medieval Urbanity', in Marc Brown and Peter Stabel (eds), *Shaping Urban Identity in Late Medieval Europe*, 3–24, Louvain, Belgium: Garant Publishers.

Hsy, Jonathan (2015), 'Disability', in David Hillman and Ulrika Maude (eds), *Cambridge Companion to the Body in Literature*, 24–40, Cambridge: Cambridge University Press.

Hudson, William, ed. (1892) *Leet Jurisdiction in the City of Norwich during the XIIIth and XIVth Centuries*, Seldon Society Publication vol. 5, London: B. Quaritch.

Hudson, William and John Cottingham Tingey, eds (1908–1910), *The Records of the City of Norwich*, Norwich: Jarrold & Sons.

Huff, Toby (2003), *The Rise of Early Modern Science: Islam, China, and the West*, 2nd edn, Cambridge: Cambridge University Press.

Huff, Toby (2010), *Intellectual Curiosity and the Scientific Revolution: A Global Perspective*, Cambridge: Cambridge University Press.

Huggon, Martin (2018), 'Medieval Medicine, Public Health, and the Medieval Hospital', in Christopher Gerrard and Alejandra Gutiérrez (eds), *The Oxford Handbook of Later Medieval Archaeology in Britain*, 759–73. Oxford: Oxford University Press.

Hunt, Tony (1990), *Popular Medicine in Thirteenth-century England*. Woodbridge: D.S. Brewer.

Huot, Sylvia (2003), *Madness in Medieval French Literature: Identities Found and Lost*, Oxford: Oxford University Press.

Hydén, Lars-Christer (1997), 'Illness and Narrative', *Sociology of Health & Illness*, 19: 48–89.

Ibn Khaldun (1958), *The Muqaddimah*, trans. Franz Rosenthal, 3 vols, Princeton: Princeton University Press.

Ingram, Hannah (2019), '"Pottes of Tryacle" and "Bokes of Phisyke": The Fifteenth-Century Disease Management Practices of Three Gentry Families', *Social History of Medicine*, 32: 751–72.

Innes, Cosmo Nelson, ed. (1868), *Ancient Laws & Customs of the Burghs of Scotland*, vol. 1: 1124–1424, Edinburgh: Printed for the Scottish Burgh Records Society.

Isabella d'Este (2017), *Selected Letters*, ed. and trans. Deanna Shemek, Toronto: Iter Press.

Isidore of Seville (1911), *Isidori Hispalensis episcopi Etymologiarym sive originum libri XX*, ed. Wallace Lindsay, Oxford: Clarendon Press.

Isidore of Seville (2006), *The Etymologies of Isidore of Seville*, ed. Stephen Barney with Muriel Hall, Cambridge: Cambridge University Press.

Ispahany, Batool, ed. (2000), *Islamic Medical Wisdom: The* Tibb al-a'imma, trans. Andrew Newman, Qom: Ansariyan Publication.

Ivo of Chartres (1854), *Opera Omnia*, Patrologia Latina 162, ed. Jacques-Paul Migne, Paris: Imprimerie Catholique.

Ivry, Alfred (2012), 'Arabic and Islamic Psychology and Philosophy of Mind', in Edward Zalta (ed.), *The Stanford Encyclopedia of Philosophy*. Available online: https://plato.stanford.edu/archives/sum2012/entries/arabic-islamic-mind/ (accessed 29 June 2020).

Izkander, Albert (1976), 'An Attempted Reconstruction of the Late Alexandrian Medical Curriculum', *Medical History*, 20: 235–58.

Jackson, Stanley (1986), *Melancholia and Depression from Hippocratic Times to Modern Times*, New Haven: Yale University Press.

Jacques, Kevin (2009), *Ibn Hajar*, New Delhi: Oxford University Press India.

Jansen-Sieben, Ria (1994), 'From Food Therapy to Cookery Book', in Erik Kooper (ed.), *Medieval Dutch Literature in its European Context*, 261–79, Cambridge: Cambridge University Press.

Janson, Horst (1952), *Apes and Ape Lore in the Middle Ages and Renaissance*, London: Warburg Institute.

Jardine, Nick (2004), 'Etics and Emics (Not to Mention Anemics and Emetics) in the History of the Sciences', *History of Science*, 42: 261–78.

Jáuregui, Clara (2018), 'Inside the *Leprosarium*: Illness in the Daily Life of Barcelona', in Erin Connelly and Stefanie Künzel (eds), *Disease, Disability and Medicine in Medieval Europe*, 78–93, Oxford: Archaeopress.

Jean Gobi (1991), *La Scala coeli*, ed. Marie Anne Polo de Beaulieu, Paris: Centre National de la Recherche Scientifique.

John of Salisbury (1990), *Policraticus: of the Frivolities of Courtiers and the Footprints of Philosophers*, ed. Cary Nederman, Cambridge: Cambridge University Press.

Johnston, Ian, trans. (2006), *Galen: On Diseases and Symptoms*, Cambridge: Cambridge University Press.

Jones, Peter Murray (1998), *Medieval Medicine in Illuminated Manuscripts*, London: British Library.

Jones, Peter Murray and Lea Olsan (2015), 'Performative Rituals for Conception and Childbirth in England, 900–1500', *Bulletin of the History of Medicine*, 89: 406–33.

Jones, Peter Murray and Lea Olsan (2019), 'Medicine and Magic', in Sophie Page and Catherine Rider (eds), *The Routledge History of Medieval Magic*, 299–311, Abingdon: Routledge.

Jones, Richard (2013), *The Medieval Natural World*, Harlow: Pearson.

Jordan, William Chester (1996), *The Great Famine: Northern Europe in the Early Fourteenth Century*, Princeton: Princeton University Press.

Jørgensen, Dolly (2008), 'Cooperative Sanitation: Managing Streets and Gutters in Late Medieval England and Scandinavia', *Technology and Culture*, 49: 547–67.

Jørgensen, Dolly (2010a), '"All Good Rule of the Citee": Sanitation and Civic Government in England, 1400–1600', *Journal of Urban History*, 36: 300–315.

Jørgensen, Dolly (2010b), 'Local Government Responses to Urban River Pollution in Late Medieval England', *Water History*, 2: 35–52.

Jørgensen, Dolly (2010c), '*The Metamorphosis of Ajax*, Jakes, and Early-Modern Urban Sanitation', *Early Modern Studies Journal*, 3. Available online, www.uta.edu/english/ees/fulltext/jorgensen3.html (accessed 29 June 2020).

Jørgensen, Dolly (2013a), 'The Medieval Sense of Smell, Stench and Sanitation', in Ulrike Krampl, Robert Beck and Emmanuelle Retaillaud-Bajac (eds), *The Five Senses of the City*, 301–13, Tours: Presses Universitaires François-Rabelais.

Jørgensen, Dolly (2013b), 'Running Amuck? Urban Swine Management in Late Medieval England', *Agricultural History*, 87: 429–51.

Jørgensen, Dolly (2014), 'Modernity and Medieval Muck', *Nature and Culture*, 9: 225–37.

Joyce, Rosemary (2005), 'Archaeology of the Body', *Annual Review of Anthropology*, 34: 139–54.

Katajala-Peltomaa, Sari (2010), 'Recent Trends in the Study of Medieval Canonizations', *History Compass*, 8/9: 1083–92.

Katajala-Peltomaa, Sari and Susanna Niiranen, eds (2014), *Mental (Dis)Order in Later Medieval Europe*, Leiden: Brill.

Kaye, Joel (2014), *A History of Balance, 1250–1375: The Emergence of a New Model of Equilibrium and its Impact on Thought*, Cambridge: Cambridge University Press.

Kaye, J[ohn] M., ed. (1966), *Placita corone; or, La corone pledée devant justices*, London: Quaritch for the Selden Society.

Keene, Derek (1982), 'Rubbish in Medieval Towns', in Allan Hall and Harry Kenward (eds), *Environmental Archaeology in the Urban Context*, 26–30, London: Council for British Archaeology.

Keil, Gundolf and Paul Schnitzer, eds (1991), *Das Lorscher Arzneibuch und die frühmittelalterliche Medizin: Verhandlungen des medizinhistorischen Symposiums im September 1989 in Lorsch*, Lorsch: Verlag Laurissa.

Kelleher, Marie (2013), 'Eating from a Corrupted Table: Food Regulations and Civic Health in Barcelona's "First Bad Year"', *E-Humanista*, 25: 51–64. Available online: www.ehumanista.ucsb.edu/volumes/25 (accessed 29 June 2020).

Kozodoy, Maud (2019), 'Late Medieval Jewish Physicians and their Manuscripts', *Social History of Medicine*, 32: 734–50.

King, Gary and Charlotte Henderson (2014), 'Living Cheek by Jowl: The Pathoecology of Medieval York', *Quaternary International*, 341: 131–42.

King, Peter (2010), 'Emotions in Medieval Thought', in Peter Goldie (ed.), *The Oxford Handbook of Philosophy of Emotion*, 167–88, Oxford: Oxford University Press.

Kingdom, Mandy (2019), 'The Past People of Exeter: Health, Social Standing and Well-being in the Middle Ages and Early Modern Period', PhD diss., University of Exeter, Exeter, UK.

Kirkham, Anne and Cordelia Warr, eds (2014), *Wounds in the Middle Ages*, Farnham: Ashgate.

Klassen, John, ed. (2001), *The Letters of the Rožmberk Sisters: Noblewomen in Fifteenth-Century Bohemia*, Cambridge: D.S. Brewer.

Klein-Franke, Felix (1980), *Die Klassische Antike in der Tradition des Islam*, Darmstadt: Wissenschaftliche Buchgesellschaft.

Kleinman, Arthur (1988), *The Illness Narratives: Suffering, Healing, and the Human Condition*, New York, Basic Books.

Kowaleski, Maryanne (2016), 'The Early Documentary Evidence for the Commercialisation of the Sea Fisheries in Medieval Britain', in James Barrett and David Orton (eds), *Cod and Herring: the Archaeology and History of Medieval Sea Fishing*, 23–41, Oxford: Oxbow.

Kristjánsdóttir, Steinunn (2010), 'The Tip of the Iceberg: The Material of Skriðuklaustur Monastery and Hospital', *Norwegian Archaeological Review*, 43: 44–62.

Kroll, Jerome and Bernard Bachrach (1984), 'Sin and Mental Illness in the Middle Ages', *Psychological Medicine*, 14: 507–14.

Krötzl, Christian, Katariina Mustakallio, and Jenni Kuuliala, eds (2015), *Infirmity in Antiquity and the Middle Ages: Social and Cultural Approaches to Health, Weakness and Care*, Farnham: Ashgate.

Krug, Ilana (2015), 'The Wounded Soldier: Honey and Late Medieval Military Medicine', in Larissa Tracy and Kelly DeVries (eds), *Wounds and Wound Repair in Medieval Culture*, 94–214, Leiden: Brill.

Kucher, Michael (2005), 'The Use of Water and its Regulation in Medieval Siena', *Journal of Urban History*, 31: 504–36.

Kurlansky, Mark (1999), *Cod: A Biography of the Fish that Changed the World*, London: Vintage.

Kunst, Günther Karl (2017), 'What Makes a Medieval Urban Animal Bone Assemblage Look Urban? Reflections on Feature Types and Recurrent Patterns from Lower Austria and Vienna', in Alice Choyke and Gerhard Jaritz (eds), *Animaltown: Beasts in Medieval Urban Space*, 9–18, Oxford: BAR Publishing.

Kuuliala, Jenni (2016), *Childhood Disability and Social Integration in the Middle Ages: Constructions of Impairments in Thirteenth- and Fourteenth-Century Canonization Processes*, Turnhout: Brepols.

Kwakkel, Erik and Francis Newton (2019), *Medicine at Monte Cassino: Constantine the African and the Oldest Manuscript of his 'Pantegni'*, Turnhout: Brepols.

Ladher, Navjoyt (2016), 'Nutrition Science in the Media: You Are What You Read', *British Medical Journal*, 353. Available online: https://doi.org/10.1136/bmj.i1879 (accessed 29 June 2020).

Lambourn, Elizabeth (2018), *Abraham's Luggage. A Social Life of Things in the Medieval Indian Ocean World*, Cambridge: Cambridge University Press.

Landgraf, Erhard (1928), 'Ein frühmittelalterlicher Botanicus', *Kyklos*, 1: 114–46.

Langermann, Tzvi and Robert Morrison, eds (2016), *Texts in Transit in the Medieval Mediterranean*, University Park: Pennsylvania State University Press.

Langslow, David (2006), *The Latin Alexander Trallianus: The Text and Transmission of a Late Latin Medical Book*, London: Society for the Promotion of Roman Studies.

Langslow, David (2007), 'The *Epistula* in Ancient Scientific and Technical Literature, with Special Reference to Medicine', in Ruth Morello and Andrew Morrison (eds), *Ancient Letters: Classical and Late Antique Epistolography*, 211–34, Oxford: Oxford University Press.

BIBLIOGRAPHY

Langum, Virginia (2016), *Medicine and the Seven Deadly Sins in Late Medieval Literature and Culture*, New York: Palgrave Macmillan.

Laurentius Rusius (1867), *La mascalcia di Lorenzo Rusio volgarizzamento del secolo XIV*, ed. Pietro Delprato and Luigi Barbieri, vol. 1, Bologna: Presso Gaetano Romagnoli.

Laurioux, Bruno (2002), *Manger au Moyen Âge*, Paris: Hachette Littératures.

Laurioux, Bruno (2006a), 'Cuisine et médecine au Moyen Âge: alliées ou ennemies?' *Cahiers de recherches médiévales*, 13: 223–38.

Laurioux, Bruno (2006b), *Gastronomie, humanisme et société à Rome au milieu du XVᵉ Siècle: autour du* De honesta voluptate *de Platina*, Florence: SISMEL/Edizioni del Galluzzo.

Laurioux, Bruno (2016), 'Cuisine, médecine et diététique: traditions, rencontres, distorsions entre le Vᵉ et le XIIᵉ siècle', in (no editor), *L'Alimentazione nell'Alto Medioevo: pratiche, simboli, ideologie*, vol. 1, 467–92, Spoleto: Fondazione Centro Italiano di Studi sull'Alto Medioevo.

Laux, Rudolf (1930), '*Ars medicinae*: Ein frühmittelalterliches Kompendium der Medizin', *Kyklos*, 3: 417–34.

LeClercq, Jean and Henri Rochais, eds (1979), *Sancti Bernardi Opera*, book 7, Rome: Editiones Cistercienses.

Le Cornec, Cécile (2006), 'Les vertus diététiques attribuées aux poissons de mer', in Chantal Connochie-Bourgne (ed.), *Mondes marins du Moyen Âge*, 271–83, Aix-en-Provence: Université de Provence.

Lee, Christina (2012), 'Disability', in Jacqueline Stodnick and Renée Trilling (eds), *A Handbook of Anglo-Saxon Studies*, 23–38, Chichester: Wiley-Blackwell.

Le Goff, Jacques (2015), *Must We Divide History into Periods?* New York: Columbia University Press.

Leguay, Jean-Pierre (1999), *La Pollution au Moyen Age*, Paris: Editions Jean-Paul Gisserot.

Leja, Meg (2016), 'The Sacred Art: Medicine in the Carolingian Renaissance', *Viator*, 47: 1–34.

Leong, Elaine (2014), '"Herbals She Peruseth": Reading Medicine in Early-Modern England', *Renaissance Studies*, 28: 556–78.

Lev, Efraim and Zohar Amar (2008), *Practical Materia Medica of the Medieval Eastern Mediterranean According to the Cairo Genizah*, Leiden: Brill.

Lewicka, Paulina (2011), *Food and Foodways of Medieval Cairenes: Aspects of Life in an Islamic Metropolis of the Eastern Mediterranean*, Leiden: Brill.

Lewicka, Paulina (2014), 'Diet as Culture: on the Medical Context of Food Consumption in the Medieval Middle East', *History Compass*, 12: 607–17.

Lewis, Carenza (2016), 'Disaster Recovery: New Archaeological Evidence for the Long-term Impact of the "Calamitous" Fourteenth Century', *Antiquity*, 90: 777–97.

Leyaker, Josef (1927), 'Zur Entstehung der Lehre von den Hirnventrikeln als Sitz psychischer Vermögen', *Archiv für Geschichte der Medizin*, 19: 253–86.

Lindberg, David (2002), 'Early Christian Attitudes toward Nature', in Gary Ferngren (ed.), *Science and Religion: A Historical Introduction*, 47–56, Baltimore: Johns Hopkins University Press.

Linden, David (1999), 'Gabriele Zerbi's *De cautelis medicorum* and the Tradition of Medical Prudence', *Bulletin of the History of Medicine*, 73: 19–37.

Lister, John, ed. (1917), *Court Rolls of the Manor of Wakefield, vol. III, 1313 to 1316, and 1286*, Leeds: Yorkshire Archaeological Society.

Litzenburger, Laurent (2016), 'La sécurité alimentaire et sanitaire à Metz à la fin du Moyen Âge', *Histoire Urbaine*, 47: 131–48.

Livingston, Michael (2015), '"The Depth of Six Inches": Prince Hal's Head-Wound at the Battle of Shrewsbury', in Larissa Tracy and Kelly DeVries (eds), *Wounds and Wound Repair in Medieval Culture*, 215–30, Leiden: Brill.

Livius (2016), 'Medieval Copper Scourge Found at Rufford Abbey', *The History Blog*, 4 April. Available online: www.thehistoryblog.com/archives/41442 (accessed 12 September 2017).

Lloyd, Geoffrey, ed. (1978), *Hippocratic Writings*, Harmondsworth: Penguin.

Lugt, Maaike van der (2011), 'Neither Ill nor Healthy: The Intermediate State Between Health and Disease in Medieval Medicine', *Quaderni Storici*, 136: 13–46.

Lydgate, John (1934), 'Tyed with a Lyne', in Henry Noble MacCracken (ed.), *The Minor Poems of John Lydgate: Part II, Secular Poems*, 832–4, London: Oxford University Press.

Maddern, Philippa (2018), '"It is Full Merry in Heaven": The Pleasurable Connotations of "Merriment" in Late Medieval England', in Naama Cohen-Hanegbi and Piroska Nagy (eds), *Pleasure in the Middle Ages*, 21–38, Turnhout: Brepols.

Magilton, John, Frances Lee and Anthea Boylston, eds (2008), *Lepers Outside the Gate: Excavations at the Cemetery of the Hospital of St James and St Mary Magdalene, Chichester, 1986–1987 and 1993*, York: Council for British Archaeology.

Maimonides, Moses (1964), 'Moses Maimonides' Two Treatises on the Regimen of Health: Fī Tadbīr al-Sihhah and Maqālah fi Bayān Ba'd al-A'rād wa-al-Jawāb 'anhā', ed. Ariel Bar-Sela, Hebbel Hoff and Elias Faris, *Transactions of the American Philosophical Society*, 54: 3–50.

Moses Maimonides (2009), *On Poisons and the Protection against Lethal Drugs*, eds Gerrit Bos and Michael McVaugh, Provo, Utah: Brigham Young University Press.

McCabe, Anne (2007), *A Byzantine Encyclopaedia of Horse Medicine: The Sources, Compilation, and Transmission of the Hippiatrica*, Oxford: Oxford University Press.

McCann, Daniel (2018), *Soul-Health: Therapeutic Reading in Later Medieval England*, Cardiff: University of Wales Press.

MacLehose, William (2013), 'Sleepwalking, Violence and Desire in the Middle Ages', *Culture, Medicine and Psychiatry*, 37: 601–24.

MacLehose, William (2020), 'Captivating Thoughts: Nocturnal Pollution, Imagination and the Sleeping Mind in the Twelfth and Thirteenth Centuries', *Journal of Medieval History*, 46: 98–131.

McCleery, Iona (2009), 'Both "Illness and Temptation of the Enemy": Melancholy, the Medieval Patient and the Writings of King Duarte of Portugal (r.1433–38)', *Journal of Medieval Iberian Studies*, 1: 163–78.

McCleery, Iona (2011), 'Medical "Emplotment" and Plotting Medicine: Health and Disease in Late Medieval Portuguese Chronicles', *Social History of Medicine*, 24: 125–41.

McCleery, Iona (2013), 'Medicine and Disease: The Female "Patient" in Medieval Europe', in Kim Phillips (ed.), *A Cultural History of Women in the Middle Ages*, 85–104, London: Bloomsbury.

McCleery, Iona (2014a), '"Christ more Powerful than Galen?" The Relationship Between Medicine and Miracles', in Matthew Mesley and Louise Wilson (eds), *Contextualizing Miracles in the Christian West, 1100–1500: New Historical Approaches*, 127–54, Oxford: *Medium Ævum*.

BIBLIOGRAPHY

McCleery, Iona (2014b), 'Medical Licensing in Late Medieval Portugal', in Wendy J. Turner and Sara Butler (eds), *Medicine and the Law in the Middle Ages*, 196–219, Leiden: Brill.

McCleery, Iona (2014c), 'Wine, Women and Song? Diet and Regimen for Royal Well-being (King Duarte of Portugal, 1433–1438)', in Sari Katajala-Peltomaa and Susanna Niiranen (eds), *Mental (Dis)Order in Later Medieval Europe*, 177–96, Leiden: Brill.

McCleery, Iona (2015), 'What is "Colonial" about Medieval Colonial Medicine? Iberian Health in a Global Context', *Journal of Medieval Iberian Studies*, 7: 151–75.

McCleery, Iona (2016), 'Getting Enough to Eat: Famine as a Neglected Medieval Health Issue', in Barbara Bowers and Linda Keyser (eds), *The Sacred and the Secular in Medieval Healing: Sites, Objects, and Texts*, 116–39, New York: Routledge.

McCormick, Michael (2001), *Origins of the European Economy: Communications and Commerce AD 300–900*, Cambridge: Cambridge University Press.

McGuire, Brian Patrick (2010), *Friendship and Community: The Monastic Experience, 350–1250*, new edn, Ithaca: Cornell University Press.

MacKinney, Loren (1942a), 'The Vulture in Ancient Medical Lore', *Ciba Symposia*, 4: 1258–71.

MacKinney, Loren (1942b), 'The Vulture in the Medieval World', *Ciba Symposia*, 4: 1272–86.

MacKinney, Loren (1952a), 'Medical Ethics and Etiquette in the Early Middle Ages. The Persistence of Hippocratic Ideals', *Bulletin of the History of Medicine*, 26: 1–31.

MacKinney, Loren (1952b), 'Multiple Explicits of a Medieval Dynamidia', *Osiris* 10: 195–205.

MacInnes, Iain (2015), 'Heads, Shoulders, Knees and Toes: Injury and Death in Anglo-Scottish Combat, *c.* 1296–*c.* 1403', in Larissa Tracy and Kelly DeVries (eds), *Wounds and Wound Repair in Medieval Culture*, 102–127, Leiden: Brill.

McIntosh, Marjorie (1998), *Controlling Misbehavior in England, 1370–1600*, Cambridge: Cambridge University Press.

McClure, George (1991), *Sorrow and Consolation in Italian Humanism*, Princeton: Princeton University Press.

McSheffrey, Shannon (2006), *Marriage, Sex and Civil Culture in Late Medieval London*, Philadelphia: University of Pennsylvania Press.

McVaugh, Michael (1993), *Medicine Before the Plague: Practitioners and their Patients in the Crown of Aragon, 1285–1345*, Cambridge: Cambridge University Press.

McVaugh Michael (1997), 'Bedside Manners in the Middle Ages', *Bulletin of the History of Medicine*, 71: 201–23.

McVaugh, Michael (2006), *The Rational Surgery of the Middle Ages*, Florence: SISMEL/ Edizioni del Galluzzo.

Magnusson, Roberta (2013), 'Medieval Urban Environmental History', *History Compass*, 11: 189–200.

Masters, Anthony (1977), *Bedlam*, London: Michael Joseph.

Meaney, Audrey (2000), 'The Practice of Medicine in England about the Year 1000', *Social History of Medicine*, 13: 221–37.

Melosi, Martin (1999), *The Sanitary City: Urban Infrastructure in America from Colonial Times to the Present*, Baltimore: Johns Hopkins University Press.

Menestò, Enrico and Silvestro Nessi (1991), *Il Processo di canonizzazione di Chiara da Montefalco*, Perugia: Regione dell'Umbria.

Menestò, Enrico (2007), *Simone da Collazzone francescano e il processo per la sua canonizzazione (1252)*, Spoleto: Fondazione Centro italiano di studi sull'alto Medioevo.

Mengel, David (2011), 'A Plague on Bohemia? Mapping the Black Death', *Past & Present*, 211: 3–34.

Metcalfe, Alex (2003), *Muslims and Christians in Norman Sicily: Arabic Speakers and the End of Islam*, New York: Routledge.

Metcalfe, Alex (2009), *The Muslims of Medieval Italy*, Edinburgh: Edinburgh University Press.

Metzler, Irina (2006), *Disability in Medieval Europe: Thinking About Physical Impairment During the High Middle Ages, c. 1100–c. 1400*, London: Routledge.

Metzler, Irina (2013), *A Social History of Disability in the Middle Ages: Cultural Considerations of Physical Impairment*, New York: Routledge.

Metzler, Irina (2016), *Fools and Idiots? Intellectual Disability in the Middle Ages*, Manchester: Manchester University Press.

Miller, H[oward] (2007), 'The Pleasures of Consumption: The Birth of Medieval Islamic Cuisine', in Paul Freedman (ed.), *Food: the History of Taste*, 135–61, London: Thames & Hudson.

Miller, Pat and David Saxby (2007), *The Augustinian Priory of St Mary Merton, Surrey: Excavations 1976–90*, London: Museum of London Archaeology Service.

Miller, Thomas and John Nesbitt (2014), *Walking Corpses: Leprosy in Byzantium and the Medieval West*, Ithaca: Cornell University Press.

Millon, Theodore (2004), *Masters of the Mind: Exploring the Story of Mental Illness from Ancient Times to the New Millennium*, Hoboken: Wiley.

Mitchell, Peter (2007), *The Purple Island and Anatomy in Early Seventeenth-century Literature, Philosophy, and Theology*, Plainsboro, NJ: Associated University Press.

Mitchell, Piers (2004), *Medicine in the Crusades: Warfare, Wounds and the Medieval Surgeon*, Cambridge: Cambridge University Press.

Mitchell, Piers (2011), 'Retrospective Diagnosis and the Use of Historical Texts for Investigating Disease in the Past', *Journal of International Palaeopathology*, 1: 81–88.

Mitchell, Piers (2015), 'Human Parasites in Medieval Europe: Lifestyle, Sanitation and Medical Treatment', *Advances in Parasitology*, 90: 389–420.

Mitchell, Piers, ed. (2015), *Sanitation, Latrines and Intestinal Parasites in Past Populations*, Farnham: Ashgate.

Moffat, Brian et al. (1986–9), *SHARP Practice 1, 2 and 3: First, Second and Third Reports on Researches into the Medieval Hospital at Soutra, Lothian Region, Scotland*, Edinburgh: SHARP.

Montanari, Massimo (2010), *Cheese, Pears and History in a Proverb*, trans. Beth Archer Brombert, New York: Columbia University Press.

Montanari, Massimo (2012), *Medieval Tastes: Food, Cooking and the Table*, trans. Beth Archer Brombert, New York: Columbia University Press.

Moorhouse, Stephen (1972), 'Medieval Distilling-Apparatus of Glass and Pottery', *Medieval Archaeology*, 16: 79–121.

Moorhouse, Stephen (1993), 'Pottery and Glass in the Late Medieval Monastery', in Roberta Gilchrist and Harold Mytum (eds), *Advances in Monastic Archaeology*, 127–48, Oxford: BAR Publishing.

Morales Muñiz, Dolores, Eufrasia Roselló Izquierdo, and Arturo Morales Muñiz (2009), 'Pesquerías medievales hispanas: las evidencias arqueofaunísticas', in (no editor) *La pesca en la Edad Media*, 145–65, Madrid: Xunta de Galicia, Sociedad Española de Estudios Medievales, Universidad de Murcia, CSIC.

BIBLIOGRAPHY

More, Alexander, and ten others (2017), 'Next-generation Ice Core Technology Reveals True Minimum Natural Levels of Lead (Pb) in the Atmosphere: Insights from the Black Death', *GeoHealth*, 1. Available online: https://agupubs. onlinelibrary.wiley. com/doi/10.1002/2017GH000064 (accessed 30 June 2020).

Morello, Ruth and Andrew Morrison (2007), 'Editors' Preface: Why Letters?' in Ruth Morello and Andrew Morrison (eds), *Ancient Letters: Classical and Late Antique Epistolography*, Oxford: Oxford University Press.

Morrison, Susan (2008), *Excrement in the Late Middle Ages: Sacred Filth and Chaucer's Fecopoetics*, New York: Palgrave Macmillan.

Müldner, Gundula (2009), 'Investigating Medieval Diet and Society by Stable Isotope Analysis of Human Bone', in Roberta Gilchrist and Andrew Reynolds (eds), *Reflections: 50 Years of Medieval Archaeology, 1957–2007*, 327–46, Leeds: Maney.

Murphy, Dominic (2015), 'Concepts of Disease and Health', in Edward Zalta (ed.), *The Stanford Encyclopedia of Philosophy*. Available online: https://plato.stanford. edu/archives/spr2015/entries/health-disease/ (accessed 29 June 2020).

Musacchio, Jacqueline (1999), *The Art and Ritual of Childbirth in Renaissance Italy*, New Haven: Yale University Press.

Neaman, Judith (1975), *Suggestion of the Devil: The Origins of Madness*, New York: Doubleday Anchor Books.

Newfield, Timothy (2009), 'A Cattle Panzootic in Early Fourteenth-Century Europe', *Agricultural History Review*, 57: 155–90.

Newton, Francis (1999), *The Scriptorium and Library at Monte Cassino, 1058–1105*, Cambridge: Cambridge University Press.

Newton, Francis (2011), 'Arabic Medicine and Other Arabic Cultural Influences in Southern Italy in the Time of Constantine the African', in F. Eliza Glaze and Brian Nance, (eds), *Between Text and Patient: The Medical Enterprise in Medieval and Early Modern Europe*, 25–55, Florence: SISMEL/Edizioni del Galluzzo.

Nichols, Stephen, Andreas Kablitz, and Alison Calhoun, eds (2008), *Rethinking the Medieval Senses: Heritage, Fascinations, Frames*, Baltimore: Johns Hopkins University Press.

Nicoud, Marilyn (2000), 'Expérience de la maladie et échange épistolaire: les derniers moments de Bianca Maria Visconti (mai-octobre 1468)', *Mélanges de l'École Française de Rome, Moyen-Âge*, 112: 311–458.

Nicoud, Marilyn (2007), *Les régimes de santé au Moyen Âge: naissance et diffusion d'une écriture médicale (XIIIe–XVe siècle)*, Rome: École Française de Rome.

Nicoud, Marilyn (2014), *Le prince et les médecins: pensée et pratiques médicales à Milan (1402–1476)*, Rome: École Française de Rome.

Nicoud, Marilyn (2015), 'L'Alimentation, un risque pour la santé? Discours médical et pratiques alimentaires au Moyen Âge', *Médiévales*, 69: 149–70.

Nicoud, Marilyn (2017), 'Nutrirsi secondo i medici nell'età antica e medievale', in Chiara Crisciani and Onorato Grassi (eds), *Nutrire il corpo, nutrire l'anima nel Medievo*, 41–68, Pisa: Edizioni ETS.

Niiranen, Susanna (2014), 'Mental Disorders in Remedy Collections: A Comparison of Occitan and Swedish Material', in Sari Katajala-Peltomaa and Susanna Niiranen (eds), *Mental (Dis)Order in Later Medieval Europe*, 151–76, Leiden: Brill.

Nikulin, Dmitri (2015), *Memory: A History*, Oxford: Oxford University Press.

Nolte, Cordula, Bianca Frohne, Uta Halle, and Sonja Kerth (2017), *Dis/ability History der Vormoderne: Ein Handbuch. Premodern Dis/ability History. A Companion*, Korb: Didymos-Verlag.

Nutton, Vivian (1992), 'Healers in the Medical Market Place: Towards a Social History of Graeco-Roman Medicine', in Andrew Wear (ed.), *Medicine in Society*, 15–58, Cambridge: Cambridge University Press.

Nutton, Vivian (1993), 'Humoralism', in William Bynum and Roy Porter (eds), *Companion Encyclopedia of the History of Medicine*, vol. 1: 281–91, London: Routledge.

Nutton, Vivian (1996), 'Medicine in Medieval Western Europe, 1000–1500', in Lawrence Conrad et al, *The Western Medical Tradition 800 BC to AD 1800*, 139–205, Cambridge: Cambridge University Press.

Nutton, Vivian (2004), *Ancient Medicine*, London: Routledge.

Nutton, Vivian (2008), 'The Fortunes of Galen', in Robert Hankinson (ed.), *The Cambridge Companion to Galen*, 355–90, Cambridge: Cambridge University Press.

Nutton, Vivian (2011), 'Pseudonymity and the Critic: Authenticating the Medieval Galen', in F. Eliza Glaze and Brian Nance (eds), *Between Text and Patient: The Medical Enterprise in Medieval and Early Modern Europe*, 481–91, Florence: SISMEL/Edizioni del Galluzzo.

Nutton, Vivian (2013), 'Byzantine Medicine, Genres, and the Ravages of Time', in Barbara Zipser (ed.), *Medical Books in the Byzantine World*, 7–18, Bologna: Eikasmós Online II.

Occhioni, Nicola (1984), *Il processo per la canonizzazione di S. Nicola da Tolentino*, Rome: Padri Agostiniani di Tolentino.

Ocker, Christopher (2002), *Biblical Poetics Before Humanism and Reformation*, Cambridge: Cambridge University Press.

O'Boyle, Cornelius (1998), *The Art of Medicine: Medical Teaching at the University of Paris, 1250–1400*, Leiden: Brill.

O'Connor, Bonnie and David Hufford (2001), 'Understanding Folk Medicine', in Erika Brady (ed.), *Healing Logics: Culture and Medicine in Modern Health Belief Systems*, 13–35, Logan: Utah State University Press.

O'Connor, Terry (2013), *Animals as Neighbors: The Past and Present of Commensal Animals*. East Lansing: Michigan State University Press.

O'Neill, Ynez (1970), 'Another Look at the "Anatomia porci"', *Viator*, 1: 115–24.

Offord, Margaret, ed. (1971), *The Book of the Knight of the Tower, Translated by William Caxton*, London: Early English Text Society.

Olsan, Lea (2003), 'Charms and Prayers in Medieval Medical Theory and Practice', *Social History of Medicine*, 16: 343–66.

Oosten, Roos van (2016), 'The Great Dutch Stink: The End of the Cesspit Era in the Pre-Industrial Towns of Leiden and Haarlem', *European Journal of Archaeology*, 19: 704–27.

Oosterwijk, Sophie (2008), 'The Medieval Child: An Unknown Phenomenon?' in Stephen Harris and Bryon Grigsby (eds), *Misconceptions about the Middle Ages*, 230–5, New York: Routledge.

Ordronaux, John (1871), *Regimen sanitatis salernitanum. Code of Health of the School of Salernum*, Philadelphia: J.B. Lippincott & Co.

Orlemanski, Julie (2019), *Symptomatic Subjects: Bodies, Medicine, and Causation in the Literature of Late Medieval England*, Philadelphia: University of Pennsylvania Press.

Osheim, Duane (1994) 'Pistoia: "Ordinances for Sanitation in a Time of Mortality"', available online: www3.iath.virginia.edu/osheim/pistoia.html (accessed 29 June 2020).

BIBLIOGRAPHY 231

Økland, Bård Gram and Knut Høiaas (2000), *Bare boss? Håntering av avfall gjennom 1000 år*. Bergen: Bryggens Museum.

Page, Sophie and Catherine Rider, eds (2019), *The Routledge History of Medieval Magic*, Abingdon: Routledge.

Palmieri, Nicoletta (2005), *Agnellus de Ravenne, Lectures galéniques: le De pulsibus ad tirones*, Saint-Etienne: Publications de l'Université de Saint-Etienne.

Palmieri, Nicoletta (2008), *L'Ars medica (Tegni) de Galien: lectures antiques et médiévales*, Saint-Etienne: Publications de l'Université de Saint-Etienne.

Patrick, Pip (2014), *The "Obese Medieval Monk": A Multidisciplinary Study of a Stereotype*, British Archaeological Reports 590, Oxford: Oxbow Books.

Paul of Aegina (1846), *The Medical Works of Paulus Aegineta, the Greek Physician*, trans. Francis Adams, vol. 2, London: The Sydenham Society.

Pender, Stephen (2010), 'Subventing Disease: Anger, Passions, and the Non-Naturals', in Jennifer Vaught (ed.), *Rhetorics of Bodily Disease and Health in Medieval and Early-Modern England*, 193–218, Farnham: Ashgate.

Pennell, Sara (2013): 'Food in History: Ingredients in Search of a Recipe', *Past and Future: The Magazine of the Institute for Historical Research*, 13: 6–9. Originally available online: www.history.ac.uk/sites/history.ac.uk/files/newsletters/past-and-future-2013-spring.pdf (accessed 29 March 2018).

Pennell, Sara and Rachel Rich (2016), 'Food the Forgotten Medicine?' introduction to *Food, Feast and Famine*, Virtual Issue 2, *Social History of Medicine*, 23 pages. Available online: https://academic.oup.com/shm/pages/virtual_issue_2 (accessed 29 June 2020).

Pereira, Olegario Nelson Azevedo (2012), 'Em torno da pesca, na costa norte de Portugal, nos séculos finais da Idade Média (1292–1493)', MA diss. University of Porto, Porto, Portugal.

Perho, Imerli (2003), 'Medicine and the Qur'ān', in Jane McAuliffe (ed.), *The Encyclopedia of the Qur'ān*, vol. 3, 349–67, Leiden: Brill.

Perho, Imerli (1995), *The Prophet's Medicine – A Creation of the Muslim Traditionalist Scholars*, Helsinki: The Finnish Oriental Society.

Peter Abelard (2013), *The Letter Collection of Peter Abelard and Heloise*, ed. and revised by David Luscombe after the trans. by Betty Radice, Oxford: Clarendon Press.

(Pseudo-) Peter of Spain (1497), *Summa experimentorum, sive Thesaurus pauperum*, Antwerp: Theodoricum Martini.

Petit, Caroline (2013), 'The Fate of a Greek Medical Handbook in the Medieval West: The *Introduction, or the Physician* Ascribed to Galen', in Barbara Zipser (ed.), *Medical Books in the Byzantine World*, 57–77, Bologna: Eikasmós Online II.

Petrarch, Francesco (1863), *Epistolae de rebus familiaribus et variae*, ed. Joseph Fracassetti, volume 2, Florence: Le Monnier.

Petrus Hispanus (1973), *Obras médicas de Pedro Hispano*, ed. Maria Helena da Rocha Pereira, Coimbra: Universidade de Coimbra.

Pfau, Aleksandra (2010a), 'Crimes of Passion: Emotion and Madness in French Remission Letters', in Wendy J. Turner (ed.), *Madness in Medieval Law and Custom*, 97–122, Leiden: Brill.

Pfau, Aleksandra (2010b), 'Protecting or Restraining? Madness as a Disability in late Medieval France', in Joshua Eyler (ed.), *Disability in the Middle Ages: Reconsiderations and reverberations*, 93–104, Farnham: Ashgate.

Pfau, Aleksandra (2008), 'Madness in the Realm: Narratives of Mental Illness in Late Medieval France', PhD diss., University of Michigan, Ann Arbor, USA.

Phillips, Joanna (forthcoming), 'Who Cared? Locating Caregivers in Chronicles of the Twelfth- and Thirteenth-Century Crusades', *Social History of Medicine*. Available online: https://doi.org/10.1093/shm/hkz100 (accessed 12 June 2020).

Pilsworth, Clare (2011), 'Beyond the Medical Text: Health and Illness in Early Medieval Italian Sources', *Social History of Medicine*, 24: 26–40.

Pilsworth, Clare (2014), *Healthcare in Early Medieval Northern Italy: More to Life than Leeches?* Turnhout: Brepols.

Pietro d'Abano (1476), *De venenis* in *Conciliator differentiarum philosophorum*, Venice: Gabriele di Pietro.

Pilsworth, Clare and Debby Banham, eds (2011), 'Medieval Medicine: Theory and Practice', special issue of *Social History of Medicine*, 24: 2–141.

Pitchon, Véronique (2016), 'Food and Medicine in Medieval Islamic Hospitals: Preparation and Care in Accordance with Dietetic Principles', *Food & History* 14: 13–33.

Plancas, Josefina (2012), 'The Zodiac and the Stars in a Treatise on Veterinary Medicine of the Crown of Aragon', *Manuscripta*, 52: 269–300.

Platearius (1994), 'Practica brevis', in Tony Hunt (ed.), *Anglo-Norman Medicine*, vol. 1, 149–315, Cambridge: D.S. Brewer.

Platina [Bartolomeo Sacchi] (1998), *On Right Pleasure and Good Health: A Critical Edition and Translation of De honesta voluptate et valetudine*, ed. Mary Ella Milham, Tempe: AMRTS.

Platt, Colin and Richard Coleman-Smith (1975), *Excavations in Medieval Southampton 1953–1969*, vol. 2, Leicester: Leicester University Press.

Pomata, Gianna (1998), *Contracting a Cure: Patients, Healers, and the Law in Early Modern Bologna*, Baltimore and London: Johns Hopkins University Press.

Pormann, Peter (2003), 'Theory and Practice in the Early Hospitals in Baghdad: Al-Kaškarī On Rabies and Melancholy', *Zeitschrift für Geschichte der Arabisch-Islamischen Wissenschaften*, 15: 197–248.

Pormann, Peter and Emilie Savage-Smith (2007), *Medieval Islamic Medicine*, Washington DC: Georgetown University Press.

Porter, Roy (1985), 'The Patient's View: Doing Medical History from Below', *Theory and Society*, 14: 175–98.

Pouchelle, Marie-Christine (1990), *The Body and Surgery in the Middle Ages*, trans. Rosemary Morris, New Brunswick: Rutgers University Press.

Powell, Hilary (2012), 'The "Miracle of Childbirth": The Portrayal of Parturient Women in Medieval Miracle Narratives', *Social History of Medicine*, 25: 795–811.

Price, Roger and Michael Ponsford (1998), *St Bartholomew's Hospital, Bristol: The Excavation of a Medieval Hospital: 1976–8*, York: Council for British Archaeology.

Prioreschi, Plinio (2003), *Medieval Medicine*, Omaha: Horatius Press.

Proctor, Caroline (2005), 'Perfecting Prevention: The Medical Writings of Maino de Maineri (d. *c.* 1368)', PhD diss., University of St Andrews, St Andrews, UK.

Proctor, Caroline (2007), 'Physician to the Bruce: Maino de Maineri in Scotland', *Scottish Historical Review*, 86: 16–26.

Proctor, Caroline (2008), 'Between Medicine and Morals: Sex in the Regimens of Maino de Maineri', in April Harper and Caroline Proctor (eds), *Medieval Sexuality: A Casebook*, 113–31, New York: Routledge.

Ragab, Ahmed (2015), *The Medieval Islamic Hospital: Medicine, Religion and Charity*, Cambridge: Cambridge University Press.

Raine, Angelo, ed. (1940), *York Civic Records*, vol. 2, York: Yorkshire Archaeological Society.

Rasmussen, Kaare Lund and eight others (2008), 'Mercury Levels in Danish Medieval Human Bones', *Journal of Archaeological Science*, 35: 2295–306.

Rawcliffe, Carole (1995), *Medicine and Society in Later Medieval England*, Stroud: Sutton Publishing.

Rawcliffe, Carole (2002a), 'Curing Bodies and Healing Souls: Pilgrimage and the Sick in Medieval East Anglia', in Colin Morris and Peter Roberts (eds), *Pilgrimage: The English Experience from Becket to Bunyan*, 108–40, Cambridge: Cambridge University Press.

Rawcliffe, Carole (2002b), '"On the Threshold of Eternity": Care for the Sick in East Anglian Monasteries', in Christopher Harper-Bill, Carole Rawcliffe and Richard Wilson (eds), *East Anglia's History: Studies in Honour of Norman Scarfe*, 41–72, Woodbridge: The Boydell Press/Centre for East Anglian Studies, University of East Anglia.

Rawcliffe, Carole (2003), 'Women, Childbirth and Religion in Medieval England', in Diana Wood (ed.), *Women and Religion in Medieval England*, 91–117, Oxford: Oxbow.

Rawcliffe, Carole (2006), *Leprosy in Medieval England*, Woodbridge: The Boydell Press.

Rawcliffe, Carole (2011), 'Medical Practice and Theory', in Julia Crick and Elisabeth van Houts (eds), *A Social History of England, 900–1200*, 391–401, Cambridge: Cambridge University Press.

Rawcliffe, Carole (2013a), *Urban Bodies: Communal Health in Late Medieval English Towns and Cities*, Woodbridge: The Boydell Press.

Rawcliffe, Carole (2013b), '"Less Mudslinging and More Facts": A New Look at an Old Debate about Public Health in Late Medieval English Towns', *Bulletin of the John Rylands Library*, 89: 203–21.

Rawcliffe, Carole and Claire Weeda, eds (2019), *Policing the Urban Environment in Premodern Europe*, Amsterdam: Amsterdam University Press.

Recio Muñoz, Victoria (2016), *La "Practica" de Plateario*, Florence: SISMEL/Edizioni del Galluzzo.

Reinarz, Jonathan (2014), *Past Scents: Historical Perspectives on Smell*, Urbana: University of Illinois Press.

Resl, Brigitte, ed. (2009), *A Cultural History of Animals in the Medieval Age*, Oxford: Berg.

Rhazes (1544), *Abubetri Rhazae Maomethi ob usum experientiamque multiplicem . . .*, Basel Henrichus Petrus

Richardson, Kristina (2012), *Difference and Disability in the Medieval Islamic World: Blighted Bodies*, Edinburgh: Edinburgh University Press.

Richer (2011), *Histories*, Volume 2, Books 3–4, ed. Justin Lake, Cambridge, MA: Harvard University Press.

Riddle, John (1965), 'The Introduction and Use of Eastern Drugs in the Early Middle Ages', *Sudhoffs Archiv*, 49: 185–98.

Riddle, John (1980), 'Dioscorides', in F. Edward Cranz and Paul Oskar Kristeller (eds), *Catalogus translationum et commentariorum: Mediaeval and Renaissance Translations and Commentaries*, vol. 4, 1–143, Washington, DC: Catholic University of America Press.

Rider, Catherine (2011), 'Medical Magic and the Church in Thirteenth-Century England', *Social History of Medicine*, 24: 92–107.

Rieder, Paula (2006), *On the Purification of Women: Churching in Northern France, 1100–1500*, New York: Palgrave.

Riley, Henry, ed. (1868), *Memorials of London and London Life in the XIIIth, XIVth, and XVth Centuries*, London: Longmans, Green & Co. Available via British History Online, www.british-history.ac.uk/no-series/memorials-london-life (accessed 29 June 2020).

Rimmon-Kenan, Shlomith (2002), 'The Story of "I": Illness and Narrative Identity', *Narrative*, 10: 9–27.

Ritchey, Sara and Sharon Strocchia, eds (2020), *Gender, Health and Healing, 1250–1550*, Amsterdam: University of Amsterdam.

Ritvo, Harriet (2007), 'On the Animal Turn', *Daedalus*, 136: 118–22.

Robb, John and Oliver Harris, eds (2013), *The Body in History: Europe from the Palaeolithic to the Future*, New York: Cambridge University Press.

Roberg, Francesco (2002), 'Studien zum *Antidotarium Nicholai* nach den ältesten Handschriften', *Würzburger medizinhistorische Mitteilungen*, 21: 73–129.

Roberg, Francesco (2007), 'Text- und redaktionskritische Probleme bei der Edition von Texten des Gebrauchsschrifttums am Beispiel des "Antidotarium Nicolai" (12. Jahrhundert): Einige Beobachtungen, mit einem Editionsanhang', *Mittellateinisches Jahrbuch*, 42: 1–19.

Roberg, Francesco (2011), 'Nochmals zur Edition des *Antidotarium Nicolai*', in Agostino Paravicini Bagliani (ed.), *Terapie e guarigioni. Convegno internazionale (Ariano Irpino, 5-7 ottobre 2008)*, 129–40, Florence: SISMEL/Edizioni del Galluzzo.

Roberts, Charlotte (2007), 'A Bioarchaeological Study of Maxillary Sinusitis', *American Journal of Physical Anthropology*, 133: 792–807.

Roberts, Charlotte (2009), 'Health and Welfare in Medieval England: The Human Skeletal Remains Contextualized', in Roberta Gilchrist and Andrew Reynolds (eds), *Reflections: 50 Years of Medieval Archaeology, 1957–2007*, 307–25, Leeds: Maney.

Roberts, Charlotte (2014), 'Surgery', in Michael Lapidge et al (eds), *The Wiley Blackwell Encyclopedia of Anglo-Saxon England*, 445–7, Oxford: Wiley Blackwell.

Roberts, Charlotte (2017), 'Applying the "Index of Care" to a Person who Experienced Leprosy in Late Medieval Chichester, England', in Lorna Tilley and Alecia Schrenk, (eds), *New Developments in the Bioarchaeology of Care*, 101–24, Basel: Springer.

Roberts, Charlotte and Keith Manchester (2005), *The Archaeology of Disease*, 3rd edn, Stroud: Sutton Publishing.

Robertson, James Craigie, ed. (1876), *Materials for the History of Thomas Becket*, 2 vols, London: Rolls Series.

Robinson, Katelynn (2020), *The Sense of Smell in the Middle Ages: A Source of Certainty*, Abingdon: Routledge.

Rodrigues, Lisbeth Oliveira and Isabel dos Guimarães Sá (2015), 'Sugar and Spices in Portuguese Renaissance Medicine', *Journal of Medieval Iberian Studies*, 7: 1–21.

Röhricht, Reinhold (1884), 'Lettres de Ricoldo de Monte-Croce sur la prise d'Acre (1291)', *Archives de l'Orient latin*, 2: 258–96.

Roffey, Simon (2012), 'Medieval Leper Hospitals in England: An Archaeological Perspective', *Medieval Archaeology*, 56: 203–33.

Roffey, Simon and Katie Tucker (2012), 'A Contextual Study of the Medieval Hospital and Cemetery of St Mary Magdalen, Winchester', *International Journal of Paleopathology*, 2: 170–80.

Rogers, Juliet and Tony Waldron (2001), 'DISH and the Monastic Way of Life', *International Journal of Osteoarchaeology*, 11: 357–65.

Rogge, Jörg, ed. (2017), *Killing and Being Killed, Bodies in Battle: Perspectives on Fighters in the Middle Ages*, Bielefeld: Transcript.

BIBLIOGRAPHY

Roosen, Joris and Daniel Curtis (2019), 'The "Light Touch" of the Black Death in the Southern Netherlands: An Urban Trick?' *Economic History Review*, 72: 32–56.

Rose, Valentin, ed. (1963), *Anecdota graeca et graecolatina: Mitteilungen aus Handschriften zur Geschichte der griechischen Wissenschaft*, first published, Berlin, 1864–79, reprinted Amsterdam: A.M. Hakkert.

Rosen, George (1964), 'The Mentally Ill and the Community in Western and Central Europe during the Late Middle Ages and the Renaissance', *Journal of the History of Medicine*, 19: 377–88.

Rosenwein, Barbara, ed. (1998), *Anger's Past: The Social Uses of an Emotion in the Middle Ages*, Ithaca: Cornell University Press.

Round, Nicholas (1980), 'La correspondencia del arcediano de Niebla en el archivo del real monasterio de Santa María de Guadalupe', *Historia. Instituciones. Documentos*, 7: 215–68.

Rubin, Jonathan (2014), 'The Use of the "Jericho Tyrus" in Theriac: A Case Study in the History of the Exchanges of Medical Knowledge between Western Europe and the Realm of Islam in the Middle Ages', *Medium Ævum*, 83: 234–53.

Rudy, Kathryn (2010), 'Dirty Books: Quantifying Patterns of Use in Medieval Manuscripts Using a Densitometer', *Journal of Historians of Netherlandish Art*, 2 (Summer), DOI: 10.5092/jhna.2010.2.1.1. Available online, https://jhna.org/articles/dirty-books-quantifying-patterns-of-use-medieval-manuscripts-using-a-densitometer/ (accessed 30 June 2020).

Sabine, Ernst (1933), 'Butchering in Mediaeval London', *Speculum*, 8: 335–53.

Sabine, Ernst (1934), 'Latrines and Cesspools of Mediaeval London', *Speculum*, 9: 303–21.

Sabine, Ernst (1937), 'City Cleaning in Mediaeval London', *Speculum*, 12: 19–43.

Sálmon, Fernando (1996), 'Academic Discourse and Pain in Medical Scholasticism (Thirteenth-Fourteenth Centuries)', in Samuel Kottek and Luis García-Ballester, (eds), *Medicine and Medical Ethics in Medieval and Early Modern Spain: An Intercultural Approach*, 136–53, Jerusalem: Magnes Press.

Salmón, Fernando (2011), 'Consumo y salud: la comida y la bebida en la medicina medieval', in (no editor), *Comer, beber, vivir: consumo y niveles de vida en la Edad Media hispânica*, 17–56, Logroño: Instituto de Estudios Riojanos.

Salmón, Fernando and Montserrat Cabré (1998), 'Fascinating Women: The Evil Eye in Medieval Scholasticism', in Roger French et al (eds), *From the Black Death to the French Disease*, 53–84, Aldershot: Ashgate.

Saunders, Corinne (2015), 'Mind, Body and Affect in Medieval English Arthurian Romance', in Frank Brandsma, Carolyne Larrington and Corinne Saunders (eds), *Emotions in Medieval Arthurian Literature: Body, Mind, Voice*, 31–46, Cambridge: D.S. Brewer.

Savage-Smith, Emilie, Simon Swain, and Gert van Gelder eds (2020), *A Literary History of Medicine*, Leiden: Brill.

Scalenghe, Sara (2014), *Disability in the Ottoman Arab World, 1500–1800*, Cambridge: Cambridge University Press.

Scarry, Elaine (1985), *The Body in Pain: The Making and Unmaking of the World*, New York: Oxford University Press.

Schmitt, Franciscus, ed. (1984), *S. Anselmi Cantuariensis Archiepiscopi, Opera Omnia*, first published 1938–1961, reprinted Stuttgart: Frommann

Scully, Terence (1985), 'The *Opusculum de saporibus* of Magninus Mediolanensis', *Medium Ævum*, 54 (1985): 178–207.

Scully, Terence (1992), 'The Sickdish in Early French Recipe Collections', in Sheila Campbell, Bert Hall and David Klausner (eds), 132–40, *Health, Disease and Healing in Medieval Culture*, Basingtoke: Macmillan.

Scully, Terence (1995), 'Mixing it Up in the Medieval Kitchen', in Mary-Jo Arn (ed.), *Medieval Food and Drink*, 1–26, Binghamton NY: Centre for Medieval and Renaissance Studies.

Scully, Terence (2005), *The Art of Cookery in the Middle Ages*. Woodbridge: The Boydell Press.

Scully, Terence (2008), 'A Cook's Therapeutic Use of Garden Herbs', in Peter Dendle and Alain Touwaide (eds), *Health and Healing from the Medieval Garden*, 60–71, Woodbridge, The Boydell Press.

Sellers, Maud (1912–1915), *York Memorandum Book, Parts I & II, Lettered A/Y in the Guildhall Muniment Room*, Durham: Andrews & Co.

Serjeantson, Dale and Christopher Woolgar (2006), 'Fish Consumption in Medieval England', in Christopher Woolgar, Dale Serjeantson and Tony Waldron (eds), *Food in Medieval England: Diet and Nutrition*, 102–30, Oxford: Oxford University Press.

Shapland, Fiona, Mary Lewis, and Rebecca Watts (2015), 'The Lives and Deaths of Young Medieval Women: The Osteological Evidence', *Medieval Archaeology*, 59: 272–89.

Shargrir, Iris (2012), 'The Fall of Acre as a Spiritual Crisis: The Letters of Riccoldo of Monte Croce', *Revue belge de philologie et d'histoire*, 90: 1107–20.

Sharpe, Reginald, ed. (1899), *Calendar of the Letter-books of the City of London: A, 1275–1298*. London: HMSO. Available via British History Online, www.british-history.ac.uk/london-letter-books/vola (accessed 29 June 2020).

Sharpe, Reginald, ed. (1905), *Calendar of Letter-books of the City of London: G, 1352–1374*, London: HMSO. Available via British History Online, www.british-history.ac.uk/london-letter-books/volg (accessed 29 June 2020).

Sharpe, Reginald, ed. (1909), *Calendar of Letter-books of the City of London: I, 1400–1422*, London: HMSO. Available via British History Online, www.british-history.ac.uk/london-letter-books/voli (accessed 29 June 2020).

Sharpe, Reginald, ed. (1911), *Calendar of Letter-books of the City of London: K, Henry VI*, London: HMSO. Available via British History Online, www.british-history.ac.uk/london-letter-books/volk (accessed 29 June 2020).

Sharpe, William, ed. (1964), *Isidore of Seville: The Medical Writings*. Transactions of the American Philosophical Society, new series, 54, pt. 2, 55–64, Philadelphia: American Philosophical Society.

Shatzmiller, Joseph (1989), *Médecine et justice en Provence médiévale: documents de Manosque, 1262–1348*, Aix-en-Provence: Publications de l'Université de Provence.

Shatzmiller, Joseph (1994), *Jews, Medicine, and Medieval Society*, Berkeley: University of California Press.

Shaw, Brent (2003), 'A Peculiar Island: Maghrib and Mediterranean', *Mediterranean Historical Review*, 18: 93–125.

Shaw, James and Evelyn Welch (2011), *Making and Marketing Medicine in Renaissance Florence*, Amsterdam: Rodopi.

Shaw, Julia and Naomi Sykes (2018), 'New Directions in the Archaeology of Medicine: Deep-Time Approaches to Human-Animal-Environmental Care', *World Archaeology*, 50: 365–83.

Shefer-Mossensohn, Miriam and Keren Abbou Hershkovitz (2013), 'Early Muslim Medicine and the Indian Context: A Reinterpretation', *Medieval Encounters*, 19: 274–99.

BIBLIOGRAPHY

Shehada, Housni Alkhateeb (2012), *Mamluks and Animals: Veterinary Medicine in Medieval Islam*, Leiden: Brill.

Shirley, Walter, ed. (1862), *Royal and Other Historical Letters Illustrative of the Reign of Henry III*, London: Longman.

Shoham-Steiner, Ephraim (2014), *On the Margins of a Minority: Leprosy, Madness and Disability Among the Jews of Medieval Europe*, trans. Haim Watzman, Detroit: Wayne State University Press.

Sigerist, Henry (1960), *Henry E. Sigerist on the History of Medicine*, ed. Felix Marti-Ibañez, New York: MD Publications.

Siraisi, Nancy (1990), *Medieval and Early Renaissance Medicine: An Introduction to Knowledge and Practice*, Chicago: Chicago University Press.

Siraisi, Nancy (1996), 'L'individuale nella medicina tra medioevo e umanesimo: I casi clinici', in Roberto Cardini and Mariangela Regoliosi (eds), *Umanesimo e medicina: Il problema dell 'individuale*, 33–62, Rome: Bulzoni.

Skemer, Don (2006), *Binding Words: Textual Amulets in the Middle Ages*, University Park: Pennsylvania State University Press.

Skinner, Patricia (1997), *Health and Medicine in Early Medieval Southern Italy*, Leiden: Brill.

Skinner, Patricia (2015), 'Visible Prowess? Reading Men's Head and Face Wounds in Early Medieval Europe to 1000 CE', in Larissa Tracy and Kelly DeVries, (eds), *Wounds and Wound Repair in Medieval Culture*, 81–101, Leiden: Brill.

Skinner, Patricia (2017), *Living with Disfigurement in Early Medieval Europe*, New York: Palgrave Macmillan.

Slavin, Philip (2012), 'The Great Bovine Pestilence and its Economic and Environmental Consequences in England and Wales, 1318–50', *Economic History Review*, 65: 1239–66.

Slavin, Philip (2019), *Experiencing Famine in Fourteenth-century Britain*, Turnhout: Brepols.

Slavin, Philip (forthcoming), 'Mites and Merchants: The Crisis of English Wool and Textile Trade Revisited, *c*. 1275–1330', *Economic History Review*. Available online https://onlinelibrary.wiley.com/doi/full/10.1111/ehr.12969 (accessed 12 June 2020).

Slavin, Philip and Sharon DeWitte (2013), 'Between Famine and Death: England on the Eve of the Black Death – Evidence from Paleoepidemiology and Manorial Accounts', *Journal of Interdisciplinary History*, 44: 37–60.

Sloane, Barney (2012), *The Augustinian Nunnery of St Mary Clerkenwell, London: Excavations 1974–96*, London: MOLA Monograph.

Smith, David Romney (2015), 'Calamity and Transition: Re-Imagining Italian Trade in the Eleventh-Century Mediterranean', *Past and Present*, 228: 15–56.

Smith, G[eorge] H. (1979), 'The Excavation of the Hospital of St Mary of Ospringe, commonly called Maison Dieu', *Archaeologica Cantiana*, 95: 81–184.

Smith, Lesley (1998), 'William of Auvergne and Confession', in Peter Biller and Alastair Minnis (eds), *Handling Sin: Confession in the Middle Ages*, 95–107, Woodbridge: York Medieval Press/The Boydell Press.

Smoller, Laura (2014), *The Saint and the Chopped-Up Baby: The Cult of Vincent Ferrer in Medieval and Early Modern Europe*, Ithaca: Cornell University Press.

Solomon, Michael (2010), *Fictions of Well-Being: Sickly Readers and Vernacular Medical Writing in Late Medieval and Early Modern Spain*, Philadelphia: University of Pennsylvania Press.

Solomon, Michael (2013), 'Non-Natural Love: Coitus, Desire and Hygiene in Medieval and Early-Modern Spain', in Elena Carrera (ed.), *Emotions and Health, 1200–1700*, 147–58, Leiden: Brill.

Solomon, Michael (2018), 'Breaking Non-Natural Bread: Alimentary Hygiene and Radical Individualism in Juan de Aviñon's *Medicina Sevillana*', in Montserrat Piera (ed.), *Forging Communities: Food and Representation in Medieval and Early-Modern Southwestern Europe*, 146–58, Fayetteville: University of Arkansas.

Sontag, Susan (1978), *Illness as Metaphor*, New York: Farrar, Straus and Giroux.

Spencer, Brian (1998), *Pilgrim Souvenirs and Secular Badges: Medieval Finds from Excavations in London*, London: HMSO.

Sprunger, David (2001), 'Depicting the Insane: A Thirteenth-Century Case Study', in Timothy Jones and David Sprunger (eds), *Marvels, Monsters, and Miracles: Studies in the Medieval and Early Modern Imaginations*, 223–41, Kalamazoo: Western Michigan University.

Staley, Lynn, ed. (1996), *The Book of Margery Kempe*, Kalamazoo: Medieval Institute Publications.

Stamp, A. E., E. Salisbury, E. G. Atkinson, and J. O'Reilly eds (1921), *Calendar of Inquisitions Post-mortem and other Analogous Documents Preserved in the Public Record Office*, volume 10: Edward III, London: HMSO.

Standley, Eleanor (2013), *Trinkets and Charms: The Use, Meaning and Significance of Dress Accessories, 1300–1700*, Oxford: Oxford University School of Archaeology.

Stannard, Jerry (1972), 'Greco-Roman Materia Medica in Medieval Germany', *Bulletin of the History of Medicine*, 46: 455–68.

Stannard, Jerry (1974), 'Medieval Herbals and their Development', *Clio Medica*, 9: 23–33.

Stearns, Justin (2009), 'New Directions in the Study of Religious Responses to the Black Death', *History Compass*, 7: 1–13.

Stearns, Justin (2011), *Infectious Ideas: Contagion in Premodern Islamic and Christian Thought in the Western Mediterranean*, Baltimore: Johns Hopkins University Press.

Stearns, Justin (2016), ''Amwās, plague of', in *Encyclopaedia of Islam Three*, 2: 28–9.

Stearns, Justin (2017), 'Public Health, the State, and Religious Scholarship: Considering Sovereignty in Idrīs al-Bidlīsī's (d.1520) Arguments for Fleeing the Plague', in Zvi Ben-Dor Benite, Stefanos Geroulanos and Nicole Jerr (eds), *The Scaffolding of Sovereignty: Global and Aesthetic Perspectives on the History of a Concept*, 163–85, New York: Columbia University Press.

Steel, Carlos, Guy Guldenstops, and Pieter Beullens, eds (1999), *Aristotle's Animals in the Middle Ages and Renaissance*, Leuven: Leuven University Press.

Stell, Philip, trans. (2003), *The York Bridgemasters' Accounts*, York: York Archaeological Trust.

Stolberg, Michael (2011), *Experiencing Illness and the Sick Body in Early Modern Europe*, New York: Palgrave Macmillan.

Stoll, Ulrich, ed. (1992), *Das Lorscher Arzneibuch: ein medizinisches Kompendium des 8. Jahrhunderts (Codex Bambergensis medicinalis 1)*, *Sudhoffs Archiv*, Supplement 28.

Stones, J[udith] A. (1989), *Three Scottish Carmelite Friaries*, Edinburgh: Society of Antiquaries of Scotland.

Strozzi, Alessandra (1997), *Selected Letters of Alessandra Strozzi, Bilingual edition*, ed. Heather Gregory, California, University of California Press.

BIBLIOGRAPHY 239

Sudhoff, Walther (1913), 'Die Lehre von den Hirnventrikeln in textlicher und graphischer Tradition des Altertums und Mittelalters', *Archiv für Geschichte der Medizin*, 7: 149–205.

Sykes, Naomi (2009), 'Animals, the Bones of Medieval Society', in Robert Gilchrist and Andrew Reynolds (eds), *Reflections: 50 Years of Medieval Archaeology 1957–2007*, 347–61, Leeds: Maney.

Taddeo Alderotti (1937), *I "Consilia"*, ed. Giuseppe Michele Nardi, Tornio: Minerva Medica.

Taillevent (1988), *The Viandier of Taillevent: An Edition of all Extant Manuscripts*, ed. Terence Scully, Ottowa: University of Toronto Press.

Talbot, Charles (1967), *Medicine in Medieval England*, London: Oldbourne.

Tanner, Norman ed. (1990), *Decrees of the Ecumenical Councils*, London: Georgetown University Press.

Temkin, Owsei (1991), *Hippocrates in a World of Pagans and Christians*, Baltimore: Johns Hopkins University Press.

Thiher, Allen (1999), *Revels in Madness: Insanity in Medicine and Literature*, Ann Arbor: University of Michigan Press.

Thomas, Carol (2010), 'Negotiating the Contested Terrain of Narrative Methods in Illness Contexts', *Sociology of Health & Illness*, 32: 647–60.

Thomas, Christopher, Barney Sloane, and Christopher Phillpotts (1997), *Excavations at the Priory and Hospital of St Mary Spital, London*, London: Museum of London Archaeology Service.

Thomas de Cantimpré (1973), *Liber de natura rerum*, ed. Helmut Boese, Berlin: Walter de Gruyter.

Thomas of Chobham (1968), *Summa Confessorum*, ed. F. Broomfield, Louvain: Éditions Nauwelaerts.

Thomason, Richard (2015), 'Hospitality in a Cistercian Abbey: the case of Kirkstall in the Later Middle Ages', PhD diss., University of Leeds, Leeds, UK.

Thorndike, Lynn (1928), 'Sanitation, Baths, and Street-Cleaning in the Middle Ages and Renaissance', *Speculum*, 3: 192–203.

Thorndike, Lynn (1934), 'A Mediaeval Sauce Book', *Speculum*, 9: 183–90.

TNA C 135, 'Inquisitions Post-mortem, Edward III', Chancery manuscripts, in The National Archive, Public Record Office division, Kew, UK.

TNA C 66, 'Patent Rolls', Chancery manuscripts, in The National Archive, Public Record Office division, Kew, UK.

Toso, Alice (2018), 'Food and Faith in Medieval Portugal', PhD diss., University of York, York, UK.

Totaro, Rebecca (2005), *Suffering in Paradise: The Bubonic Plague in English Literature from More to Milton*, Pittsburgh: Duquesne University Press.

Totelin, Laurence (2004), 'Mithridates' Antidote: A Pharmacological Ghost', *Early Science and Medicine*, 9: 1–19.

Totelin, Laurence (2011), 'Old Recipes, New Practice? The Latin Adaptations of the Hippocratic *Gynaecological Treatises*', *Social History of Medicine*, 24: 74–91.

Tracy, Larissa and Kelly DeVries, eds (2015), *Wounds and Wound Repair in Medieval Culture*, Leiden: Brill.

Trevisa, John (1975), *On the Properties of Things: John Trevisa's translation of Bartholomæus Anglicus De Proprietatibus Rerum*, ed. Michael Seymour, Oxford: Clarendon Press.

Tuke, Daniel Hack (1882), *Chapters in the History of the Insane in the British Isles*, London: Kegan Paul, Trench & Co.

Turner, Bryan (1995), *Medical Power and Social Knowledge*, written with Colin Samson, London: SAGE Publications.

Turner, Marion, ed. (2016), 'Medical Discourse in Premodern Europe', special issue of *Journal of Medieval and Early Modern Studies*, 46: 1–188.

Turner, Marion (2016), 'Illness Narratives in the Later Middle Ages: Arderne, Chaucer and Hoccleve', *Journal of Medieval and Early Modern Studies*, 46: 61–88.

Turner, Wendy J. (2010), 'Silent Testimony: Emotional Displays and Lapses in Memory as Indicators of Mental Instability in Medieval English Investigations', in Wendy J. Turner (ed.), *Madness in Medieval Law and Custom*, 81–95, Leiden: Brill.

Turner, Wendy J. (2013a), *Care and Custody of the Mentally Ill, Incompetent and Disabled in Medieval England*, Turnhout: Brepols.

Turner, Wendy J. (2013b), 'Defining Mental Affliction in Medieval English Administrative Records', in Cory James Rushton, (ed.), *Disability and Medieval Law: History, Literature, Society*, 134–56, Newcastle-upon-Tyne: Cambridge Scholars.

Turner, Wendy J. (2018), 'Mental Health and Homicide in Medieval English Trials', *Open Library of Humanities*, 4. Available online: https://olh.openlibhums.org/articles/10.16995/olh.295/ (accessed 30 June 2020).

Turner, Wendy, J. ed. (2010), *Madness in Medieval Law and Custom*, Leiden: Brill.

Turner, Wendy J. and Sara Butler, eds (2014), *Medicine and the Law in the Middle Ages*, Leiden: Brill.

Turner, Wendy J. and Tory Pearman, eds (2010), *The Treatment of Disabled Persons in Medieval Europe: Examining Disability in the Historical, Legal, Literary, Medical, and Religious Discourses of the Middle Ages*, Lewiston: Edwin Mellen Press.

Turner, Wendy J. and Christina Lee, eds (2018), *Trauma in Medieval Society*, Leiden: Brill.

Tymms, Samuel, ed. (1850), *Wills and Inventories from the Registers of the Commissary of Bury St. Edmund's and the Archdeacon of Sudbury*, London: J.B. Nichols & Son for the Camden Society.

Tyson, Rachel (2000), *Medieval Glass Vessels Found in England*, c. *AD 1200–1500*, York: Council for British Archaeology.

Ugo Benzi (1518), *Consilia Ugonis Senensis saluberrima ad omnes egritudines*, Venice: impensa heredum Octauiani Scoti ac sociorum.

Ullman, Manfred (1978), *Islamic Medicine*, Edinburgh: Edinburgh University Press.

Van Arsdall, Anne (2005), 'Reading Medieval Medical Texts with an Open Mind', in Elizabeth Lane Furdell (ed.), *Textual Healing: Essays on Medieval and Early Modern Medicine*, 9–29, Leiden: Brill.

Van Arsdall, Anne (2007), 'Challenging the "Eye of Newt" Image of Medieval Medicine', in Barbara Bowers (ed.), *The Medieval Hospital and Medical Practice*, 195–205, Aldershot: Ashgate.

Van Arsdall, Anne (2011), 'The Transmission of Knowledge in Early Medieval Medical Texts: an Exploration', in F. Eliza Glaze and Brian Nance (eds), *Between Text and Patient: The Medical Enterprise in Medieval and Early Modern Europe*, 201–15, Florence: SISMEL/Edizioni del Galluzzo.

Van Ess, Josef (2001), *Der Fehltritt des Gelehrten: Die "Pest von Emmaus" und ihre theologischen Nachspiele*, Heidelberg: C. Winter.

Varlık, Nükhet (2015), *Plague and Empire in the Early Modern Mediterranean World: The Ottoman Experience, 1347–1600*, Cambridge: Cambridge University Press.

Vaught, Jennifer, ed. (2010), *Rhetorics of Bodily Disease and Health in Medieval and Early Modern England*, Farnham: Ashgate.

BIBLIOGRAPHY

Ventura, Iolanda (2005), 'The "Curae ex animalibus" in the Medical Literature of the Middle Ages: The Example of the Illustrated Herbals', in Baudouin Van den Abeele (ed.), *Bestiaires médiévaux: Nouvelles perspectives sur les manuscrits et les traditions textuelles*, 213–48, Louvain-la-Neuve: Université Catholique de Louvain, Institut d'Etudes Médiévales.

Ventura, Iolanda (2010), 'Medicina, Magia e *Dreckapotheke* sull'uso della sostanze animali nella letteratura farmceutica tra XII e XV secolo', in Agostino Paravicini Bagliani (ed.), *Terapie e guarigioni*, 303–62, Florence: SISMEL/Edizioni del Galluzzo.

Ventura, Iolanda (2012), 'Sulla diffusione del *Circa instans* nei manoscritti e nelle biblioteche del tardo medioevo: ricenzione e letteratura di un'opera medica', in Giuseppe de Gregoria and Maria Galante (eds), *La Produzione Scritta Tecnica e Scientifica nel Medioevo: Libro e Documento tra Scuole e Professioni*, 465–549, Spoleto: Fondazione Centro Italiano di Studi sull'alto Medioevo.

Voigts, Linda (1976), 'A New Look at a Manuscript Containing the Old English Translation of the *Herbarium Apulei*', *Manuscripta*, 20: 40–61.

Voigts, Linda (1978), 'The Significance of the name Apuleius to the *Herbarium Apulei*', *Dumbarton Oaks Papers*, 52: 214–27.

Voigts, Linda (1979), 'Anglo-Saxon Plant Remedies and the Anglo-Saxons', *Isis*, 70: 250–68.

Wakefield, Jerome (1992), 'The Concept of Mental Disorder', *American Psychologist*, 47: 373–88.

Waines, David (1999), 'Dietetics in Medieval Islamic Culture', *Medical History*, 43: 228–40.

Walker, Sue Sheridan, ed. (1983), *The Court Rolls of the Manor of Wakefield from October 1331 to September 1333*, Leeds: Yorkshire Archaeological Society.

Walker-Meikle, Kathleen (2012), *Medieval Pets*, Woodbridge: The Boydell Press.

Walker-Meikle, Kathleen (2013–2014), 'Toxicology and Treatment: Medical Authorities and Snake-bite in the Middle Ages', *Korot*, 22: 85–104.

Walker-Meikle, Kathleen (2017), 'Animal Venoms in the Middle Ages', in Philip Wexler (ed.), *Toxicology in the Middle Ages and Renaissance*, 151–58, Amsterdam: Elsevier.

Wallis, Faith (2005), 'Bartholomaeus of Salerno', in Steven Livesey, Thomas Glick and Faith Wallis (eds), *Medieval Science, Technology and Medicine: An Encyclopedia*, 77–80, London: Routledge.

Wallis, Faith (2011), 'Why was the *Aphorisms* of Hippocrates Re-Translated in the Eleventh Century?' in Carlos Fraenkel et al (eds), *Vehicles of Transmission, Translation and Transformation*, 179–99, Turnhout: Brepols.

Wallis, Faith, ed. (2010), *Medieval Medicine: A Reader*, Toronto: University of Toronto Press.

Watson, Gemma (2013), 'Roger Machado: A Life in Objects', PhD diss., University of Southampton, Southampton, UK.

Watt, John (2014), 'Why Did Ḥunayn, the Master Translator into Arabic, Make Translations into Syriac? On the Purpose of the Syriac Translations of Ḥunayn and his Circle', in Jens Scheiner and Damien Janos (eds) *The Place to Go: Contexts of Learning in Baghdād, 750–1000 CE*, 363–88, Princeton: The Darwin Press.

Weiss Adamson, Melitta (2004), *Food in Medieval Times*, Westport CT: Greenwood Press.

Weiss Adamson, Melitta (1995), *Medieval Dietetics: Food and Drink in* Regimen sanitatis *Literature from 800 to 1400*, Frankfurt-am-Main: Peter Lang.

West, John (2008), 'Ibn al-Nafīs, the Pulmonary Circulation, and the Islamic Golden Age', *Journal of Applied Physiology*, 105: 1877–80.

Wiethaus, Ulrike (1993), '"If I had an Iron Body": Femininity and Religion in the Letters of Maria de Hout', in Karen Cherewatuk and Ulrike Wiethaus (eds), *Dear Sister: Medieval Women and the Epistolary Genre*, 172–91, Philadelphia: University of Pennsylvania Press.

Wheatley, Edward (2010), *Stumbling Blocks before the Blind: Medieval Constructions of a Disability*, Ann Arbor: University of Michigan Press.

Whitaker, Cord (2019), *Black Metaphors*, Philadelphia: University of Pennsylvania Press.

Whitaker, Elaine (1993), 'Reading the Paston Letters Medically', *English Language Notes*, 31: 19–27.

Whitney, Elspeth (2011), 'What's Wrong with the Pardoner? Complexion Theory, the Phlegmatic Man, and Effeminacy', *The Chaucer Review*, 4: 357–89.

Wickersheimer, Ernest (1909), 'Les secrets et les conseils de Maître Guillaume Boucher et de ses confrères: contribution à l'histoire de la médecine à Paris vers 1400', *Bulletin de la société française d'histoire de la médecine*, 8: 200–306.

Wickersheimer, Ernest (1939), 'Faits cliniques observés a Strasbourg et à Haslach en 1362 et suivis de formules de remèdes', *Bulletin de la société française d'histoire de la médecine*, 33: 85–108.

Willows, Marlo (2017), 'Prayers and Poultices: Medieval Health Care at the Isle of May, Scotland, *c*. 430–1580 AD', in Lindsay Powell, William Southwell-Wright and Rebecca Gowlands (eds), *Care in the Past: Archaeological and Interdisciplinary Perspectives*, 141–66, Oxford: Oxbow.

Wilson, Brett (2007), 'The Failure of Nomenclature: The Concept of "Orthodoxy" in Islamic Studies', *Comparative Islamic Studies*, 3: 169–94.

Winer, Rebecca (2017), 'The Enslaved Wetnurse as Nanny: The Transition from Free to Slave Labor in Childcare in Barcelona after the Black Death (1348)', *Slavery & Abolition: A Journal of Slave and Post-Slave Studies*, 38: 303–19.

Winter, Johanna van (2007), *Spices and Comfits: Collected Papers on Medieval Food*, Totnes: Prospect Books.

Wolf, Kenneth (2011), *The Life and Afterlife of St Elizabeth of Hungary: Testimony from her Canonization Hearing*, New York: Oxford University Press.

Woolgar, Christopher (1999), *The Great Household in Late Medieval England*, New Haven and London: Yale University Press.

Woolgar, Christopher (2000), '"Take this Penance Now, and Afterwards the Fare Will Improve": Seafood and Late Medieval Diet', in David Starkey, Chris Reid and Neil Ashcroft (eds), *England's Sea Fisheries: The Commercial Sea Fisheries of England and Wales Since 1300*, 36–44, London: Chatham Publishing.

Woolgar, Christopher (2006), *The Senses in Late Medieval England*, New Haven: Yale University Press.

Woolgar, Christopher (2007), 'Feasting and Fasting: Food and Taste in Europe in the Middle Ages', in Paul Freedman (ed.), *Food: The History of Taste*, 163–95, London: Thames & Hudson.

Woolgar, Christopher (2010), 'Food and the Middle Ages', *Journal of Medieval History*, 36: 1–19.

Woolgar, Christopher (2016), *The Culture of Food in England, 1200–1500*, New Haven: Yale University Press.

Woolgar, Christopher (2018), 'Medieval Food and Colour', *Journal of Medieval History*, 44: 1–20.

Woolgar, Christopher, Dale Serjeantson, and Tony Waldron, eds (2006), *Food in Medieval England: Diet and Nutrition*, Oxford: Oxford University Press.

World Health Organisation (2000), *General Guidelines for Methodologies on Research and Evaluation of Traditional Medicine*, Geneva. Originally available online: http://apps.who.int/medicinedocs/en/d/Jwhozip42e/ (accessed 29 March 2018).

Wray, Shona Kelly (2004), 'Boccaccio and the Doctors: Medicine and Compassion in the Face of Plague', *Journal of Medieval History*, 30: 301–22.

Wray, Shona Kelly (2009), *Communities and Crisis: Bologna during the Black Death*, Leiden: Brill.

Yearl, Mary (2007), 'Medieval Monastic Customaries on *Minuti* and *Infirmi*', in Barbara Bowers (ed.), *The Medieval Hospital and Medical Practice*, 175–94, Aldershot: Ashgate.

Yearl, Mary (2014), 'Medicine for the Wounded Soul', in Cordelia Warr and Anne Kirkham (eds), *Wounds in the Middle Ages*, 109–28, Abingdon: Routledge.

Yoeli-Tlalim, Ronit (2019), 'Galen in Asia?' in Petros Bouras-Vllianatos and Barbara Zipser (eds), *Brill's Companion to the Reception of Galen*, 594–608, Brill: Leiden.

Yoshikawa, Naoë Kukita (2009), 'Holy Medicine and Disease of the Soul: Henry of Lancaster and *Le Livre de Seyntz Medicines*', *Medical History*, 53: 397–414.

Yoshikawa, Naoë Kukita, ed. (2015), *Medicine, Religion and Gender in Medieval Culture*, Cambridge: D.S. Brewer.

Ysebaert, Walter (2015), 'Medieval Letters and Letter Collections as Historical Sources: Methodological Questions, Reflections, and Research Perspectives (Sixth-Fifteenth Centuries)', in Christian Høgel and Elisabetta Bartoli (eds), *Medieval Letters between Fiction and Document*, 33–62, Turnhout: Brepols.

Ziegler, Joseph (1998), *Medicine and Religion, c. 1300: The Case of Arnau de Vilanova*, Oxford: Oxford University Press.

Ziegler, Joseph (1999), 'Practitioners and Saints: Medical Men in Canonization Processes in the Thirteenth to Fifteenth Centuries', *Social History of Medicine*, 12: 191–225.

Zipser, Barbara, ed. (2009), *John the Physician's "Therapeutics:" A Medical Handbook in Vernacular Greek*, Leiden: Brill.

Zipser, Barbara, ed. (2013), *Medical Books in the Byzantine World*, Bologna: Eikasmós Online II.

Zupko, Ronald and Robert Laures (1996), *Straws in the Wind: Medieval Urban Environmental Law – The Case of Northern Italy*, Boulder, CO: Westview Press.

CONTRIBUTORS

Naama Cohen-Hanegbi is Senior Lecturer in History at Tel Aviv University in Israel. She researches the relationship between medicine and religion in the Late Middle Ages and the history of the emotions. She edited a special cluster on Jews and medicine in the later Middle Ages for *Social History of Medicine* (2019). She has two books: *Caring for the Living Soul: Emotions, Medicine and Penance in the Late Medieval Mediterranean* (2017) and a co-edited volume *Pleasure in the Middle Ages* (2018).

Roberta Gilchrist is Professor of Archaeology and Research Dean at the University of Reading in the UK. She has published widely on the archaeology of burial, religious communities and magic, with a particular focus on gender and belief. Her books include *Medieval Life: Archaeology and the Life Course* (2012), *Glastonbury Abbey: Archaeological Investigations, 1904–79* (2015) and *Sacred Heritage: Monastic Archaeology, Identities, Beliefs* (2020).

F. Eliza Glaze is Professor of History at Coastal Carolina University in the USA. She researches medical textuality in the early and central Middle Ages, especially in Italy, with keen interests in the dissemination of medical knowledge across Europe during the eleventh and twelfth centuries. She co-edited *Between Text and Patient: The Medical Enterprise in Medieval and Early Modern Europe* (2011) and is a contributing author to *Medicine at Monte Cassino* (2019). Her latest article appears in *Early Science & Medicine* (2018).

Dolly Jørgensen is Professor of History at the University of Stavanger in Norway. She is an environmental historian who researches the history of sanitation, sensory history and human–animal relations, spanning from the Middle Ages to today. She was President of the European Society for Environmental History

(2013–2017). She is author of is *Recovering Lost Species in the Modern Age: Histories of Longing and Belonging* (2019) and co-editor of *New Natures: Joining Environmental History with Science and Technology Studies* (2013), *Northscapes: History, Technology and the Making of Northern Environments* (2013) and *Visions of North in Premodern Europe* (2018).

Iona McCleery is Associate Professor of Medieval History at the University of Leeds in the UK. She researches the history of medicine, the cult of the saints and food, with a focus on late-medieval Portugal and its early empire in the Atlantic and West Africa. Recent publications include articles on famine, the effects of medieval colonialism on health, miracles and public engagement. She is co-editor of the forthcoming *Reading Medieval Sources: Miracle Collections*.

Justin Stearns is Associate Professor in Arab Crossroads Studies at New York University's campus in Abu Dhabi in the United Arab Emirates. He researches the relationships between law, science, medicine and theology in the pre-modern Islamicate world. He is author of *Infectious Ideas: Contagion in Pre-Modern Islamic and Christian Thought in the Western Mediterranean* (2011). He is currently writing a book on the natural sciences in early-modern Morocco.

Wendy J. Turner is Professor of History at Augusta University in the USA. She researches medieval mental health, the history of disabilities and the relationship between medicine and law. Her (co-)edited books include *Madness in Medieval Law and Custom* (2010), *The Treatment of Disabled Persons in Medieval Europe* (2010), *Medicine and the Law* (2013) and *Trauma in Medieval Society* (2018). She is the author of *The Care and Custody of the Mentally Ill, Incompetent and Disabled in Medieval England* (2013).

Kathleen Walker-Meikle is Postdoctoral Research Fellow at King's College London in the UK. She has wide experience of collaborating on research projects relating to manuscript studies, medieval medicine and digital humanities. She researches the history of animals, especially animal bites, toxicology and pets and is currently investigating animal skin and skin diseases. She is the author of *Medieval Pets* (2012) and two newly reissued popular history books: *Cats in Medieval Manuscripts* (2019) and *Dogs in Medieval Manuscripts* (2020).

Gemma L. Watson is a Senior Research Manager at the University of Oxford in the UK. She was previously Postdoctoral Research Assistant in Medieval Archaeology at the University of Reading. She researches material culture, the archaeology of magic and belief, the relationship between archaeology and documentary history, and the relationship between things and people, especially in early Tudor England. She is co-editor of *Writing the Lives of People and Things, AD 500–1700* (2015) and *Medieval Archaeology* (2016).

INDEX

Italic numbers are used for illustrations.

Abelard, *Historia calamitatum* 142
Adela of Blois 144
air 24–7, 29, 75, 94
Alan of Lille 100, 153 n.3
Albala, Ken 58
albarellos 117
Albertus Magnus 100
    De animalibus (On Animals) 96–7
Alcuin, Abbot of St. Martin at Tours 183–4
Aldobrandino of Siena 45
Alexander II, Pope 140
Alfanus of Salerno 195, 196, 198
'Alī b. al-'Abbās al-Majūsī 41
    Kitāb Kāmil aṣ-ṣinā 'a aṭ-ṭibbīya (The
        Complete Book of the Medical
        Art) 13, 196
almanacs 188–9
alopecia 90
Alvastra Abbey, Sweden 116
ambergris 101
amputations 112
amulets 124
anatomy
    of animals 104
    brain anatomy *25*, 157–61, *161–3*,
        163–4
anima 156–7
animal turn 87

animals, use and meaning in medicine
    87–105
    conclusion 105
    introduction 87
    as medical metaphors 88–91, *93*
    nourishing or healing by 100–2
    parallels between human and animal
        medicine 102, 104–5
    as source of ill health and disease
        93–100
Anselm of Canterbury 140, 141, 143
Anthimus 44–5, *45–6*
Anthony, Saint *95*
Anthropocene Age 11
Antidotarium Nicolai 199
Antonio de Verceil 144
aqua vitae 113
Aquinas, Thomas 54, 56
archaeology of fish 52
archaeology of healing 107–29
    archaeology and cultural history
        108–10
    body and soul 123–8, *125*, *127*
    conclusion 128–9
    hospitals and monasteries 110–14, *113*
    introduction 107–8
    materials 119–22, *119*, *121–2*
    medical objects 114–19, *115*, *118*

archaeology of sanitation 23
Aretaeus of Cappadocia 90
Arnau de Vilanova 45, 58
    De esu carnium (On Meat Eating) 54
Articella (Little Art of Medicine) 198
Arundel, West Sussex 119
al-'Asqalānī, Ibn Ḥajar 63, 64
astrology 102, *103*, 104
Augustine 78
authority. *See* texts, authority of
Avebury, Wiltshire 116
Avicenna. *See* Ibn Sīnā

Baldwin I, King of Jerusalem 104–5
barber-surgeons 114–16, *115*, 118, 119
Barnwell Observances 111
Barrett, James 56
Bartholomew the Englishman 25, 159, 168
    De proprietatibus rerum 24, 88
battle injuries 166
Baviera, Baverio 147
bears 104–5
Beatrice of Villa 141
Beaumanoir, Philippe de 172–3
beavers 101
Beccaria, Augusto 186
Belgium 37, 125, *125*
Benzi, Ugo 147, 148
Bergen, Norway 32
Bergqvist, Johanna 123
Bernard of Clairvaux 141
Bernard de Gordon 89, 97, 98
Berwick, Scotland 32
Bible 54, 68, 69–70
al-Bidlīsī, Idrīs 77
bioarchaeology
    and fish 40, 52
    of skeletal remains 111–14
biomedicine 5
biopolitics 17–18
birthing amulets 124
bites, animal 95–8, *96*, 99
Black Death 10–12, 26–7, 73–8, 120–1
Blanche of Brittany 143
blood
    circulation of 159, 163–4
    as marker of injury 138
bloodletting
    bowls for 118
    of horses 102

and the humours 13
    milk, avoidance of after 101
    plague, treatment of 76
    in religious communities 111
Boccaccio, *Decameron* 135
body
    history of 108–9
    organization of 164
body and soul 123–8, *125, 127*
body politic 42
body worlds 109
Bologna, Italy 29–30, 33, 36, 137
Bonfield, Christopher 50
Bonne of Savoy, Duchess of Milan 142,
    143
Books of Hours 92, 93
Boucher, Guillaume 88, 147
bowls 118, *118*, 122, *122*
brain. *See* mind/brain concepts
Brody, Saul 68
building rules 31–2, 35–6
butchery waste 26, 27, 28–9, 94
Bynum, Caroline Walker 126

Caelius Aurelianus, *On Acute and Chronic
    Diseases* 181
Caesarius of Heisterbach 143–4
Calendrier des Bergers 93
Campbell, Bruce 11
cancer 88
canonization inquest testimonies 145–6,
    149–52
capacity, lack of 172–4
Carolingian period 183–6
Carruthers, Mary 158, 174
Carthusian Order 54
case histories 146–9
Cassiodorus, *Institutes of Divine and
    Human Learning* 180
castoreum 101
cats, dead 26
Cavallo, Sandra 16–17
Celestine III, Pope 143
cell theory of the brain 158, 159–60, 174
cemeteries, populations in 111–14
cess pits 32–3
    See also latrines
Chadwick, Edwin 26
Charles VI, King of France 29
charms 124–5, 125–6

INDEX

249

Chaucer, Geoffrey 170
cheese 101
Chiara de Montefalco, Saint 151
childbirth 122, 124
Chiquart 47, 48, 50, 60
Christianity
    burials, objects found with 110
    dietary practices in 54, 56–9
    disease, views of 69–71, 78–81, 177
Circa instans 199
Cistercians 56
Clarke, Edwin 157–8
Cockayne, Emily 24
cod 52
Cohen, Esther, *The Modulated Scream* 135
comfits 41
common sense 160
complexio 134
Condrau, Flurin 7
consilia 44, 145–6, 148, 149
Constantine the African 25, 196, 198
    Pantegni 13, 89, 196
    Viaticum 89–90
consultations. *See consilia*
contagion 71, 77
context of objects 109–10
contra-naturals 15
contracts between patients and healers
    137–8
cookery books 40, 48, 50, 57–8, 59–60
copper 120–1, *121*, 126–7, 128
coral 121–2
corpses, preparation of 110, 125–6
correspondence about illness 140–3,
    148–9, 185–6
corruption of the air 26, 29, 75
Coventry, Warwickshire 27–8, 30, 33, 35,
    36
crab 88
crayfish 47
criminals 173
Crispin, Gilbert 144
crucifixion, pain of 144
cultural history, definition of 108
culture, concept of 6–7
cynomancy 179

dairy products 101
De Groote, Koen 125
dead bodies, preparation of 125–6

death, fear of 151
deformities 69
Denmark 30, 32, 120
Desiderius of Benevento 195
devotional treatises 144–5
Dewhurst, Kenneth 157–8
diagnosis, process of 146–9
Díaz de Toledo, Fernando 142, 145,
    153 n.4
Díes, Manuel, *Libre de cavalls* (Book of the
    Horse) 102, *103*, 104
diet, reconstruction of 112
digestion 41–2
Dioscorides 180
disabilities 69, 165, 167, 168, 171
Disability Studies 10
disease 63–81
    Christian attitudes towards 69–71,
        78–81, 177
    conclusion 79–81
    definition of 132
    introduction 63–4
    Islamic attitudes towards plague in
        Egypt 73–8
    knowledge of 65–6, 68
    Mediterranean sphere 64–5
disease and environment. *See* environment
    and disease
disease man 160, *162*
distilling 113, *113*
divorce 172
dogs 98–100, 102, 104, 179
Dols, Michael 73
donkeys 90
dormouse 104
Douglas, Mary 24
drug jars 117
drugs. *See* medicine; pharmacology
drunkenness 91, 93, 170
Duarte, King of Portugal 42
    Leal Conselheiro (Loyal Counsellor)
        144–5
dung carts 33
dung, disposal of 26, 27, 36, 37
dyeing 29, 31

eating 42–3
Ebner, Margaret 144
Edinburgh, Scotland 126
Edmund, Brother 143

education of physicians 107, 146, 181–2, 183–4, 186, 198–9
Edward III, King of England 26, 29, 30
eels 50, 52, 101
Eleanor of Aquitaine 143
elephantia 89–90
Elizabeth of Hungary, Saint 150
emic and *etic* approaches 6–7
emotional states 143–5, 148
emotions, location of 156
England, Old English texts 190–3
Enrique I, King of Castile 166
environment. *See* sanitation
environment and disease 10–11
environmental data 114
epidemics. *See* plague epidemics
Eraclius, Bishop of Liège 89
Erasistratus of Ceos 158–9
Etheldreda, Saint 126
ex votos 104
Exeter, Devon *119*, 120
experiences of ill health 131–53
 conclusion 152–3
 correspondence about illness 140–3
 emotional pain 143–5
 introduction 131–2
 methodology 132–5
 patients' histories 145–52
 sickness, definition of 135–40, *136–7*
experiments on animals 104–5
eyes 30–1

Fagan, Brian 54
famines 112
fantasy 160
fasting 54
feeding bottles 118
feelings, location of 156
Ferrer, Vincent 63, 64, 78–81
fines 35
finger rings 124–5
fireflies 97
Fischer, Klaus-Dietrich 70
fish
 archaeology of 52
 consumption and supply 46–50, *51*, 52, *53*, 54
 in regimen texts 43–6
 religiosity versus digestibility 54, *55*, 56–9

sauces for 45, 46, 58–9
sauces of 44
types of 44–6, 48, *49*, 50, *51*
fish ponds 48
fishing
 illegal 48, 50
 methods of 52, *53*, 54
Fissell, Mary 6–7, 108
fleas 100
folk medicine 109–10, 129 n.1
food 39–60
 animals, good and bad 101
 conclusion 59–60
 contamination of 31
 debates and theories 40–3
 fish
  archaeology of 52
  consumption and supply 46–50, *51*, 52, *53*, 54
  in regimen texts 43–6
  religiosity versus digestibility 54, *55*, 56–9
  sauces for 45, 46, 58–9
  sauces of 44
  types of 44–6, 48, *49*, 50, *51*
 introduction 39
 leprosy, causes of 90–1
Forme of Cury 47
Foucault, Michel 17–18
four-segment theory of the brain 160
foxes 90
frameworks, medieval 12–18
Frantzen, Allen 56
Fredericus of St George 151
frenesy 167
frogs 98
Frugard, Roger 166
fruit 41, 42
Fulbert of Chartres 140

Galen
 on blood 163–4
 on the brain 158
 on disease 65–6
 on fish 44
 on leprosy 90–1
 texts of 179, 180, 181, 198
Galenism 66, 68
Gariopontus of Salerno 194–5
Gasper, Giles 46, 57, 58, 59, 140

INDEX 251

Gell, Alfred 127
Geltner, Guy 12, 23
gems 121
gender differences 123
Gentilcore, David 47
Gentile da Foligno 44, 99
Geoffrey de la Tour Landry, *The Book of the Knight of the Tower* 123
Gesta Romanorum (Deeds of the Romans) 91
al-Ghazālī, *Iḥyā 'ulūm al-dīn* (Revival of the Religious Sciences) 71–3
Ghent, Belgium 37
Ghost of Anantis 128, 129 n.3
Gilbert, Abbot of St Étienne 143
Gilbertus Anglicus 168–9
    Compendium medicinae 89, 90
Gilles de Corbeil 90
Glastonbury Abbey, Somerset 117
Glaze, Eliza 5–6
Gloucester, Gloucestershire 26
gluttony 42, 56
Gonzaga, Chiara 142
Goodich, Michael 152
Gordon, Stephen 126–7, 127–8
Gower, John 170
Gratian 172
Green, Monica 5, 8–9
Gregory of Nazianzos 69
grief 143
grooming, personal 123
guardianship 172–3
Guibert of Nogent 104–5
gutters 33, 35
Guy de Chauliac 88, 116

ḥadīth 71
hair 123
Hansen's disease. *See* leprosy
Harington, John 27
head injuries 165–7
health
    concept of 1, 5
    definitions of 132, 138–40
healthscaping 12
heart
    functions of 159
    and mind 156, 158
    and plague 74, 76
Hebrew Bible 68

Henry III, King of England 140, 143
Henry of Grosmont, 1st Duke of Lancaster, *Le Livre de Seyntz Medicines* (Book of Holy Medicines) 144
Herbarium complex 180–1, 190–2
heretical belief 69–70
hernia truss 126, *127*
Herophilus of Chalcedon 158–9
herpes estiomenus 89
herring 45, 50
Hippocrates 65, 180
Hippocratic works, *The Nature of Man* 12
Hoeniger, Cathleen 60
Horden, Peregrine 18
horses 102, *103*, 104
Hospital Brothers of St Anthony 95
hospitals 110, 112, 116, 117, 118, 126
Howell, Martha 35
human remains 111–14, 125–6
human waste. *See* latrines
humouralism
    definition 12–13, 15
    and disease 66
    and food 41–2, 44, 58
    and mental health 168
humours
    and disease 65, 66
    and health 139
    and leprosy 89, 90
    and senses 91, 93
    treatments for 121
    types of 12
Ḥunayn ibn Isḥāq 15
hydrophobia 98
hygiene, bodily 123

Ibn al-Athīr 74
Ibn Butlan 1, *2–3*, 17, 28, 49, 51
Ibn Ezra, Abraham 171
Ibn Ḥajar al-'Asqalānī,, *An Offering of Kindness on the Virtue of the Plague* 73–8
Ibn al-Jazzār, *Kitab Zād al-musāfir wa-qūt al-ḥāḍir* (Provision for the Traveller and Sustenance for the Settled) 196
Ibn al-Nafīs 159
Ibn Sīnā
    al-Qānūn (The Canon)
        influence of 67, 68

on leprosy 89, 90
on the plague 74, 76
on rabies 98
on venomous snakes 96
Kitāb al-Najāt, on the brain 160, *161*, 163
Iceland 116
idiota 171
illness, attitudes towards 135–7, 164
illness narratives 132–4
images
    authority of 179
    of the brain 160–1, *161–3*, 163
imagination 160
incapacity 172–4
indigenous medicine 129 n.1
innocents 169–70
inscriptions 124–5, *125*
intromission 30–1
Isabella d'Este 142
Isagoge Sorani 182
Ishāq al-Isrā'īlī 196
Isidore of Seville 3–4
    Etymologies 182–3
Islam
    disease, views of 71–3, 80
    foods in 45
    plague in Egypt, attitudes towards 74–8
Ivo of Chartres 144

Jedburgh Observantine Friary, Scotland 114
Jesus 69, 70–1, 78, 80
jet 122, *122*
jinn, and plague 75, 76
job titles for sanitation duties 36
Johannitius. *See* Ḥunayn ibn Isḥāq
John, King of England 42
John of Gaddesden 127
John of Salisbury 42
Juan of Aviñón 144
Judaism
    and disease 68–9, 79–80
    foods in 45

Kalender of Shepherdes 14, 93
Kaye, Joel 58
Kempe, Margery 145
Kleinman, Arthur, *The Illness Narratives* 132–3

knives 114
knots 127
knowledge transmission 8
Kowaleski, Maryanne 56
Krakow, Poland 35, 36
Kucher, Michael 35

Lacnunga (Remedies) 127, 192
Lacy, Edmund, Bishop of Exeter 104
lamprey 46
Lanfranc of Bec 140, 144
latrines
    laws for 32–3, 36–7
    and odours 29–30
    public provision of 33
Laurentius Rusius, *Hippiatrica sive marescalia* 102
Laurioux, Bruno 58
law and mental health 172–4
laws
    food 40, 50
    and mental health 172–4
    sanitation 22, 31–2, 32–3, 35–6, 36–7
learning disorders 165, 167, 168, 171
Leechbooks (Physicians' Books) 192
legal cases 137–8
Leiden, Netherlands 32–3
leprosy 68, 69, 76, 80, 89–91, 120
lethargy 168–9
letters about illness 140–3, 148–9, 185–6
Libellus de imaginibus deorum (Little Book on the Images of the Gods) 91, 93
Liber passionalis (The Book of Diseases) 188
ligatures 120, 126–8
Lincoln, Lincolnshire 120
lions 90, 91, *92*, 93
living conditions 112
London, England
    Assize of Nuisance 36–7
    birthing amulets 124
    butchery waste 27, 28–9, 94
    coral working 122
    feeding bowl 118, *118*
    hospitals 113
    human remains 112
    jet bowl 122, *122*
    latrines 30, 33
    pigs in 95

INDEX

253

sanitation 26, 35, 36
urinals 116–17
See also St Mary Spital, London
Lorsch Book of Remedies 70–1, 184
Louis, Duke of Orleans 104
Lucca, Italy 26, 29–30, 31, 36, 37
lupus 89
Lydgate, John 170

Maddern, Philippa 145
madness 145, 168, 170
See also mental health
Magdeburg, Germany 32
magic 127
Maimonides, Moses 45
Maino de Maineri 46, 59, 60
Malmö, Sweden 30
mania 167–8
manuals 186–90, 194–5, 199
manure 94
See also dung, disposal of
manuscripts 8, 188
See also texts, authority of
Marcellus of Bordeaux 186
Marguerite of Provence, Queen of France
140
Martin of Germany 131, 134
martyrdom, and plague 75
martyrs 178
Mary Rose 114–16, *115*, 118, 119
material culture. *See* archaeology of
healing
Matilda of Scotland, Queen of England
141
Mattiolo de Mattioli 131, 134
McIntosh, Marjorie 22
medical tools 114
medici 193
medicine
folk medicine 109–10, 129 n.1
food as 41
ideas of 3–4, 5–6
at monastic and hospital sites 113–14,
113
study of medieval 8–10
See also pharmacology
melancholia 167–8, 169
memory 156, 160, 171, 174
mental health 165, 167, 167–71, 172–4
mental pain 143–5

mercury 113–14, 119–20, *119*
miasmas 24–6, 94
Middle Ages, concept of 4–5
midwives 126, 129 n.2
milk 101
mind/brain concepts 155–75
brain anatomy 25, 157–61, *161–3*,
163–4
brain/head injuries 165–6
brain malfunctions 167–9
conclusion 174–5
consent, legal positions 171–4
introduction 155–7
learning disabilities 171
mental health 165, 167, 169–71
miracle tales 143–4
miracles 56–7, 150–2
monasteries
fish, eating of 54, 56
gendered material culture 123
libraries of 180, 181, 183, 184–5, 188,
189, *189*, 195
medical equipment 116, 117
medical practice in 110–14
scratched-mark pottery 125, *125*
Mondeville, Henri de 88, 97, 99
monkeys 91, *92*, 93, 102
Montagnana, Bartolomeo de 147
Monte Cassino Abbey, Italy 184–5, 189,
189, 195, 196, 198
Monte, Giovanni Batista de 147–8
More, Thomas 27
mortars 118–19
Muḥammad, Prophet 71
Muscio, *Gynaecology* 179
music, as a cure 97
mystical writings 144

Narbonne, France 31
narratology 7
naturalism 132
naturals 15
al-Nawawī 74
nervous system 159
neutrum/neutralitas 138–9
Niccolo, Bishop of Viterbo 144
Nicholas of Poland 101
Nicholas of Salerno 199
Nicholas of Tolentino, Saint 150, 151
Nicoud, Marilyn 43, 60

nighttime-only waste disposal 31
Niiranen, Susanna 167
non compos mentis 171
non-naturals 15–18, 66, 168, 174
non sanus memoria 171
normativism 132
Norway 32
Norwich, Norfolk 26, 33, 35, 37
notebooks 189–90
Nottingham, Nottinghamshire 29, 37
nuisance laws 31–2, 35–6

objects. *See* archaeology of healing
odours 24–30
    and disease 24–6
    from latrines 29–30
    organic waste 27–9
    and plague 26–7
Old English texts 190–3
Øm, Denmark 120
organic wastes 24, 26, 27–9
Oribasius, *Collectiones medicae* (Medical
    Collections) 180
Origen 69
Oviedo, Spain 50

pain
    emotional 143–5
    physical 135, 141, 142, 143
Paisley Abbey, Renfrewshire 114
panthers 91
parasites 100
Paris, France 31, 50, 52
Paston family 142, 143, 153 n.4
patients' histories
    experiences of ill health 145–52
    in health studies 132–4
Paul of Aegina 98
paving 33, 35
penitents 139
Petegem, Belgium 125, *125*
Peter Abelard, *Historia calamitatum* 142
Peter of Blois 89
Petrarch 141, 144
Petrus Hispanus 44, 45
pets 102
pharmacology
    animals, use of 101–2
    ingredients 40–1
    metals, gems and stone 119–22

plants, use of 114, 118
    texts about 180–1, 190–1, 195–6, 199
    See also medicine
philosophy, study of 182
physicians
    Carolingian 183–4
    case histories and letters of 146–9
    education of 107, 146, 181–2, 183–4,
        186, 198–9
    food, advice on 47, 57
    urinals, use of 116–17
physiology 159, 163–4
Pietro d'Abano 99
pigs 91, *92*, *93*, *94–5*, 104
pilgrimages 123–4
pious religiosity 123
Pistoia, Italy 27
plague epidemics 10–12, 26–7, 52, 73–8
Planet Man *92*, *93*
plants, pharmaceutical use of 40–1, 114
Platearius, Johannes 167–8, 199
plates, medical 120, *121*
Platina 58
    De honesta voluptate et valetudine (On
        Right Pleasure and Good Health)
        40, 47
Pliny the Elder, *Natural History* 179
pneuma 158, 163–4
poisonous animals 97–8
Poland 35, 36
political models 42
pollution 24
porpoise 45
Porter, Roy 133
Porto, Portugal 50
pottery
    for medicinal use 117–18
    scratched-mark 125, *125*
preventative measures 120–1, 123–5
priests, as physicians 139
Priscianus, Theodorus 190
Proctor, Caroline 47
Prophetic Medicine 71
Pseudo-Dioscorides, *Book of Medicine from
    Feminine Herb*s 180
public services 33
punishment and disease 68–9, 169

quid pro quo 190
Qur'an 71

INDEX

rabies 98–100
Raunds, Northamptonshire 126
Rawcliffe, Carole 50
al-Rāzī, Muhammad ibn Zakariyyā 98
Reggio Emilia, Italy 138
regimen texts 26, 43–6, 101
regulations
    food 40, 50
    and mental health 172–4
    sanitation 22, 31–2, 32–3, 35–6, 36–7
Reisch, Gregor, *Margarita Philosophica*
        160–1, *163*
religious attitudes towards disease 68–73
religious institutions. *See* monasteries
religious practices. *See* Christianity; Islam;
        Judaism
revenants 128
Ribe, Denmark 32
Riccoldo of Monte Croce 143
Richard II, King of England 47
Richard of Durham 102
Richer of Rheims 193
rivers
    latrines over 33
    waste disposal in 27–8, 29, 30
Robert I, King of Scotland 47
Roger de Baron, *Practica* 90
Rogerius Frugardi 89
Roland of Parma 88, 89
Rusius, Laurentius, *Hippiatrica sive*
        marescalia 102

saints
    animals, healing of 104
    humans, healing of 149–52
Salerno, Italy 194–6, 198–9, 201
Salmón, Fernando 60
Salutati, Coluccio 141
sanitas 1, 21
sanitation, urban 21–38
    animals and 93–5
    conclusion 37–8
    enforcement 35–7
    infrastructure 31–5
    introduction 21–3
    sensory perceptions 24–31
sapphire 121
schools of medicine 181, 198–9
scorpions 97
scourges 120

Scully, Terence 58
self-help manuals 186–90
Seni, Croatia 30
senses and humours 91, 93
sensory perceptions 24–31
sheep 91, *92*, 93
shellfish 47
Shoham-Steiner, Ephraim 68–9, 173–4
shrines 104, 123–4, 150
sick people
    attitudes towards 135–7
    feeding vessels for 118, *118*
    food for 41, 47
    types in monastic infirmaries 111
sickness, definition of 135–40, *136–7*
Siena, Italy 35
sight
    and animals 91
    and the brain 161, *161*
    and unhealthy situations 30–1
sin
    and disease 68–9, 70, 139, 144, 145,
        151
    and mental health 169
Skriðuklaustur, Iceland 116
slugs 90
smell, sense of 91
smells. *See* odours
snakes 89, 90, 96, *96*
Solomon, Michael 58
Soranus of Ephesus 179
soul, connection with body 126–8, *127*,
        156–7
sound minds 173
sources 22
Southampton, Hampshire 117
Soutra Hospital, Scotland 118
souvenirs 123–4
Spain 50
spatial context 109–10
sperm whales 101
spices 41, 61 n.2
spiders 97
St Amand Abbey, France 188
St Andrew's Gilbertine Priory, York 120
St Antony's fire 95
St Bartholomew's Hospital, Bristol 118
St Claire Monastery, Petegem 125, *125*
St Giles by Brompton Bridge, North
        Yorkshire 114

St James Priory, Bristol 124
St John's Priory, Pontefract 113
St Mary Magdalen, Winchester 112, 118
St Mary Magdalene Hospital, Reading 120, *121*
St Mary Merton Priory, Surrey 117, 126, *127*
St Mary of Ospringe Hospital, Kent 118–19
St Mary Spital, London 112, 113, 116–17, 118, *118*, 124
St Nicholas' Hospital, Fife 117
stable isotope analysis 112
stigmata 144
stockfish 45, *50*, *51*, 52
stomach 42
stone mortars 118–19
Stonor, Sir Edmund 143
street cleaners 35
streets 33, 35, 36
Strozzi family 142, 143, 153 n.4
sturgeon 45, 48
al-Subkī, Tāj al-Dīn 76
surgery
    evidence for 112
    for head injuries 166–7
    texts about 187–8, *187*
surgical instruments 114, 116
Sweden 30, 35, 116, 123
swine. *See* pigs
symptoms 146–9
syphilis 120

Tacuinum sanitatis (Tables of Health) 1, *2–3*, *17*, *28*, *49*, *51*, *60*
Taillevent 47, 48, 50
tanning 29, 31
tarantulas and tarantism 97
taste 31
Tereoperica (Therapeutics) 188
testimonies, canonization 145–6, 149–52
texts, authority of 177–202
    authority, definitions of 177
    Carolingian centres 183–6
    conclusion 201
    introduction 177–8
    late antiquity to the early middle ages 178–83
    Old English texts 190–3

Salerno, texts from 194–6, 198–9, 201
self-help manuals 186–90
textual birthing amulets 124
theoretical approaches 7–8
therapeutics. *See* pharmacology
theriac 101–2
Thomas of Aquinas 54, 56
Thomas Becket 56–7
Thomas Cantilupe, Saint 104
Thomas de Cantimpré 91
thoughts, location of 156
three-cell theory of the brain 158, 159–60, 174
Three Magi 124–5
Tillman de Syberg 147
tools, medical 114, 116
towns. *See* sanitation, urban
traditional medicine 109–10, 129 n.1
trepanation/trephination 112, 116, 166–7
Trevisa, John 88
Trota of Salerna 199, *200*, 201
Trotula 199
Tuke, Daniel Hack 165
Turner, Marion 134
tyria 90

uncleanliness 24
universities 198–9
urban environment. *See* sanitation, urban
urinals 116–17
urine 90, 97, 98, 99

venomous animals 95–7, *96*
vermin 97
vernacular texts 190–3
Verona, Italy 31
Vesalius, Andreas 164
vessels, medical 117–18, 122, *122*
veterinary medicine 102, *103*, 104
Visconti, Bianca Maria, Duchess of Milan 142, 143, 144, 148

Wakefield, West Yorkshire 48, 50
Walahfrid Strabo, Abbot of Reichenau 189–90
Wallis, Faith 46, 57, 58, 59
wardship 172–3
waste collection services 33

INDEX

257

waste disposal 26, 27–9, 31
water
  contamination of 31
  and odours 27, 29
  and rabies 98, 99
  See also rivers
Wellcome Trust 9
whales 101
William of Marra 97, 99–100
William of Norwich 104
wills 173
Winchester, Hampshire 31, 112, 118
Winter, Johanna van 57–8

wolves 89
women 123, 126, 193, 199, *200*, 201
  See also childbirth; midwives
Woolgar, Christopher 47, 50, 59
words, written 124–5, *125*
working conditions 112
worms 100
wounds, assessment of 138

York, North Yorkshire 30, 31, 33, 120
Yperman, Jehan 160

zodiac horse 102, *103*, 104